Ovarian Cancer 3

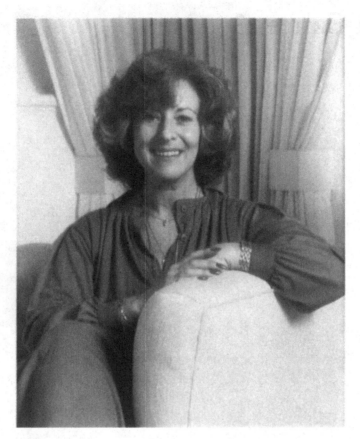

Helene Harris

Ovarian Cancer 3

Edited by

Frank Sharp

Department of Obstetrics and Gynaecology,
Northern General Hospital, Sheffield University, Sheffield, UK

Peter Mason

The Samaritan Hospital for Women,
St Mary's Hospital Medical School, London, UK

Tony Blackett

Department of Obstetrics and Gynaecology
Northern General Hospital, Sheffield University, Sheffield, UK, and

Jonathan Berek

Division of Gynecologic Oncology
UCLA School of Medicine, Los Angeles, USA

CHAPMAN & HALL MEDICAL

London · Glasgow · Weinheim · New York · Tokyo · Melbourne · Madras

Published by
Chapman & Hall, 2-6 Boundary Row, London SE1 8HN, UK

Chapman & Hall, 2-6 Boundary Row, London SE1 8HN, UK

Blackie Academic & Professional, Wester Cleddens Road, Bishopbriggs, Glasgow G64 2NZ, UK

Chapman & Hall GmbH, Pappelallee 3, 69469 Weinheim, Germany

Chapman & Hall USA, One Penn Plaza, 41st Floor, New York NY 10119, USA

Chapman & Hall Japan, ITP-Japan, Kyowa Building, 3F, 2-2-1, Hirakawacho, Chiyoda-ku, Tokyo 102, Japan

Chapman & Hall Australia, Thomas Nelson Australia, 102 Dodds Street, South Melbourne, Victoria 3205, Australia

Chapman & Hall India, R. Seshdri, 32 Second Main Road, CIT East, Madras 600 035, India

First edition 1995

©1995 Chapman & Hall
Softcover reprint of the hardcover 1st edition 1995

Typeset in 10/12 pt Palatino by EXPO Holdings, Malaysia.

ISBN 978-1-4757-0138-8   ISBN 978-1-4757-0136-4 (eBook)
DOI 10.1007/978-1-4757-0136-4

A catalogue record for this book is available from the British Library

Library of Congress Catalog Card Number: 94-71818

∞ Printed on acid-free text paper, manufactured in accordance with ANSI/NISO Z39.48-1992 (Permanence of Paper).

Contents

Contents

Part Three EARLY OVARIAN CANCER AND BORDERLINE TUMOURS

Part Four CHEMOTHERAPY, RADIOTHERAPY AND ETHICS

Contributors

V. Abeler
Dept of Pathology, The Norwegian Radium Hospital, Montebello, N–0310 Oslo, Norway

G.M. Abu-Jawdeh
Dept of Pathology, Beth Israel Hospital, Boston, MA 02215, USA

N. Auersperg
Dept of Anatomy, University of British Columbia, 2177 Westbrook Mall, Vancouver, British Columbia V6T 1Z3, Canada

F.R. Balkwill
Imperial Cancer Research Fund, 44 Lincoln's Inn Fields, London WC2A 3PX, UK

A. Barber
Dept of Biochemistry, University of Glasgow, Glasgow G12 8QQ, Scotland

R.C. Bast Jr
Division of Medicine, Box 092, MD Anderson Cancer Center, 1515 Holcombe Blvd, Houston, TX 77030, USA

D.A. Bell
Dept of Pathology, Massachusetts General Hospital, Boston, MA 02114, USA

A. Berchuck
Dept of Obstetrics and Gynecology, Duke University Medical Center, Durham, NC 27710, USA

J.S. Berek
Professor and Vice-Chair, Chief of Gynecology and Gynecologic Oncology, UCLA School of Medicine, The Jonsson Comprehensive Cancer Center, Los Angeles, CA 90024–1740, USA

K.R. Berend
Duke University Medical Center, Durham, NC 27710, USA

M. Berman
Dept of Obstetrics and Gynecology, Clinical Cancer Center, University of California, Irvine Medical Center, Orange, CA, USA

P. Beverley
ICRF Tumour Immunology, Courtauld Institute of Biochemistry (UCH), 91 Riding House St., London W1P 8BT, UK

D.M. Black
Beatson Institute for Cancer Research, Garscube Estate, Switchback Rd, Bearsden, Glasgow G61 1BD, UK

B. Bonavida
Dept of Microbiology and Immunology, UCLA School of Medicine, University of California, 10833 Le Conte Avenue, Los Angeles, CA 90024, USA

Contributors

M.A. Bookman
Fox Chase Cancer Center, 7701 Burholme Avenue, Philadelphia, PA 19111, USA

C.M. Boyer
Dept of Medicine, Duke University Medical Center, Durham, NC 27710, USA

M. Brandely
Roussel-Uclaf, Romainville, France

R. Bugat
Purpan Hospital, Toulouse, France

J. Burchell
Imperial Cancer Research Fund, 44 Lincoln's Inn Fields, London, WC2A 3PX, UK

R. Burger
Dept of Obstetrics and Gynecology, Clinical Cancer Center, University of California, Irvine Medical Center, Orange, CA, USA

F. Burke
Imperial Cancer Research Fund, 44 Lincoln's Inn Fields, London WC2A 3PX, UK

I.G. Campbell
University of Southampton, Dept of Obstetrics and Gynaecology, Princess Anne Hospital, Southampton, UK

L. Cannon-Albright
Dept of Internal Medicine, University of Utah, 420 Chipeta Way, Salt Lake City, UT 84108, USA

B. Chesak
Dept of Gynecologic Oncology, M.D. Anderson Cancer Center, 1515 Holcombe Blvd, Houston, TX 77030, USA

D. Clarke-Pearson
Dept of Obstetrics and Gynecology, Duke University Medical Center, Durham, NC 27710, USA

B.B. Cohen
MRC Human Genetics Unit, Western General Hospital, Edinburgh, Scotland

M.I. Colnaghi
Division of Experimental Oncology, Istituto Nazionale Tumori, Via G. Venezian 1, Milan, Italy

N. Colombo
San Gerardo Hospital, Monza, Italy

M. Conaway
Dept of Community and Family Medicine, Duke University Medical Center, Durham NC 27710, USA

L. Daly
Dept of Medicine, Duke University Medical Center, Durham, NC 27710, USA

M. Daly
Fox Chase Cancer Center, 7701 Burholme Avenue, Philadelphia, PA 19111, USA

B. Davies
Imperial Cancer Research Fund, 44 Lincoln's Inn Fields, London WC2A 3PX, UK

K. De Sombre
Dept of Medicine, Duke University Medical Center, Durham, NC 27710, USA

P. Devillier
Roussel-Uclaf, Romainville, France

J.M. DiMaio
Dept of Surgery, Box 3551, Duke University Medical Center, Durham, NC 27710, USA

P. DiSaia
Dept of Obstetrics and Gynecology, Clinical Cancer Center, University of California, Irvine Medical Center, Orange, CA, USA

L. Dubeau
Dept of Pathology, Kenneth Norris Jr Comprehensive Cancer Center, 1441 Eastlake Avenue, Los Angeles, CA 90033, USA

D.F. Easton
Institute of Cancer Research, 15 Cotswold Rd, Belmont, Surrey, UK

D.M. Eccles
CRC Genetic Epidemiology Research Group, Dept of Child Health, University of Southampton, Southampton, UK

E.A. Eisenhauer
NCIC Clinical Trials Group, Queen's University, 82–84 Barrie St., Kingston, Ontario K7L 3N6, Canada

O.J. Finn
Dept of Molecular Genetics and Biochemistry, University of Pittsburgh School of Medicine, Pittsburgh, PA 15213, USA

B. Fisk
Dept of Gynecologic Oncology, M.D. Anderson Cancer Center, 1515 Holcombe Blvd, Houston, TX 77030, USA

D. Ford
Institute of Cancer Research, 15 Cotswold Rd, Belmont, Surrey, UK

W.D. Foulkes
Division of Medical Genetics, McGill University, Montreal General Hospital, 1650 Avenue Cedar, Montreal, Quebec, H3G 1A4, Canada

E. Francois
Centre François Lacassagne, Nice, France

R.S. Freedman
Dept of Gynecologic Oncology, M.D. Anderson Cancer Center, 1515 Holcombe Blvd, Houston, TX 77030, USA

P. Fumoleau
Centre René Gauducheau, Nantes, France

H. Gabra
ICRF Medical Oncology Unit, Western General Hospital, Edinburgh, Scotland

T. Gatanaga
Dept of Molecular Biology and Biochemistry, University of California, Irvine, CA

L.A. Getts
Fox Chase Cancer Center, 7701 Burholme Avenue, Philadelphia, PA 19111, USA

K. Gholami
Dept of Medical Informatics, University of Utah, 420 Chipeta Way, Salt Lake City, UT 84108, USA

B.J. Giantonio
Fox Chase Cancer Center, 7701 Burholme Avenue, Philadelphia, PA 19111, USA

A.K. Godwin
Fox Chase Cancer Center, 7701 Burholme Avenue, Philadelphia, PA 19111, USA

D.E. Goldgar
Dept of Medical Informatics, University of Utah, 420 Chipeta Way, Salt Lake City, UT 84108, USA

J. Gosewehr
Dept of Gynecologic Oncology, Kenneth Norris Jr Comprehensive Cancer Center, 1441 Eastlake Avenue, Los Angeles, CA 90033, USA

G. Granger
Dept of Molecular Biochemistry, University of California, Irvine, CA 92717-3900, USA

E. Grosen
Dept of Obstetrics and Gynecology, Clinical Cancer Center, University of California, Irvine Medical Center, Orange, CA, USA

Contributors

L. Gruber
MRC Human Genetics Unit, Western General Hospital, Edinburgh, Scotland

J.P. Guastalla
Centre Léon Bérard, Lyon, France

K. Hamaguchi
Fox Chase Cancer Center, 7701 Burholme Avenue, Philadelphia, PA 19111, USA

T.C. Hamilton
Fox Chase Cancer Center, 7701 Burholme Avenue, Philadelphia, PA 19111, USA

M. Hogan
Fox Chase Cancer Center, 7701 Burholme Avenue, Philadelphia, PA 19111, USA

J.A. Hurteau
Dept of Obstetrics and Gynecology, Duke University Medical Center, Durham, NC 27710, USA

C.G. Ioannides
Dept of Gynecologic Oncology, M.D. Anderson Cancer Center, 1515 Holcombe Blvd, Houston, TX 77030, USA

T. Irimura
Dept of Tumor Biology, M.D. Anderson Cancer Center, 1515 Holcombe Blvd, Houston, TX 77030, USA

K. Jackson
Fox Chase Cancer Center, 7701 Burholme Avenue, Philadelphia, PA 19111, USA

I. Jacobs
Dept of Obstetrics and Gynaecology, Rosie Maternity Hospital, Cambridge CB2 2SW, UK

K.R. Jerome
Dept of Molecular Genetics and Biochemistry, University of Pittsburgh School of Medicine, Pittsburgh, PA 15213, USA

S.W. Johnson
Fox Chase Cancer Center, 7701 Burholme Avenue, Philadelphia, PA 19111, USA

T.A. Jones
Imperial Cancer Research Fund, 44 Lincoln's Inn Fields, London WC2A 3PX, UK

P.B. Jordan
Dept of Surgery, Box 3551, Duke University Medical Center, Durham, NC 27710, USA

J. Kaern
Dept of Gynecology, Norwegian Radium Hospital, Montebello, N-0310 Oslo, Norway

S. Kassim
Dept of Medicine, Duke University Medical Center, Durham, NC 27710, USA

T.M. Kim
Dept of Pathology, Kenneth Norris Jr Comprehensive Cancer Center, 1441 Eastlake Avenue, Los Angeles, CA 90033, USA

E.C. Kohn
Laboratory of Pathology, National Cancer Institute, 9000 Rockville Pike, Bethesda, MD 20892, USA

P.A. Kruk
Gerontology Research Center, Laboratory of Molecular Genetics, 4940 Eastern Avenue, Baltimore, MD 21224, USA

S. Langdon
ICRF Medical Oncology Unit, Western General Hospital, Edinburgh, Scotland

S. Larbaoui
Roussel-Uclaf, Romainville, France

E.J. Latimer
Palliative Care Program, Henderson General Hospital, 711 Concession St East, Hamilton, Ontario L8V IC3, Canada

R. Leake
Dept of Biochemistry, University of Glasgow, Glasgow G12 8QQ, Scotland

R.C.F. Leonard
ICRF Medical Oncology Unit, Western General Hospital, Edinburgh, Scotland

A. Lessels
Dept of Pathology, Western General Hospital, Edinburgh, Scotland

L. Levin
London Regional Cancer Center, 790 Commissioners Rd East, London, Ontario N6A 4L6, Canada

C.M. Lewis
Dept of Medical Informatics, University of Utah, 420 Chipeta Way, Salt Lake City, UT 84108, USA

B.M. Longenecker
Dept of Immunology, Faculty of Medicine, University of Alberta T6G 2H7, Canada

H.K. Lyerly
Dept of Surgery, Box 3551, Duke University Medical Center, Durham, NC 27710, USA

G.D. MacLean
Medical Oncology Unit, Cross Cancer Institute, 11560 University Avenue, Edmonton, Alberta T6G 1Z3, Canada

S.L. Maines-Bandiera
Dept of Anatomy, University of British Colombia, 2177 Westbrook Mall, Vancouver, British Colombia T6G 1Z3, Canada

F. Maloisel
Centre Paul Strauss, Strasbourg, France

O. Martínez-Maza
Dept of Microbiology and Immunology, UCLA Medical School, Los Angeles, USA

F.E. Matthews
Institute of Cancer Research, 15 Cotswold Rd, Belmont, Surrey, UK

M. McDonald
Dept of Medical Informatics, University of Utah, 420 Chipeta Way, Salt Lake City, UT 84108, USA

L. Mignot
Foch Hospital, Suresnes, France

B. Miller
ICRF Medical Oncology Unit, Western General Hospital, Edinburgh, Scotland

G.B. Mills
Oncology Research, Toronto General Hospital, Toronto, Ontario M5G 2C4, Canada

Y. Mizutani
Department of Urology, Faculty of Medicine, Kyoto University, Kyoto 606, Japan

A. Monnier
A. Boulloche Hospital, Montbéliard, France

H. Morimoto
Mayo Clinic Scottsdale, S.C. Johnson Medical Research Building, 13400 East Shea Blvd., Scottsdale, AZ 85259, USA

J.M. Morsman
Dept of Obstetrics and Gynecology, Plymouth General Hospital, Devon, UK

M. Mousseau
La Tronche Hospital, Grenoble, France

M.S. Naylor
Institute of Cancer Research, Haddow Laboratories, South Surrey, SM2 5NG, UK

M.A. Nooy
Academisch Ziekenhuis, Leiden, Netherlands

Contributors

G. Netter
Clinique Courlancy, Reims, France

K. O'Briant
Dept of Medicine, Duke University Medical Center, Durham, NC 27710, USA

P.J. O'Dwyer
Fox Chase Cancer Center, 7701 Burholme Avenue, Philadelphia, PA 19111, USA

C.M.D. Oliveira
Coimbra Hospital, Coimbra, Portugal

D. Oram
Dept of Obstetrics and Gynaecology, University of London Hospital, London, UK

O. Owens
Dept of Biochemistry, University of Glasgow, Glasgow G12 8QQ, Scotland

R.F. Ozols
Fox Chase Cancer Center, 7701 Burholme Avenue, Philadelphia, PA 19111, USA

N. Peat
Imperial Cancer Research Fund, 44 Lincoln's Inn Fields, London WC2A 3PX, UK

J. Peto
Institute of Cancer Research, 15 Cotswold Rd, Belmont, Surrey, UK

E.O. Pettersen
Dept of Tissue Culture, Norwegian Radium Hospital, Montebello, N-0310 Oslo, Norway

M.J. Piccart
Institut Jules Bordet, Rue Heger-Bordet 1, Brussels 1000, Belgium

L.G. Poels
Dept of Cell Biology and Histology, Catholic University of Nijmegen, 6500 HB Nijmegen, Netherlands

E. Pujade-Lauraine
Hôtel Dieu Hospital, Paris, France

W.R. Robinson
Dept of Obstetrics and Gynecology, Tulane University School of Medicine, 1430 Tulane Avenue, New Orleans, LA 70112, USA

G. Rodriguez
Dept of Obstetrics and Gynecology, Duke University Medical Center, Durham, NC 27710, USA

N. Rosenblum
Fox Chase Cancer Center, 7701 Burholme Avenue, Philadelphia, PA 19111, USA

K. Rowe
Dept of Medical Informatics, University of Utah, 420 Chipeta Way, Salt Lake City, UT 84108, USA

J.T. Safrit
Aaron Diamond AIDS Research Center, 455 First Avenue, 7th Floor, New York, NY 10016, USA

H. Salazar
Fox Chase Cancer Center, 7701 Burholme Avenue, Philadelphia, PA 19111, USA

J. Schultz
Fox Chase Cancer Center, 7701 Burholme Avenue, Philadelphia, PA 19111, USA

R.E. Scully
Dept of Pathology, Massachusetts General Hospital, Boston, MA 02114, USA

M. Skolnick
Dept of Medical Informatics, University of Utah, 420 Chipeta Way, Salt Lake City, UT 84108, USA

M. Smith
Imperial Cancer Research Fund, 44 Lincoln's Inn Fields, London WC2A 3PX, UK

E. Solomon
Imperial Cancer Research Fund, 44 Lincoln's Inn Fields, London WC2A 3PX, UK

J. Soper
Dept of Obstetrics and Gynecology, Duke University Medical Center, Durham, NC 27710, USA

C.M. Steel
MRC Human Genetics Unit, Western General Hospital, Edinburgh, Scotland

K.D. Swenerton
BC Cancer Agency, Vancouver Clinic, 600 West 10th Avenue, Vancouver, British Columbia V5Z 4E6, Canada

J. Taylor-Papadimitriou
Imperial Cancer Research Fund, 44 Lincoln's Inn Fields, London WC2A 3PX, UK

J. Taylor Wharton
Dept of Gynecologic Oncology, M.D. Anderson Cancer Center, 1515 Holcombe Blvd, Houston, TX 77030, USA

J.R. Testa
Fox Chase Cancer Center, 7701 Burholme Avenue, Philadelphia, PA 19111, USA

G.M. Thomas
Division of Radiation Oncology, Toronto-Bayview Regional Cancer Center, 2075 Bayview Avenue, Toronto, Ontario M4N 3MJ, Canada

C.G. Tropé
Dept of Gynecologic Oncology, Norwegian Radium Hospital, Montebello, 0310 Oslo, Norway

J. Trowsdale
Imperial Cancer Research Fund, 44 Lincoln's Inn Fields, London WC2A 3PX, UK

M. Velicescu
Dept of Pathology, Kenneth Norris Jr Comprehensive Cancer Center, 1441 Eastlake Avenue, Los Angeles, CA 90033, USA

D.F. Via
Dept of Surgery, Box 3551, Duke University Medical Center, Durham, NC 27710, USA

M. Wallace
MRC Human Genetics Unit, Western General Hospital, Edinburgh, Scotland

M. Wan
Dept of Pathology, Kenneth Norris Jr Comprehensive Cancer Center, 1441 Eastlake Avenue, Los Angeles, CA 90033, USA

J. Wiener
Dept of Obstetrics and Gynaecology, Duke University Medical Center, Durham, NC 27710, USA

R. Woolas
Dept of Obstetrics and Gynaecology, Northern General Hospital, Sheffield, UK

S. Wu
Dept of Medicine, Duke University Medical Center, Durham, NC 27710, USA

F.J. Xu
Dept of Medicine, Duke University Medical Center, Durham, NC 27710, USA

Y. Xu
Oncology Research, Toronto General Hospital, Toronto, Ontario M5G 2C4, Canada

S. Yonehara
Biotechnology Institute, Tokyo Metropolitan Institute of Medical Sciences, Tokyo, Japan

Y. Yu
Dept of Medicine, Duke University Medical Center, Durham, NC 27710, USA

J. Zheng
Dept of Pathology, Kenneth Norris Jr Comprehensive Cancer Center, 1441 Eastlake Avenue, Los Angeles, CA 90033, USA

S. Zweizig
Dept of Gynecologic Oncology, Kenneth Norris Jr Comprehensive Cancer Center, 1441 Eastlake Avenue, Los Angeles, CA 90033, USA

Preface

The Helene Harris Memorial Trust has become recognized as providing one of the most important international fora for the presentation of research in ovarian cancer. Four biennial meetings have taken place, the most recent of which was held between May 11–14, 1993, in Toronto, Canada. This forum has grown in stature from its inception in 1987 and has brought together interdisciplinary clinical and scientific researchers from around the world who are endeavouring to perform 'cutting edge' studies in the field. The assembled group of prestigious investigators met on this occasion to present their data, to exchange ideas, and to arrange collaborations with the goal of developing new means of detection, treatment and cure of ovarian cancer.

The incentive for the establishment of the Trust and its international forum was the premature loss through ovarian cancer of Helene Harris, the wife of Mr John Harris. Mr Harris and the Trustees looked for a meaningful way to honour the memory of Helene and to advance the noble cause of gaining an increase in the scientific knowledge of the subject. For those of us who spend most of our waking hours assisting patients and their families who are devastated by this disease, the Trust's generosity provides inspiration, hope and the opportunity for their practical application in a unique professional forum.

The excitement and enthusiasm of the scholars who have met to discuss their research on ovarian cancer is remarkable. New levels of knowledge in many aspects of the basic sciences and their clinical application have been reached during the past several years, and the Trust has made an important contribution to this achievement. Over the years, the meetings have become more innovative in their approach to the subject, as the participants have extended themselves in this special collaboration and debate. Whereas the programme of the very first Trust Forum contained only one brief session on the biology of ovarian cancer, the results of the most recent forum, contained herein, fully reflect the burgeoning biological research now influencing clinical practice. Most notably, research inquiries have developed a greater emphasis on the molecular genetics of ovarian cancer. These efforts have engendered presentations that help to focus our attention on the most fundamental methods of achieving control of aberrant ovarian growth. The programme has fostered interdisciplinary international research, as well as improved understanding of the genetics and inheritance of familial susceptibility to ovarian cancer and this, in turn, has led to considerable co-operative research into molecular control of the disease.

Collating the research information and translating it into a form that can be applied in the clinic for the welfare of the patient is a critical part of the work of the Trust. This book summarizes the topics covered in the Fourth Helene Harris Memorial Trust Biennial International Forum on Ovarian Cancer together with its conclusions and recommendations. The book also documents the Trust's commitment to support the finest efforts of all of those who are combating this disease.

Frank Sharp, Sheffield
Peter Mason, London
Tony Blackett, Sheffield
Jonathan Berek, Los Angeles

Helene Harris Memorial Trust Introduction

The Helene Harris Memorial Trust was formed in 1986 to promote communication, discussion and research into ovarian cancer on an international scale. The dialogue between scientists and clinicians covering all departments of the work has proved to be a most successful innovation. It is pleasing to note that parallel bodies using a similar format are now being set up for other types of cancer.

This is the third book published for the H. H. M. T. on ovarian cancer by Chapman & Hall; they have produced yet another fine volume and I would like to express my gratitude on behalf of the H. H. M. T. The three books in the series taken together represent the largest body of work on research and current treatment of ovarian cancer available anywhere in the world and I believe that scientists, clinicians, hospitals and medical schools will find them invaluable.

I would like to thank our editors, Professor Frank Sharp, Mr Peter Mason, Professor Jonathan Berek and Dr Anthony Blackett for their dedicated work which has provided a volume which will prove indispensable to everyone involved in the latest treatment and research into ovarian cancer.

My thanks also to our many distinguished contributors who have voluntarily donated the presentations from which this book is compiled. A further debt of gratitude is owed to Mrs Shirley Claff and Mrs Geraldine Presland for their fine efforts in administering, liaising and transcribing the work of our varied contributors from many countries.

I would also like to extend my appreciation to the Toronto Group in Academic Gynaecological Oncology and Dr Denny DePetrillo, who were our hosts for the Toronto Forum. Toronto has been in the forefront of the research work and the latest clinical practice for ovarian cancer and it was a privilege to hold our 4th Forum in Toronto and enjoy the strong input into the work and the fine cooperation of Dr DePetrillo and his colleagues.

J.E. Harris

Part One
Genetics of Ovarian Cancer

Chapter 1

The genetic epidemiology of ovarian cancer

D.F. EASTON, D. FORD, F.E. MATTHEWS and J. PETO

1.1 INTRODUCTION

Anecdotal evidence for familial clustering of ovarian cancer dates back many years, ovarian tumours occurring in more than one member of the same family being reported as early as 1877 [1]. Since then a number of families containing multiple cases of ovarian cancer have been reported [2,3]. Many of these families also segregate early onset breast cancer [4] or other cancers [5] and the families have generally been suggestive of an autosomal dominant gene conferring a high lifetime risk of disease. Over the past few years more rapid progress has been made in understanding the possible inherited basis of ovarian cancer, firstly through population based epidemiological studies of familial risks and secondly through genetic linkage studies which have demonstrated that many breast–ovarian cancer families are the result of a predisposing gene on chromosome 17q known as BRCA1 [6,7]. In this paper we review some of the epidemiological evidence on genetic susceptibility to ovarian cancer and the 17q linkage studies. We also consider the risks of ovarian cancer conferred by mutations in the BRCA1 gene and examine the likely contribution of BRCA1 to familial

ovarian cancer and to ovarian cancer in general.

1.2 SYSTEMATIC STUDIES OF FAMILIAL OVARIAN CANCER

Most of the systematic evidence for familial clustering of ovarian cancer derives from case–control studies. To date there have been seven published case–control studies with information on family history [8–14]. These are summarized in Table 1.1. All seven studies show some familial effect, with a higher proportion of cases than controls reporting a family history. Combining the results from these studies, the overall familial relative risk is estimated to be 5.0 [15].

Despite the consistency of this evidence, however, there are limitations with the case–control data. One major difficulty is that information on family history is usually obtained by interview and it is likely that some cancers in relatives will be missed or misclassified. This introduces the possibility of serious bias. A second limitation is that the number of cases with affected relatives is small, with the estimated familial risks consequently imprecise, and it is therefore

3

Table 1.1 Numbers of ovarian cancer patients and controls reporting a positive first degree family history of ovarian cancer. Total number of affected relatives is given in brackets, where reported

Study	Cases			Controls		
Casagrande *et al.* (1979)	4/150	(2.7%)	(4)	0/450	(0%)	(0)
Hildreth *et al.* (1981)	4/62	(6.5%)		4/1036	(0.4%)	
Cramer *et al.* (1983)	4/215	(1.9%)		0/150	(0%)	
Tzonou *et al.* (1984)	9/146	(6.2%)	(10)	0/146	(0%)	
Booth (1986)*	4/235	(1.7%)		1/451	(0.2%)	
Schildkraut and Thompson (1989)	16/493	(3.2%)	(16)	26/2465	(1.1%)	(26)
Koch *et al.* (1989)†	10/197	(5.1%)	(10)	4/210	(1.9%)	(4)

* Ovarian cancer *deaths* only
† Included aunt

impossible to make any reliable inferences concerning the mode of inheritance.

1.3 THE OPCS GENETICS STUDY

These difficulties have been overcome to a large extent in the study of Easton *et al.* [16] known as the OPCS genetics & study. This is a population based cohort study of mortality in the first degree relatives of 1203 ovarian cancer patients in the UK. Since it is based on national mortality records, problems of recall bias are avoided. This study confirms that there is an excess familial risk of ovarian cancer but the relative risk was found to be only 2.3-fold (Table 1.2), suggesting that some of the case–control studies may have exaggerated the familial risk. The study also found significant excess mortality from cancers of the stomach, colon, rectum, pancreas and prostate (Table 1.2). There was an excess of breast cancer (relative risk 1.30) which, though not significant, is in line with the relative risk obtained in the CASH (Cancer and Steroid Hormone) study (relative risk 1.6 based on 45 cases) [17] and that obtained for ovarian cancer in the relative & of breast cancer patients in the companion OPCS study (relative risk 1.31 based on 55 deaths).

One interesting result from the OPCS study is that the risk of ovarian cancer was significantly higher in the sisters of cases than in their mothers (Table 1.3). This is true even after adjusting for the age of the index case and the age of the relative. A significantly higher risk in siblings was also seen for breast cancer. Part of this difference in risk can be explained by the known association between ovarian and breast cancers and parity. Since families are ascertained on the basis of the presence of an affected individual, the mothers

Table 1.2 Cancer mortality in relatives of ovarian cancer patients†

Cancer	Observed	Expected	Relative risk
Ovary	34	14.74	2.31***
Stomach	68	45.95	1.48**
Colon	48	35.23	1.36*
Rectum	32	20.94	1.53*
Pancreas	27	18.03	1.50*
Lung	127	115.24	1.10
Breast	57	43.93	1.30
Endometrial	6	4.52	1.33
Prostate	21	14.59	1.44*
Bladder	17	13.37	1.27
Unspecified	26	14.30	1.82**
Other	97	104.55	0.93
Total	560	445.39	1.26***

* $p<.05$ ** $p<.01$ *** $p<.001$
† From Easton *et al.* [16]

Table 1.3 Cancer mortality in first degree relatives of ovarian cancer patients, by type of relative[+]

Type of relative	Site affected in relative			
	Ovary Obs/Exp	Breast Obs/Exp	Stomach Obs/Exp	Colorectal Obs/Esp
Parent	15/10.66	28/30.87	53/39.88	62/47.12
Sibling	19/ 4.06	28/12.75	15/ 6.06	19/ 9.93
Relative risk sibling *vs* parents (95% CI)	2.36 (1.10–5.09)	2.09 (1.15 - 3.78)	1.46 (0.77–2.78)	1.33 (0.74–2.38)

[+] From Easton *et al.* [16]

in this study are likely to have had a greater number of children and hence their expected ovarian and breast cancer risks will be lower than those based on national rates. Assuming that the effects of parity on ovarian cancer risk are as given by the CASH study [18], Easton *et al.* [16] estimated that the true ratio of risks in sisters to mothers in this study was 1.77 for ovarian cancer and 2.09 for breast cancer. The remaining difference in risk could be due to environmental factors shared between sisters or to some recessive gene or genes conferring susceptibility to ovarian cancer.

Much more striking results are obtained by examining the cancer mortality in individuals with more than one affected relative (Table 1.4). For example, individuals with two relatives affected with ovarian cancer had a relative risk of 27. This excess was based on four families with three cases of ovarian cancer,

three in which the mother and a sister of the index case were affected and one in which two sisters were affected in addition to the index case. In fact, of the nine women who had both a mother and a sister affected, three died from ovarian cancer. This massive risk suggests strongly the presence of a highly penetrant ovarian cancer gene.

Table 1.4 also provides stronger support for the familial association between ovarian cancer and colorectal cancer. In individuals having relatives affected with both ovarian and colorectal cancers, there were 11 colorectal cancer deaths compared with 1.23 expected. These excesses are probably the result of families with the autosomal dominant 'Lynch II syndrome', in which colorectal cancer occurs in association with endometrial, ovarian and a number of other cancers [19]. Disease in some Lynch II fami-

Table 1.4 Cancer mortality in individuals with two affected relatives[+]

Sites affected in relatives	Site affected in index case			
	Ovary Obs/Exp	Breast Obs/Exp	Stomach Obs/Exp	Colorectum Obs/Exp
Ovary+ovary	4/0.15	2/0.62	0/1.04	4/1.17
Ovary+breast	2/0.40	1/0.68	5/1.66	3/1.93
Ovary+stomach	0/0.62	5/1.85	1/1.03	2/2.27
Ovary+colorectum	4/0.66	3/1.96	2/1.88	11/1.23

[+] From Easton *et al.* [16]

lies has now been shown by linkage analysis to be due to genes on chromosome 2p and 3p [20].

In view of the familial association between ovarian and breast cancers, another interesting group are the relatives of those individuals with both breast and ovarian cancer. Thirty such cases could be identified in this study and the corresponding study of breast cancer index cases [21]. Of the 60 female relatives of such cases, six died from ovarian cancer compared with 0.38 expected at national rates and eight died from breast cancer compared with 1.12 at national rates. These results suggest that a high proportion of such double primary cases are the result of a gene conferring a high risk of both cancers.

From the point of view of genetic counselling, the results from this study suggest that an important distinction should be made between those individuals with just one affected close relative and those with two or more affected close relatives. Women in the former group have a risk by age 70 of the order of 2–3%, probably not justifying management distinct from women without a family history (although they might be a useful group for randomized trials to evaluate the efficacy of screening), whereas women in the latter group may have a lifetime risk of 20% or more.

1.4 LINKAGE ANALYSIS

Until 1990, none of the genes predisposing to ovarian cancer had been identified or even localized. However in 1990, Hall *et al.* [6] demonstrated genetic linkage in some early onset breast cancer families between the disease and the marker D17S74 on chromosome 17q21. This breast cancer locus has been named BRCA1. That this gene also predisposes to ovarian cancer was demonstrated by Narod *et al.* [7], who found evidence of linkage to D17S74 in some families segregating both early onset breast cancer and ovarian cancer.

Following these two publications and some conflicting unpublished results, an international linkage consortium was established by 13 research groups in an attempt to localize the BRCA1 gene more precisely and to evaluate the extent of heterogeneity and the characteristics of linked families. This consortium analysed linkage data on six genetic markers on chromosome 17q in 214 families. The families included 57 families with at least one case of ovarian cancer in addition to breast cancer [22].

Multipoint linkage analysis using this set of families was able to localize the position of BRCA1 to a region defined by the markers D17S588 (42D6) and D17S250 (mfd15), an interval whose genetic length is approximately 8 centiMorgans (cM) in males and 18 cM in females, with odds of better than 66:1 over other orders. More recent typing of other markers in informative recombinants from linked families has further localized BRCA1 to the interval RARA-D17S78, an interval of less than 4 cM [23].

One of the most striking results from the consortium study was that a clear difference emerged between the breast–ovarian cancer

Table 1.5 Multipoint linkage analysis of breast–ovarian cancer to D17S588 and D17S250ˑ

Group	Number of families	LOD score	Proportion linked*
Breast–ovary	57	20.79	1.00
Breast only**	153	6.01	0.45

Breast only, by number of cases diagnosed below aged 45:

At most 2	110	1.46	0.44
3–4	36	1.89	0.39
5 or more	7	2.88	0.72

ˑ From Easton *et al.* [16]
* All estimates assume that BRCA1 is located 9 cM proximal to D17S588 on the female genetic map, its most likely position in this analysis
** Four families with male breast cancer cases were excluded

families and those segregating breast cancer alone (Table 1.5). In the multipoint heterogeneity analysis, the estimated proportion of linked breast–ovarian families (defined as those containing at least one ovarian cancer in addition to breast cancer cases) was in fact 1.0 with a lower 95% confidence limit of 0.79. In contrast, the families segregating breast cancer alone showed clear evidence of heterogeneity, the estimated proportion of linked families being 0.45 with 95% confidence limits 0.25–0.66.

In fact, the proportion of 'breast–ovarian' cancer families linked to 17q is almost certainly not 100%. A few breast–ovarian families have been reported in which one of the affected individuals does not share the putative disease chromosome. Some of these families contain more recent marker typings not included in the consortium analyses. Perhaps the most convincing example of an unlinked breast–ovarian cancer family has been

reported by Goldgar *et al.* [24]; this family contains six cases of breast cancer in women diagnosed under the age of 50, one male breast cancer case and four ovarian cancer cases. In this family at least three affected individuals (one ovarian cancer and two female breast cancers) do not share the putative 17q linked haplotype. Other breast–ovarian cancer families which are probably not linked to BRCA1 have been noted by Smith *et al.* [25] and Feunteun *et al.* [26].

1.5 THE PENETRANCE OF THE BRCA1 GENE

From the point of view of managing women with a high risk of ovarian cancer, it is important to be able to provide estimates of the age specific risks of cancer to gene carriers. Ultimately it should be possible to obtain such

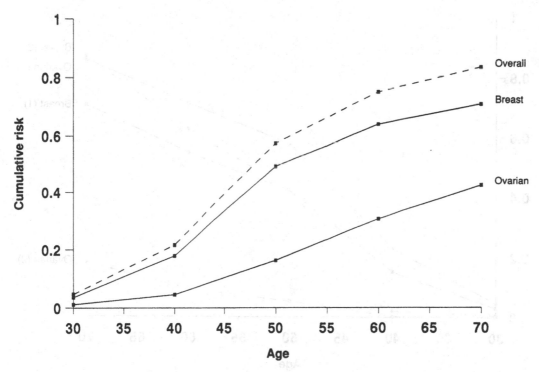

Figure 1.1 Estimated cumulative risks of breast and ovarian cancers and overall risk of either cancer, in BRCA1 mutation carriers, assuming no allelic heterogeneity.

estimates through population based studies of gene carriers, but at the moment the only source of data is from linked families. Such families are not ideal for estimating penetrance, because they have been selected for the occurrence of multiple cases of breast and ovarian cancer and this ascertainment must be allowed for in the analysis. Easton *et al.* [22] overcame this ascertainment problem by maximizing the LOD score over all possible penetrance functions. This gave an estimated cumulative risk of breast or ovarian cancer of 59% by age 50 and 82% by age 70.

A crude estimate of the disease specific risks can be obtained by dividing up the overall estimated incidence by the observed age specific proportions of both breast and ovarian cancer [27]. The resulting age specific penetrances of breast and ovarian cancers are shown in Figure 1.1; the risks of breast and ovarian cancers by age 70 are estimated to be 71% and 41% respectively.

An interesting feature of the ovarian cancer risks in BRCA1 gene carriers is that, in contrast to breast cancer, the risk of ovarian cancer appears to be very low below age 40 (there were in fact only three cases of ovarian cancer below age 40 in this study and none below age 30); above age 40 the estimated risk is about 2% per annum. In fact the pattern of age specific incidence rates is reasonably comparable to that in the general population. Although the ratio of the estimated incidence of ovarian cancer in gene carriers to that in the general population declines from about 100-fold at ages 40–49 to about 40-fold at ages 60–69, these age specific rates are based on relatively small numbers and the decline is

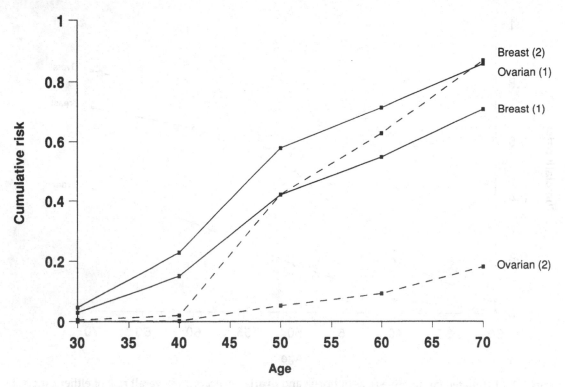

Figure 1.2 Estimated cumulative risks of breast cancer (solid lines) and ovarian cancer (dashed lines) in BRCA1 mutation carriers assuming two susceptibility alleles, indicated by (1) (high ovarian cancer risk) and (2) (moderate ovarian cancer risk).

not nearly as dramatic as for breast cancer, where the incidence ratio declines from 100-fold below age 40 to 11-fold at ages 60–69. A potentially important practical implication of these ovarian cancer incidence rates is that, if prophylactic oophorectomy in a woman at high risk is being considered, an operation in the late thirties might be as effective at reducing the risk of ovarian cancer as an operation at an earlier age.

One major limitation with the above estimates is that they assume that the same risks apply to all families. A simple examination of the linked families suggests that this is unlikely to be true; in many families, the risk of ovarian cancer appears to be low in comparison with the breast cancer risk, whereas in other families the ovarian cancer risk is as high if not higher than the breast cancer risk. For example, one family in the consortium dataset contained nine breast cancers diagnosed under the age of 60 with no ovarian cancers, whilst another contained two breast cancers and eight ovarian cancers. Easton *et al.* [27] have shown that the consortium results are in fact more compatible with a model having two mutant BRCA1 alleles, one conferring a cumulative risk by age 70 of 71% for breast cancer and 87% for ovarian cancer and the other a cumulative risk of 86% for breast cancer and 18% for ovarian cancer (Figure 1.2). Under this model, the first ('high ovarian cancer risk') allele would comprise 11% of BRCA1 mutations in the population, with the second ('moderate ovarian cancer risk') allele comprising the remaining 89%. It will be interesting to see if this allelic heterogeneity can be confirmed by correlating types of BRCA1 mutation with observed cancer risk in the family once the gene has been identified. If it were true, it would obviously have important management implications, since a woman might only opt for prophylactic oophorectomy if she were known to be carrying a high ovarian cancer risk mutation.

1.6 OVARIAN CANCER ONLY FAMILIES

Although there are anecdotal reports of families with an apparent predisposition to ovarian cancer but not early onset breast cancer, few such families have been studied for linkage to BRCA1 and the families which have been studied are generally too small to provide definitive evidence for or against linkage. Steichen-Gersdorf *et al.* [28] have studied 17q linkage in eight families containing three or more cases of ovarian cancer but no cases of premenopausal breast cancer or colorectal cancer (which would suggest a Lynch II syndrome family). In six of the eight families the ovarian cancer cases all shared a consistent 17q haplotype, although only two of the families gave a LOD score of greater than 1.0. In two families one affected individual did not share the putative linked haplotype, so that these families either contain a sporadic ovarian cancer case or are unlinked. Thus evidence to date, weak though it is, suggests that the majority of such 'ovarian cancer only' families are also due to BRCA1 mutations.

1.7 THE GENE FREQUENCY OF BRCA1

It is not possible to estimate the gene frequency for BRCA1, or its contribution to ovarian cancer incidence, directly from the genetic linkage studies. However, a reasonable estimate may be obtained by combining the penetrance estimates for BRCA1 with the results of population based studies such as the OPCS study.

To do this, we assume that the excess mortality from ovarian cancer in the relatives of breast cancer patients is entirely due to BRCA1. In the OPCS breast cancer study there were 47 deaths below age 70 compared with 32.1 expected, or an excess of 14.9 deaths. If this excess were entirely due to BRCA1 and given the penetrance estimates for BRCA1 in Figure 1.2 (i.e. allowing for allelic heterogeneity), the overall population gene frequency for BRCA1 can be estimated to be 0.0007 [29]. A similar analysis can also be conducted using the excess breast cancer mortality observed in the OPCS ovarian cancer study (37 observed as compared with 31.8 expected below age 70) which gives a similar gene frequency estimate.

Assuming a gene frequency of 0.0007, BRCA1 would account for an estimated 2.6% of ovarian cancer incidence below the age of 70, including 4.7% of cases below the age of 50. The corresponding estimates for breast cancer are 2.3% of cases below age 70 and 5.2% of cases below age 50.

1.8   THE CONTRIBUTION OF BRCA1 TO FAMILIAL OVARIAN CANCER

Another issue is the extent to which BRCA1 explains the overall familial clustering of ovarian cancer and whether there are other major ovarian cancer susceptibility genes to be identified. This remains unclear, but various observations suggest that the BRCA1 gene may in fact account for a high proportion of the familial risk. Given the estimated gene frequency of 0.0007 required to explain the breast–ovarian familial association, one can compute that the relative risk of ovarian cancer (up to age 60) in the first degree relatives of ovarian cancer patients due to BRCA1 alone would be approximately 1.6. Thus BRCA1 would account for about half the overall excess familial risk of ovarian cancer (which is 2.3-fold in the OPCS study). Moreover, this could be an underestimate since it does not take account of mutations conferring a high risk of ovarian cancer but a low risk of breast cancer, which would not have been represented in the breast cancer linkage studies. Furthermore, the results from the OPCS study suggest that most if not all of the familial effect can be explained in terms of highly penetrant susceptibility genes and the

linkage results shown above suggest that most families with at least three ovarian cancer cases are due to BRCA1.

The proportion of the ovarian cancer familial risk (though perhaps not the overall proportion of ovarian cancer) due to the Lynch II syndrome gene(s) is probably quite small. This is suggested particularly by the fact that the overall excess mortality from colorectal cancer in the relatives of ovarian cancer patients is only about one half of the ovarian cancer excess, whereas the risk of ovarian cancer in 'Lynch II' gene carriers is clearly low compared to the colorectal cancer risk, both from this study and from anecdotal Lynch II pedigrees.

The above arguments are clearly very approximate. A precise estimate of the proportion of ovarian cancer cases and families due to different predisposing genes will only be obtained using population based studies of mutations in ovarian cancer cases, once the genes have been identified. However, in the meantime, the issue of whether BRCA1 accounts for the majority of familial ovarian cancers could be resolved fairly straight-forwardly by a systematic study of 17q haplotype sharing in affected sister pairs with ovarian cancer, using the methodology of Risch [30]. The power of such an analysis could be improved by additionally considering the loss of alleles in ovarian tumours from such families; this is because 17q allele loss, which has been shown to occur in over 50% of ovarian cancer tumours [31], invariably involves the wild type (non-mutation bearing) chromosome in linked families [32].

1.9   DISCUSSION

Linkage analysis has now been successful at mapping two genes causing important cancer syndromes with ovarian involvement, namely the BRCA1 gene and the hMSH2 and hMCH1 genes on chromosomes 2p and 3p, and it is likely that these genes will be identified in the near future. Although the majority of breast–ovarian cancer families (and possibly 'high risk' ovarian cancer families) appear to be linked to BRCA1, there may be a sufficient number of families unlinked to BRCA1 to map the responsible gene in those families, provided that genetic heterogeneity is not too extensive.

The population based studies suggest that these 'high penetrance' genes are probably responsible for a substantial fraction of the familial effect in ovarian cancer. However, it is probable that other genes conferring a lower risk of ovarian cancer exist; these genes, if common, could in principle account for a higher proportion of ovarian cancer than BRCA1. Such genes would be difficult to detect using linkage analysis, since they would not account for much familial clustering and would instead require allelic association studies in candidate genes to identify them.

Once the BRCA1 gene has been identified, it should be possible to determine the age specific risks in gene carriers, the gene frequency and the extent of allelic heterogeneity with more certainty, using population based studies.

A major question concerns the effect of other risk factors in predisposed individuals. For ovarian cancer there are two well established non-genetic risk factors, namely parity and oral contraceptive use. Case–control studies have consistently demonstrated a protective effect of long term oral contraceptive use. In the most comprehensive study, the CASH study, the relative risk associated with 10 or more years use was 0.2 [18]. (Oral contraceptives could not at this stage be safely advised as a therapeutic measure in BRCA1 gene carriers, however, as their long term use also increases the risk of breast cancer in younger age groups.) Ovarian cancer risk is inversely related to familial size; in the CASH study, the risk for women with four or more children was estimated to be 32%

of the risk to nulliparous women. There are as yet no reliable estimates as to the effects of such risk factors in gene carriers, but an international collaborative epidemiological study of BRCA1 mutation carriers is attempting to address these issues. This study will also be useful for testing the benefits of various therapeutic interventions, such as prophylactic oophorectomy, in high risk women.

REFERENCES

1. Olshausen (1877). *Die Krankheiten der Ovarian*, F. Enke, Stuttgart.
2. Liber, A.F. (1950) Ovarian cancer in mother and five daughters. *Arch. Pathol.*, **49**, 280–90.
3. Fraumeni, J.F. Jr, Grundy, G.W., Creagan, E.T. and Everson, R.B. (1975) Six families prone to ovarian cancer. *Cancer*, **36**, 364–9.
4. Lynch, H.T., Harris R.E., Guirgis, H.A. *et al.* (1978) Familial association of breast/ovarian cancer. *Cancer*, **41**, 1543–9.
5. Lynch, H.T., Albano, W.A., Lynch, J.F. *et al.* (1982) Surveillance and management of patients for high risk of ovarian carcinoma. *Obstet. Gynecol.*, **59**, 589–96.
6. Hall, J.M., Lee, M.K., Morrow, J. *et al.* (1990) Linkage analysis of early onset familial breast cancer to chromosome 17q21. *Science*, **250**, 1684–9.
7. Narod, S.A., Feuteun, J., Lynch, H.T. *et al.* (1991) Familial breast–ovarian cancer locus on chromosome 17q12-q23. *Lancet*, **338**, 82–3.
8. Casagrande, J.T., Pike, M.C., Ross, R.K. *et al.* (1979) 'Incessant ovulation' and ovarian cancer risk. Lancet, **ii**, 170–3.
9. Hildreth, N.G., Kelsey, S.L., Li Volsi, V. *et al.* (1981) An epidemiologic study of epithelial carcinoma of the ovary. *Am. J. Epidemiol.*, **114**, 398–405.
10. Cramer, D.W., Hutchinson, G.B., Welch, W.R. *et al.* (1983) Determinants of ovarian cancer risk I: reproductive experiences and family history. *J. Natl. Cancer Inst.*, **71**, 711–16.
11. Tzonou, A., Day, N.E., Trichopolous, D. *et al.* (1984) The epidemiology of ovarian cancer in Greece: a case–control study. *Eur. J. Cancer Clin. Oncol.*, **20**, 1045–52.

12. Booth, M.A. (1986) Aspects of the epidemiology of ovarian cancer. PhD Thesis, University of London.

13. Schildkraut, J.M. and Thompson, W.D. (1988) Familial ovarian cancer: a population based case–control study. *Am. J. Epidemiol.*, **128**, 456–66.

14. Koch, M., Gaedke, H. and Jenkins, H. (1989) Family history of ovarian cancer: a case–control study. *Int. J. Epidemiol.*, **18**, 782–5.

15. Easton, D.E. and Peto, J. (1990) The contribution of inherited predisposition to cancer incidence. *Cancer Surveys*, **9**, 395–416.

16. Easton, D.F., Matthews, F., Swerdlow, A.J. and Peto, J. (1994) Cancer risks to relatives of ovarian cancer patients. Submitted.

17. Schildkraut, J.M., Risch, N. and Thompson, W.D. (1989) Evaluating genetic association among ovarian, breast and endometrial cancer: evidence for a breast ovarian relationship. *Am. J. Hum. Genet.*, **45**, 521–9.

18. Cancer and Steroid Hormone Study (1987) The reduction in the risk of ovarian cancer associated with oral contraceptive use. *N. Engl. J. Med.*, **316**, 650–5.

19. Lynch, H.T., Kimberling, W., Albano, W.A. *et al.* (1985) Hereditary non polyposis colrectal cancer (Lynch syndrome I and syndrome II) 1. Clinical description of the resource. *Cancer*, **56**, 934–8.

20. Peltomaki, P., Aaltonen, L.A., Sistonen, P. *et al.* (1993) Genetic mapping of a locus predisposing to human colorectal cancer. *Science*, **260**, 810–12.

21. Peto, J., Easton, D.F., Matthews, F. and Swerdlow, A.J. (1994) Cancer risks to relatives of breast cancer patients. Submitted.

22. Easton, D.F., Bishop, D.T., Ford, D. *et al.* (1993) Genetic linkage analysis in familial breast and ovarian cancer – results from 214 families. *Am. J. Hum. Genet.*, **52**, 678–701.

23. Simard, J., Feunteun, J., Lenoir, G. *et al.* (1993) Genetic mapping of the breast–ovarian cancer syndrome to a small interval on chromosome 17q12–21: exclusion of candidate genes EDH17B2 and RARA. *Hum. Mol. Genet.*, **2**, 1193–9.

24. Goldgar, D.E., Rowe, K., Cannon-Albright, L. *et al.* (1994) Genetic epidemiology of familial ovarian cancer in Utah. In *Ovarian Cancer 3*, (eds F. Sharp, P. Mason, J. Berek, A.D. Blackett), Chapman & Hall, London.

25. Smith, S.A., Easton, D.F., Ford, D. *et al.* (1993) Genetic heterogeneity and localisation of a familial breast–ovarian cancer gene on chromosome 17q12-q21. *Am. J. Hum. Genet.*, **52**, 767–76.

26. Feunteun, J., Narod, S.A., Lynch, H.T. *et al.* (1993) A breast–ovarian cancer susceptibility gene maps to chromosome 17q21. *Am. J. Hum. Genet.*, **52**, 736–42.

27. Easton, D.F., Ford, D., Bishop, D.T. *et al.* The risks of breast and ovarian cancer in BRCA1 gene carriers. In preparation.

28. Steichen-Gersdorf, E., Smith, S.A., Ponder, M.A. *et al.* (1994) Analysis of eight families with familial epithelial ovarian cancer for linkage to BRCA1 on 17q12-21; prospects for genetic diagnosis. Submitted.

29. Ford, D., Peto, J., Easton, D.F. *et al.* Estimates of the gene frequency of BRCA1, and its contribution to breast and ovarian cancer incidence. In preparation.

30. Risch, N. (1987) Assessing the role of HLA-linked and unlinked determinants of disease. *Am. J. Hum. Genet.*, **40**, 1–14.

31. Jacobs, I.J., Smith, S.A., Wiseman, R.W., *et al.* (1993) A deletion unit on chromosome 17q in epithelial ovarian tumors distal to the familial breast/ovarian cancer locus. *Cancer Res.*, **53**, 1218–21.

32. Smith, S.A., Easton, D.F., Evans, D.G.R. and Ponder, B.A.J. (1992) Allele losses in the region 17q12-q21 in familial breast and ovarian cancer involve the wild type chromosome. *Nature Genet.*, **2**, 128–33.

Chapter 2

Genetic epidemiology of familial ovarian cancer in Utah

D.E. GOLDGAR, K. ROWE, C.M. LEWIS, M. McDONALD, K. GHOLAMI, L. CANNON-ALBRIGHT and M. SKOLNICK

2.1 INTRODUCTION

Ovarian cancer is the fifth most common cancer in American women but their fourth leading cause of cancer death. Ovarian cancer will strike an estimated 1% of women in their lifetime and is usually fatal. Because of the high mortality associated with ovarian cancer, identification of individuals at increased risk is particularly important. Individuals at very high risk due to genetic susceptibility might consider prophylactic oophorectomy to prevent development of ovarian tumors.

Ovarian cancer among first degree rela-tives is recognized to be predictive of risk of ovarian cancer in the proband [1,2]. Schildkraut and Thompson [2] reported odds ratios for ovarian cancer in first and second degree relatives of 3.6 and 2.9 respectively, compared with women having no family history of ovarian cancer. Interest in the gen-etics of ovarian cancer has substantially increased with the localization of a breast cancer susceptibility locus [3], denoted BRCA1, to the long arm of chromosome 17, and the subsequent finding that ovarian cancers in some breast–ovarian families were due to this locus [4]. The Breast Cancer Linkage Consortium's analysis of 214 breast and breast–ovarian families indicated that virtually all breast–ovarian families were due to BRCA1 [5] and this has been further verified by Feunteun *et al.* [6]. We have however reported several apparently unlinked families [7] and feel it unlikely that all ovarian cancer families are due to BRCA1. As well as the BRCA1 locus, locations of other genes for ovarian cancer sus-ceptibility have been suggested through tumor deletion studies [8–10]. These locations include chromosomes 3p, 6q, 11p and 17p.

In addition to family history, a number of reproductive and hormonally related factors convey increased risk for ovarian cancer. Nulliparity has been consistently related to higher risk for ovarian cancer, as have low numbers of pregnancies. A clear dose-response relationship exists where increasing numbers of pregnancies decrease the risk for ovarian cancer [11]. In contrast to breast cancer, age at first pregnancy does not appear to have a significant effect on ovarian cancer.

The basis of many of our genetic epidemio-logical studies of ovarian cancer in Utah is the Utah Population Database (UPDB). The UPDB is composed of two key linked resources: the Utah Genealogy, consisting of 1.5 million Utah descendants of approx-imately 10 000 Mormon pioneers [12] and the Utah Cancer Registry (UCR) which has had complete statewide incidence data since 1966

13

and now contains more than 113 000 cases. Links have been created between the genealogy and the cancer registry whenever unique identity could be established. Currently, over 45 000 cancer cases in the Utah Cancer Registry have been linked to the genealogical resource. The UPDB allows us to compare the average genealogical relationship between cases of cancer at a given site with sets of suitably matched controls, as well as providing a method of ascertaining large cancer-prone kindreds from a well-defined population.

In this chapter we examine familiality of ovarian cancer in Utah using two distinct approaches. The first approach identifies specific 'families' which contain an excess of ovarian cancer. Here a 'family' refers to all descendants of a single individual who is at the top of the genealogy. These families can then be characterized by age of onset and by the presence or absence of excess frequencies of cancer at other sites. From our second approach, we report on the results of 17q linkage analysis of a group of families identified from the UPDB and subsequently expanded by our group.

2.2 METHODS

2.2.1 IDENTIFICATION OF INDIVIDUAL FOUNDERS WITH EXCESS OVARIAN CANCER AMONG THEIR DESCENDANTS

For a given founder (individual without parents in the genealogy) identified in the UPDB, the following procedure was used to define whether or not an excess of cancer was present at any (or all) site(s). First, the number and types of cancers found among all descendants of the specified founder were tabulated. Next, for each site, we calculated the expected number of cancers based on the birth-year cohort, sex and birthplace distribution (Utah *vs.* non-Utah) of these descendants and cohort specific incidence figures found in

the UPDB as a whole. A statistical comparison between the observed and expected numbers of cancers at each site was obtained by computing the *p*-value associated with the observed numbers of each type of cancer, assuming a Poisson distribution with parameter equal to the expected number.

Ideally, in searching for families with excess numbers of ovarian cancers, we would perform this 'observed/expected' procedure on the descendants of all 10 000 founders in the UPDB. Unfortunately, computational and storage considerations did not permit this approach. Instead, the following approach was used to reduce the number of founders to investigate. For each founder in the genealogy, the number of cancers at each site was tabulated. Based upon the relative frequency of each cancer site in the entire genealogy, we calculated the expected number of cancers at each site found among the descendants. A similar ad hoc Poisson probability calculation was used to identify all founders in whom there was a significant excess of cancer among descendants at any one of the 20 sites studied (at a *p*-value of less than 0.01) with at least five cases of cancer being observed at that site. Computationally this was much more feasible since we have constructed ancestral trees for each cancer case linked to the UPDB. This procedure resulted in a total of 426 founders and was further reduced to 254 founders by requiring that there be at least seven cases for a common site (i.e. prostate, breast, colorectum, melanoma, lung) and five cases for a rare site in which the significant excess was observed. The observed/expected calculations were then performed using the cohort distribution of the descendants of these 254 founders.

2.2.2 ASCERTAINMENT OF FAMILIES

The kindreds reported in this paper were ascertained from two sources. Kindreds 2082 and 2044 were originally ascertained through the UPDB as part of a series of families which

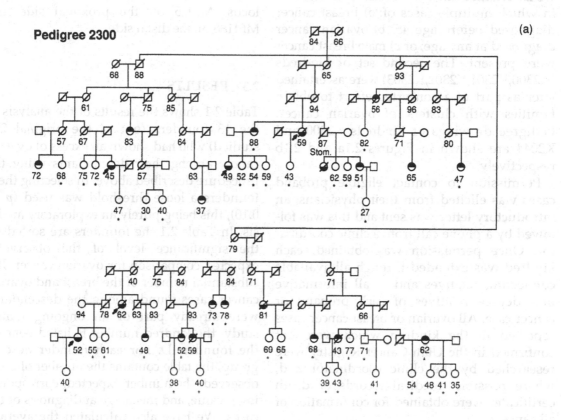

Pedigree 2300 (a)

Pedigree 2044 (b)

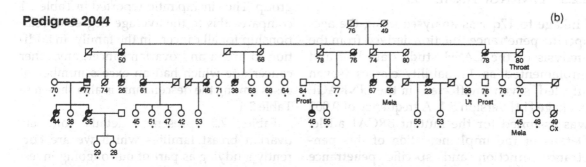

Figure 2.1(a) and (b) Pedigree drawings of kindreds K2300 and K2044. Males who do not have cancer and who are not necessary to connect other parts of the pedigree have been omitted. The arrows designate the probands through whom the family was ascertained. Women diagnosed with breast cancer are denoted by upper-half shaded symbol, ovarian cancer by lower-half shaded symbol. Numbers beneath each symbol represent age at diagnosis, age at death or age at last observation for affected, deceased and living unaffected individuals, respectively.

met certain criteria for sampling. Specifically, we ascertained clusters of related individuals in which multiple cases of: a) breast cancer diagnosed before age 45; b) ovarian cancer diagnosed at any age; or c) male breast cancer were present. The second set of kindreds (K2300,K2301,K2302,K2303) were ascertained later as part of a concerted effort to obtain families with clusters of ovarian cancer. Pedigree drawings of kindreds K2300 and K2044 are shown in Figures 2.1a and 2.1b respectively.

Permission to contact eligible proband cases was elicited from their physicians, an introductory letter was sent and this was followed by a phone call from a clinic coordinator. Once permission was obtained, each kindred was extended through all available connecting relatives and to all informative first degree relatives of each proband or cancer case. All ovarian or breast cancer cases reported in the kindred which were not confirmed in the Utah Cancer Registry were researched by the clinic coordinator and, where possible, medical records or death certificates were obtained for confirmation of all cancers.

2.2.3 LINKAGE ANALYSIS

Linkage to 17q was analysed using the age-specific penetrance function derived from the analysis of the CASH study data [13] and implemented as 14 liability classes (seven affected, seven unaffected) in the LINKAGE package [14] version 5.1. A frequency of 0.003 was assumed for the mutant BRCA1 allele. Details of the implementation of this penetrance function and specific penetrance values can be found in [5]. As in the BCLC analysis, ovarian cases were given the same penetrance as for women in the earliest onset breast cancer group (age less than 30). Men were assumed to be in the youngest unaffected liability class and thus treated essentially as being of unknown phenotype. LOD

scores were calculated between BRCA1 and two markers known to flank the BRCA1 locus, Mfd15 on the proximal side and Mfd188 on the distal side.

2.3 RESULTS

Table 2.1 shows the results of the analysis of the 13 founders (out of the original 254 studied) who had shown an excess of ovarian cancer among their descendants using the procedure described above. In selecting these founders a loose threshold was used ($p < 0.10$), this being purely an exploratory analysis. In Table 2.1 the founders are sorted by the significance level of the observed/ expected comparison for ovarian cancer. If a substantial number of the breast and ovarian cancer cases found among the descendants were already part of an ongoing family study, the kindred number is listed beneath the founder ID. For each founder descent group, the table contains the number of cases observed, the number expected, corresponding p value, and mean age at diagnosis of the cases. We have also calculated the average degree of relationship between the ovarian–breast cases within each founder descent group. The kinship ratio reported in Table 2.1 compares this to the average degree of relationship for all cancers in the family. In addition to breast and ovarian cancer, any other cancer site which had an excess number of cases among the descendants is also shown in Table 2.1.

Table 2.2 presents details on six ovarian–breast families which we are currently studying as part of our ongoing investigations of the BRCA1 locus. Of the six families studied, one is definitely linked to 17q, two more exhibit LOD scores for at least one of the two markers and the other three appear unlinked to 17q. Our largest and most extensively studied family, K2082, is the largest 17q linked family yet identified (in

16

terms of number of cases and LOD score); this family is described in detail elsewhere [16]. Although the LOD scores are quite modest, we believe that based on haplotype analysis, kindreds K2300 and K2301 will eventually prove to be linked to 17q. If kindred K2044 is linked to chromosome 17q, three out of the 16 cancer cases must be termed sporadic, including an ovarian cancer diagnosed at age 46 and three breast cancers diagnosed at ages 38, 56 and 23. Although genotyping is at an early stage in family K2302, it contains three ovarian cancer cases which do not share a common 17q haplotype in the BRCA1 region.

2.4 DISCUSSION

It is well known that there is a strong familial component to ovarian cancer. In this paper we have investigated related individuals with excess ovarian cancer in order to characterize this familiality.

The analysis of individual founder groups produced some interesting results. Of the seven 'families' with clearly significant differences ($p < 0.01$) between observed and expected numbers of ovarian cancers among their descendants, three had mean ages at diagnosis which were significantly younger than the mean of all cases in the UPDB. Similarly, only three of these founders contained significant excesses of breast cancers among their descendants. It is noteworthy that these are the three families which have shown evidence of 17q linkage.

When examining other cancer sites which were also observed to be in excess in the descendants of the 13 founders with excess ovarian cancer, the most commonly observed site was the prostate. In two of these cases, these actually appeared to be prostate cancer families which had a slightly elevated incidence of ovarian cancer. Melanoma, multiple myeloma and lung/respiratory cancers also appeared to be in excess in at least two of these 13 founder groups. In addition, the frequency of individuals who had multiple tumors was elevated among descendants of three founders.

The finding that two out of the six families for which some linkage data were available were apparently unlinked to 17q calls into question the previous finding that virtually all breast–ovarian families are due to the BRCA1 gene [5,6]. Moreover, another breast–ovarian family containing four cases of ovarian cancer, which is not included in this report, also appears unlinked to 17q. More rigorous family studies are necessary to obtain an accurate estimate of the proportion of ovarian and breast–ovarian cancer families which are due to the BRCA1 gene.

One of the goals of this research was to evaluate the approach outlined in this paper as a tool for identifying kindreds suitable for linkage analysis of ovarian cancer. It is comforting that the use of this approach did identify the large linked family, K2082, as well as two other potentially linked kindreds. Our results thus far have also found a number of difficulties with this type of population-based sampling of families. Chief among these is that, even in the case of the descendants of the founder of K2082, one would expect eight breast cancer cases and one or two ovarian cancer cases simply by virtue of sheer numbers of descendants. If, by chance, genotyping was performed early on in a higher proportion of these cases, the family would have appeared unlinked and the kindred might not have been expanded further. Coincidentally, now that genotyping has been largely completed in K2082, we have identified eight breast cancer cases and one ovarian case which do not share the 17q haplotype common to the other cases in this family. Secondly, in studying large groups of descendants in this way, one can never be sure what the 'family' actually consists of, i.e. what is the precise origin of the BRCA1 mutation. It may be that the mutation was actually

Table 2.1 Analysis of founders from the Utah Population Database who have an excess number of cases of ovarian cancer among their descendants

Founder ID (Kindred)	Ovarian cancer					Breast cancer					Other sites			
	No. cases			Age at diagnosis+	KR**	No. cases			Age at diagnosis	KR	Site	No. cases		
	Obs	Exp	p			Obs	Exp	p				Obs	Exp	p
756023 (2082)	9	1.2	.0001	54++	1.4	19	8.0	.0007	51+++	0.9	Endocrine	4	1.5	0.059
1159935 (2301)	9	1.3	.0001	58	0.9	18	9.1	.006	59	0.8	Lymphoma	9	2.8	.003
											Multiple	11	4.6	.008
363442 (2302)	6	0.8	.0002	56+	2.4	6	5.6	.48	57	1.1				
367006 (2300)	6	1.1	.0008	59	1.7	14	7.1	.014	62	1.3	Multiple	12	3.7	.0005
											Prostate	17	9.0	.012
											Uterus	5	2.2	.07
354311	4	0.6	.003	49+	1.3	8	4.0	.052	69	2.0				
322781	4	0.6	.004	61	0.3	6	4.2	.24	64	0.6	Colon	5	2.2	.07
459798	9	3.2	.005	62	0.8	9	21.1	.999	58	0.8	Lung	14	8.0	.03
755683 (2303)	5	1.6	.025	68	1.0	6	11	.96	52	1.0	Soft tissue	3	0.5	.02
											Testes	3	0.9	.07
											Lung	7	3.6	.08
335606	4	1.3	.045	65	2.7	13	8.7	.033	70	1.4	Prostate	24	9.3	.0001

Founder										Cancer			
757776	4	1.5	.06	46+	0.2	0.9	8	9.8	.76	57	Lip	4	1.3	.04
											Multiple myeloma	3	0.8	.048
331033	5	2.1	.06	56	0.8	1.1	14	13.9	.53	66	Multiple myeloma	6	1.3	.002
											Prostate	23	14	.019
											Stomach	5	1.8	.03
324751	4	1.7	.086	66	1.1	0.9	8	11.0	.86	60	Melanoma	9	3.5	.009
											Stomach	4	1.5	.062
341230	5	2.4	.09	61	0.6	1.1	12	15.7	.85	63	Vaginal	5	0.7	.0008
											Respiratory	14	7.1	.014
											Multiple	15	8.0	.018
											Testes	4	1.0	.021
											Melanoma	10	4.7	.023

† Mean age at diagnosis of cases found among descendants of the specified founder is reported. When individual had more than one breast cancer, only the first cancer is used in calculation. Number of +'s after age indicates p value for comparison with average age at diagnosis for 933 cases of ovarian cancer and 6365 cases of breast cancer

‡ KR is the kinship ratio. Values greater than 1.0 indicate that the average degree of relationship between ovarian or breast cases is greater than that observed for all cancers found among descendants of the founder

Table 2.2 Description of the six ovarian–breast cancer families

| Kindred | Ovarian cancer | | | | Breast cancer | | | 17q LOD scores | | | |
| | Number sampled | No. affected | Age at diagnosis | | No. affected | Age at diagnosis | | Mfd15 | | Mfd188 | |
			Med	Min		Med	Min	$\theta = 0.00$	0.05	0.00	0.05
K2044	42	4	56	47	12	49	24	−1.66	−1.16	−0.72	−0.29
K2082	182	18	51	32	29	47	28	2.79	3.68	3.88	4.46
K2300	73	7	53	45	15	63	38	0.28	0.41	0.24	0.55
K2301	14	6	63	58	14	59	33	−0.93	−0.57	0.37	0.24
K2302	30	6	57	48	6	52	36	−0.48	−0.32	−1.26	−0.83
K2303	70	5	68	57	7	48	30	−0.63	−0.20	−0.60	−0.28

brought into the family by a married-in individual. In K2082 we were fortunate because the founder at the top of the pedigree had two wives and the same rare 17q haplotype could be found in breast–ovarian cancer cases in descendants of both marriages. Lastly, we always have to recognize the possibility that there may be more than one BRCA1 or other cancer gene segregating within the family.

In summary, we have found that, although this method is fraught with hazards, when it does work, the rewards are great. One then has a large sample of both unaffected and affected individuals who share a common mutation for genetic epidemiologic studies of the phenotypic effects of that mutation.

ACKNOWLEDGEMENTS

This work was supported by grants CA-55914, CA-48711, CN-05222 and RR-00064 from the National Institutes of Health.

REFERENCES

1. Hildreth, N.G., Kelsey, J.L., Li, V.A. *et al.* (1991) An epidemiologic study of epithelial carcinoma of the ovary. *Am. J. Epidemiol.*, **114**, 398–405.
2. Schildkraut, J.M. and Thompson, W.D. (1988). Familial ovarian cancer: a population-based case–control study. *Am. J. Epidemiol.*, **128**, 456–66.
3. Hall, J.M., Lee, M.K., Newman, B. *et al.* (1990) Linkage of early-onset familial breast cancer to chromosome 17q21. *Science*, **250**, 1684–9
4. Narod, S.A., Feunsteun, J., Lynch, H.T. *et al.* (1991) Familial breast–ovarian cancer locus on chromosome 17q12-q23. *Lancet*, **338**, 82–3.
5. Easton, D.F., Bishop, D.T., Ford, D. *et al.* (1993) Genetic linkage analysis in familial breast and ovarian cancer – results from 214 families. *Am. J. Hum. Genet.*, **52**, 678–701.
6. Feunteun, J., Narod, S.A., Lynch, H.T. *et al.* (1993) A breast–ovarian susceptibility gene maps to chromosome 17q21. *Am. J. Hum. Genet.*, **52**, 736–42.
7. Goldgar, D.E., Cannon-Albright, L.A., Oliphant, A.R. *et al.* (1993) Chromosome 17q linkage studies of 18 Utah breast cancer kindreds. *Am. J. Hum. Genet.*, **52**, 743–8.
8. Eccles, D., Cranston, G., Steel, C.M. *et al.* (1990) Allele losses on chromosome 17 in human epithelial ovarian carcinoma. *Oncogene*, 5, 1599–601.
9. Ehlen, T. and Dubeau, L. (1990) Loss of heterozygosity on chromosomal segments 3p, 6q and 11p in human ovarian carcinomas. *Oncogene*, **5**, 219–22.
10. Lee, J.H., Kavanagh, J.J., Wildrick, D.M. *et al.* (1990) Frequent loss of heterozygosity on chromosomes 6q, 11 and 17 in human ovarian carcinomas. *Cancer Res.*, **50**, 2724–8.
11. Daly, M.B. (1992) The epidemiology of ovarian cancer. *Hematol. Oncol. Clin. N. Am.* , **6**, 729–38.

12. Skolnick, M. (1980) The Utah genealogical data base: a resource for genetic epidemiology. In *Banbury Report No 4: Cancer Incidence in Defined Populations*, (eds J. Cairns, J.L. Lyon, M. Skolnick), Cold Spring Harbor Laboratory, New York, pp 285–97.

13. Claus, E.B., Risch, N. and Thompson, W.D. (1991) Genetic analysis of breast cancer in the Cancer and Steroid Hormone Study. *Am. J. Hum. Genet.*, **48**, 232–42.

14. Lathrop, G.M., Lalouel, J.M., Julier, C. *et al.* (1985) Multilocus linkage analysis in humans: detection of linkage and estimation of recombination. *Am. J. Hum. Genet.*, **37**, 482–98.

15. Goldgar, D.E., Fields, P., Lewis, C.M. *et al.* (1992) A large kindred with 17q-linked susceptibility to breast and ovarian cancer: relationship between genotype and phenotype. *Am. J. Hum. Genet.*, (Suppl.), A96.

16. Goldgar, D.E., Fields, P., Lewis, C.M. *et al.* (1994) A large kindred with 17q-linked breast and ovarian cancer: genetic, phenotypic and genealogical analysis. *J. Nat. Cancer Inst.* **86**, 200–9.

Chapter 3

Isolating tumour suppressor genes relevant to ovarian carcinoma – the role of loss of heterozygosity

W.D. FOULKES and J. TROWSDALE

3.1 INTRODUCTION

Despite the increasing use of chemotherapeutic regimens that achieve high rates of response, the long term outlook for patients with ovarian carcinoma remains dismal. The all-stage five year survival is about 28% and has not improved in the last decade or more [1]. It has become clear that new strategies are required and uncovering genes whose aberrant function can be demonstrated in ovarian carcinoma may have important diagnostic and therapeutic implications.

Here we restrict our discussion to the identification of tumour suppressor genes (TSGs), which in the simplest terms act recessively at the cellular level. This is in contradistinction to oncogenes, which are generally considered to be dominant to the wild type. Since the 1960s there has been accumulating evidence that fusing normal with malignant cells results in some fused cells reverting to a less malignant phenotype [2]. This tumour suppressing activity of normal cells has been localized to specific chromosomes by using microcell transfer of single chromosomes to tumours *in vitro* and selecting for reversion [3]. It is now clear that some transferred chromosomes are able to revert complex malignant phenotypes and therefore may contain important differentiation inducing genes.

However, as yet this technique has not led directly to the discovery of new TSGs.

Over the last 20 years, there has been a number of conceptual and technological advances in human genetics that have made the laborious task of isolating TSGs considerably easier. Experiments that were performed in order to clone the gene responsible for retinoblastoma (RB) provide a useful example. Retinoblastoma, a paediatric eye tumour, can occur in two forms: sporadic, where the tumour is unilateral and the condition is not inheritable, and familial, where usually bilateral (sometimes multiple) tumours are seen rather than unilateral ones, and the disease can be traced through families. RB was the first TSG to be isolated in this fashion and serves as a model against which all other TSGs are assessed. We have used some of the techniques described below to look for regions of the genome that might harbour TSGs relevant to ovarian carcinoma.

3.1.1 CHROMOSOMES AND CANCER

The idea that cancer is a disorder of chromosomes had been considered for many years (Boveri, 1911, quoted in [4]) and with the discovery of chromosomal banding, the description of the normal and abnormal appearance of the complement of chromosomes (a kary-

23

otype) was made possible. Regions of chromosomes that were deleted, duplicated or translocated in various human cells could be discerned. Constitutional deletions (e.g. in lymphocytes) within the long arm of chromosome 13, band 14 (13q14) were seen in children with retinoblastoma [5]. Analysis of a unique retinoblastoma family with a balanced translocation involving 13q14 [6] together with other cytogenetic data [7] suggested strongly that RB was a recessive cancer gene. This idea of cancer genes being recessive to the wild type gene was first put forward by DeMars [8].

3.1.2   THE TWO HIT HYPOTHESIS

Clinical and epidemiological data had shown that in the familial form of retinoblastoma, bilateral tumours occur. In the sporadic non-familial form single, unilateral tumours are the rule. From a statistical analysis of sporadic and inherited forms Knudson hypothesized that only two mutations were rate limiting [9]. This hypothesis was later refined to suggest that mutations were occurring in both alleles of the same, unidentified gene [10, 11]. In the bilateral cases of retinoblastoma, one mutation was inherited and one occurred somatically (the retinoblasts), whereas in sporadic cases both mutations occurred in the somatic cells. This 'two hit' hypothesis explained why children inheriting a mutant copy of the putative gene would suffer multiple tumours and at an earlier age: the first of two necessary mutations had already occurred. This fitted with the cytogenetic data, implying that in the deletion cases, the seemingly normal chromosome 13 contained a cryptic abnormality in the putative gene at band q14. In the non-deletion cases, both 'hits' were submicroscopic. It also implied that one normal gene was sufficient to suppress tumourigenesis, since only those cells with two 'hits' actually developed into cancers. Hence these genes acted recessively, one normal copy being sufficient to suppress the development of cancers. In most adult cancers, many more than one gene have to be knocked out to initiate a tumour, which would explain why the incidence of cancer rises markedly with increasing age.

3.1.3   POLYMORPHISM, LINKAGE AND DISEASE GENE TRACKING

Although protein polymorphisms in the enzyme esterase D were shown to be co-inherited with retinoblastoma [12], such polymorphisms are insufficiently informative (i.e. too many homozygotes) for their general use in tracking diseases. Esterase D has no biological relationship to the development of this disease and it is this non-functional or positional aspect of the marker that is at the centre of genetic linkage analysis. In the late 1970s it had been shown that the human genome contained minor interindividual sequence variation or polymorphism [13]. It was soon appreciated that this might have important implications for human genetics [14]. DNA probes that recognized these restriction fragment length polymorphisms (RFLPs) could be used to track diseases through families. If the probe was sufficiently close to the disease in question then, by linkage disequilibrium, the particular RFLP might be coinherited within a family. Using statistical techniques it became possible to estimate the likelihood that any marker was a certain genetic distance from the disease locus. The number of probes that could be assigned to specific genomic loci was at that time very low, but the use of somatic cell hybrids and the discovery of hypervariable regions of the genome gradually overcame this problem. Using this genomic approach it was possible to show tight linkage between anonymous, accurately localized markers and specific diseases and thus narrow down the region within which the gene must lie.

3.1.4 NORMAL–TUMOUR PAIRS: LOSS OF HETEROZYGOSITY

The cloning of RB was assisted by the analysis of DNA from the retinoblastomas and corresponding normal tissue. If a particular probe recognizes sequence differences between the maternally and paternally inherited DNA then such probes can be used for linkage analysis. They can also be used to study the differences between DNA extracted from tumours and that from uninvolved tissues. In order to look for such differences, the constitutional DNA and tumour DNA are studied in the same experiment. First the DNA is digested with endonucleases which reveal the polymorphisms, then the digested DNA is size fractionated through an agarose gel by electrophoresis. The DNA is transferred to a solid support (filter) and this filter is hybridized with a radiolabelled probe of known localization. Providing that there is endonuclease-recognized sequence variation within the genomic region hybridized with the probe, then the two versions (alleles) can be distinguished by autoradiography, as they will have migrated to different places on the gel. Thus in the normal tissue there may be two bands seen on an autoradiograph. If only one band is seen in the tumour then this is referred to as reduction to homozygosity or loss of heterozygosity (LOH). Large deletions of course may be seen by cytogenetic analysis but submicroscopic deletions, non-disjunction with reduplication or mitotic recombination (see below) will not be detected. The molecular approach can identify and distinguish between these events if a sufficient number of well-spaced markers mapping to the same chromosome is used. This is important because it appears that the latter two mechanisms are common ways in which TSGs are inactivated: in this recessive

model, even two doses of an abnormal gene cannot compensate for the absence of a normal gene.

3.1.5 CLONING OF TUMOUR SUPPRESSOR GENES: A SYNTHESIS

The use of RFLPs led to the identification of a minimally deleted region within 13q14 that was consistent with the cytogenetic and linkage data and which supported the hypothesis of Knudson [15]. This subsequently led to the isolation of RB, which was shown to be aberrant in retinoblastoma [16]. Thus the cloning of RB depended upon clinical and epidemiological data, cytogenetics, somatic cell hybrid and DNA probe resources, linkage analysis in familial retinoblastoma, LOH studies in normal–tumour pairs and finally expression and mutation analysis of candidate cDNAs from the region within which RB was known to lie.

3.2 SOME PROBLEMS IN OVARIAN CANCER GENETICS

The cloning of RB provided a huge stimulus to all those working in cancer genetics and has been followed by the characterization of a number of TSGs which have been shown to be aberrant in both hereditary and sporadic forms of cancer (Table 3.1). It can be seen from this that little is known about the role of many of the known TSGs in ovarian carcinoma. Furthermore, no TSGs specific to this cancer have been isolated. Some of the reasons for this are listed below.

1. Until quite recently it was not appreciated that ovarian carcinoma formed part of definable familial cancer syndromes, despite much evidence that hereditary forms of the disease did exist.
2. Linkage analysis in such rare families can be complicated by the relatively late onset

Table 3.1 Human tumour suppressor genes: involvement in ovarian cancer

Gene[†]	Aberrant in the germ line in hereditary cancer syndromes?	Somatic mutations?[‡]	Aberrant in ovarian cancer?	References
APC	Yes, familial adenomatous polyposis	Yes	No evidence of mutations, 26–50% LOH on 5q	27, 49
DCC	No	No	No published reports, 43% LOH on 18q	28
NF1	Yes, neurofibromatosis type 1	Yes	No published reports, 54% LOH on 17q	24
NF2	Yes, neurofibromatosis type 2	Yes	No published reports, 33% LOH on 22q	
TP53	Yes, Li-Fraumeni syndrome and variants	Yes	Yes, deletions, nonsense and missense mutations. Positive immunohistochemistry	30, 31
RB	Yes, retinoblastoma	Yes	One case of probable homozygous deletion, 44% LOH on 13q	23, 25, 26, 27
VHL	Yes, von Hippel–Lindau syndrome	Not tested	No published reports, 23% LOH	
WT1	Not in familial Wilms' tumour, but seen in association with genital and other congenital abnormalities	No	No, but up to 50% LOH on 11p	29, 50

† This includes inherited cancer predisposing genes that are not formally proven to be TSGs as well as putative TSGs that do not appear to be associated with an inherited predisposition to cancer. At present it is unclear whether NME1, MCC and ERBA should be included in this list
‡ In cancers other than the tumour type in which the mutation was originally reported

of this disease. When ovarian carcinoma does occur, it may be difficult to exclude affected but unlinked individuals (phenocopies).

3. The pathogenesis of ovarian carcinoma is less well understood than that of colorectal carcinoma, where a stepwise progression from benign adenoma to malignant carcinoma has been demonstrated. This has been accompanied by a description of the molecular events that underlie these pathological changes [17]. However, there have been some recent advances in our understanding of the natural history of ovarian carcinoma [18] which will hopefully lead to a similar description of molecular events in the disease.

4. Cytogenetic studies have shown that aneuploidy and qualitative abnormalities such as deletions and translocations are extremely common in ovarian carcinoma, probably reflecting the fact that most detected tumours are late stage. It has not been possible to find chromosomal areas consistently involved in all tumours. This has somewhat limited the specificity of a molecular approach.

3.3 THE CANDIDATE GENE APPROACH

The cloning of genes by position only is very laborious. In the recent example of the gene responsible for Huntingdon's disease, it took an international consortium a decade or so to clone the gene, starting from a closely linked marker. Although there were special problems with the cloning of this gene, it serves to demonstrate that positional cloning can be extremely difficult and labour-intensive. True candidate gene cloning is relatively straightforward: genes encoding enzymes known to be aberrant in a disease process can be analysed for mutations. Thus the gene is cloned on the basis of function. As more genes are cloned and accurately mapped, it is highly likely that a modified form of positional cloning will become more prevalent. In this 'positional candidate cloning' approach [19], genes mapping to a large region (perhaps 5 million base pairs) known to be linked to a familial disease may be analysed for mutations directly, without waiting for more accurate information on the precise position of the candidate. The gene is chosen as a candidate because of its relevance to the disease process. This combined approach is typified by autosomal dominant retinitis pigmentosa. The gene encoding rhodopsin was localized to 3q and several years later, retinitis pigmentosa was genetically linked to the same region. As rhodopsin is expressed in rod photoreceptors which are affected early in the course of the disease, there was an *a priori* reason to suspect that this gene might be implicated. Soon after the linkage data were published, mutations were reported in the rhodopsin gene in affected members from a number of different families, indicating that these mutations were causal [20]. Thus accurate positional information was not required for the identification of the correct gene.

In breast and ovarian carcinoma, the positional candidate gene approach has been used to try to find BRCA1. A number of genes regulating oestrogen and its derivatives, such as oestradiol 17β dehydrogenase type 2 (17HSD2), are known to map near to BRCA1. Although no abnormalities have been noted in 17HSD2 in inherited or sporadic breast

cancer (D.M. Black, personal communication), other candidate genes within the limits of the linked region are under intense investigation.

3.4 CHROMOSOMAL MECHANISMS OF LOSS OF HETEROZYGOSITY

In the early 1980s cytogenetic studies had demonstrated both qualitative and quantitative chromosomal abnormalities in ovarian carcinoma. However, it was not possible using conventional banding techniques to discriminate between sequences from the maternal and paternal chromosomes. By using Southern blotting and a large number of RFLPs per chromosome arm, it became possible to show that there are several different chromosomal mechanisms causing LOH. These studies have shown that breakage of a chromosome with subsequent loss of genetic material is not necessarily the commonest mechanism by which LOH occurs. Other mechanisms such as non-disjunction and mitotic recombination have been shown to be important as well.

Mitotic recombination, first noted in *Drosophila*, had not previously been noted in human cancer cells before the work of Cavenee *et al.* showed that it occurred in retinoblastoma on chromosome 13 [15]. Recombination normally occurs during meiosis, where homologous chromosomes exchange sequences. The significance of mitotic recombination for TSGs is that the chromosomes will be identical below the crossover point resulting in LOH and therefore any crossover centromeric to the TSG will result in homozygosity at that locus. Thus there is no requirement for two mutations in the TSG or for a deletion of the wild type gene. This also applies to non-disjunction, which occurs when paired chromosomes fail to separate at cell division. Again, this can occur during mitosis, resulting in a cell where both chromosomes are derived from the same parent. Thus there will be LOH over the whole chromosome. Examples from our own work of mitotic recombination and non-disjunction are illustrated in Figure 3.1. Where data exist, non-disjunction and mitotic recombination appear to be common mechanisms of LOH in all cancers studied. Other mechanisms of LOH such as deletion (terminal or interstitial), gene conversion and

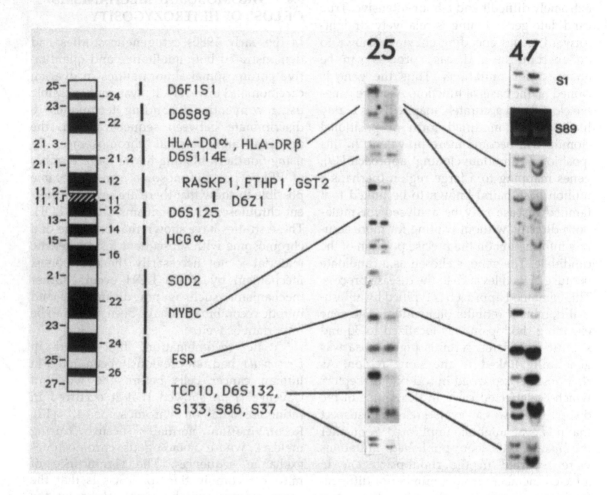

Figure 3.1 Loss of heterozygosity on chromosome 6. On the left is a karyogram of chromosome 6 with the probes used in our publication [39] marked. A selection of the autoradiographs and one ethidium bromide stained polyacrylamide gel is shown. The tumours are numbers 25 and 47. In both cases the lymphocyte DNA is shown on the left and the tumour DNA on the right. Tumour 25 demonstrates LOH at all informative markers on chromosome 6. This is probably accounted for by nondisjunction. Tumour 47 shows LOH at all markers on 6q, but retention at all markers on 6p. Due to loading differences, the intensity of the retained bands varies between autoradiographs. From comparison with other autoradiographs not shown here, mitotic recombination is probably the mechanism of LOH in this case. The lines connecting the autoradiographs signify common chromosomal locations. The autoradiographs represents, from top to bottom, HLA-DQα, RASKP1, MYBC, ESR, D6S133, D6S132 (tumour 25) and D6F1S1, D6S89, HLA-DQα, D6S114E, ESR, D6S86, TCP 10 (tumour 47). D6F1S1 and D6S89 have been abbreviated to S1 and S89 respectively. The upper allele for S89 is faint but has equal intensity in the lymphocyte and tumour lanes.

translocation are also seen, but unfortunately these methods appears to be less common than recombination and non-disjunction. In particular, very few cases of small deletions in ovarian carcinoma (interstitial or otherwise) have been seen. However, looking for these unusual cases is a very worthwhile task, because they may precisely localize the position of a TSG and render cloning the gene a far more manageable operation.

3.5 LOSS OF HETEROZYGOSITY IN OVARIAN CARCINOMA

The numerous studies of LOH in ovarian carcinoma have all been published since 1989 and are all largely based on techniques described by Cavenee *et al.* [15] using normal–tumour pairs to look for LOH. There are five basic reasons for choosing particular chromosomes on which to look for LOH:

1. The position of known TSGs that may be implicated, such as p53 on chromosome 17p.
2. LOH reported on that chromosome in other tumours.
3. The presence of clonal cytogenetic lesions on that chromosome in tumours, e.g. 3p, 6q and 11.
4. Linkage in families with ovarian carcinoma to a particular region of one chromosome, for example 17q.
5. The systematic approach – one or more marker(s) on each arm (usually telomeric) to define an 'allelotype' for that tumour.

These five types of studies have been carried out for ovarian carcinoma and have enabled the construction of a provisional 'cumulative allelotype' based on all the published studies of LOH up to April 1993. The data from these studies are listed chromosome by chromosome in Table 3.2. A histogram (Figure 3.2) has been constructed from this table. While this figure contains a large amount of useful data, it is important to note that there are a number of biases with this type of accumulative analysis. A breakdown of the data into sets with chromosome arms having 0–20% LOH, 20–30% LOH and >30% LOH demonstrates one potential bias. In these three sets there was an average of 28.4, 83.8 and 98.5 tumours studied per classification, as regions of the chromosome where a particular group have shown high LOH are likely to attract further studies. Clearly a more systematic approach would limit this bias. The chromosomal location of known TSGs is marked on Figure 3.2 and it is no surprise that frequent LOH is seen on chromosomal arms known to harbour TSGs. Despite this, there are relatively few studies of the TSGs themselves (Table 3.1) and so the conclusion that the LOH on a particular arm can be accounted for by a known TSG mapping to that arm must remain speculative. Another problem is that this data are compiled from studies where only one probe per arm was used, as well as studies where more serious attempts to map LOH were made, sometimes using up to 20 probes per chromosome. These latter studies are effectively underrepresented as they take much more time. LOH mapping studies may end up with lower LOH frequency overall but usually provide more information about events along the whole chromosome. If only one probe per chromosome is used (as was often the case in the earlier studies) then LOH on one arm may actually reflect LOH on the other arm, which will not show in the results.

Figure 3.2 shows that 14 chromosomal arms show greater than 30% LOH. This figure is generally regarded, somewhat arbitrarily, as the level of significance for LOH, implying that TSGs are likely to be located within regions showing 30% LOH or more. Does this mean that there are at least 14 TSGs of importance to ovarian carcinoma? Probably not. One problem is that of cause and effect. Whilst LOH at a site known to be linked to a

Table 3.2 Compilation of published data on LOH in ovarian carcinoma: a provisional allelotype

Chromosomal arm	Frequency of LOH (%)*	Smallest region of LOH (reference)	References (listed as in order in column 2)
1p	1/14 (7), 1/15 (7), 7/18 (39)	—	[32], [26], [28]
1q	0/5 (0), 4/14 (29), 1/15 (7)	—	[33], [32], [26]
2p	0/11 (0)	—	[32]
2q	1/5 (20), 4/29 (14)	—	[33], [32]
3p	4/7 (57), 6/15 (40), 6/33 (18), 2/4 (50), 5/22 (23)	3p22-21.1 [36] 3p24.1-22 [35]	[34], [35], [32], [36], [38]
3q	1/18 (6)	—	[32]
4p	10/24 (42)	—	[32]
4q	1/16 (6)	—	[32]
5p	0/9 (0), 0/18 (0)	—	[34], [35]
5q	0/8 (0), 0/15 (0), 6/12 (50)	—	[33], [32], [27]
6p	0/9 (0), 6/12 (50), 8/29 (28)	6pter-p22.3, 6p22-12 [39]	[33], [32], [39]
6q	4/7 (57), 9/14 (64), 5/9 (56), 5/29 (17), 17/33 (52), 4/19 (21), 16/29 (55), 2/13 (15)	6q27 [34, 35, 37], 6q24-qter [33], [38]	[34], [33], [35], [32], [37], [38], [39], [23]
7p	3/7 (43)	—	[32]
7q	0/11 (0), 4/19 (21), 1/5 (20), 2/18 (11)	—	[29], [32], [33], [40]
8p	—	—	
8q	5/16 (31)	—	[32]
9p	—	—	
9q	1/10 (10), 2/20 (10)	—	[35], [32]
10p	3/27 (11), 4/18 (22)	—	[32], [39]
10q	2/16 (13), 5/24 (21), 4/13 (31)	—	[35], [32], [38]
11p	5/10 (50), 5/11 (46) 4/9 (44), 8/23 (35), 7/29 (24), 18/44 (41), 2/13 (15), 10/19 (53), 10/25 (40), 5/15 (33), 5/10 (50)	11p13, 11p15.5 [41] 11p15.5-11p13 [40]	[29], [33], [34], [35], [32], [41], [42], [40], [23], [43], [27]
11q	0/5 (0), 0/12 (0), 1/19 (5), 14/27 (52)	11q23.3-qter [42]	[33], [26], [32], [42]
12p	0/7 (0), 3/8 (38)	—	[33], [32]
12q	5/15 (33)	—	[32]
13p	—	—	

Table 3.2 contd

Chromosomal arm	Frequency of LOH (%)*	Smallest region of LOH (reference)	References (listed as in order in column 2)
13q	6/20 (30), 1/17 (6), 6/27 (22), 22/42 (52), 18/31 (58), 10/14 (71)	13q33-34 [38]	[26], [35], [32], [38], [23], [27]
14p	—	—	
14q	5/28 (18), 3/9 (33)	—	[32], [28]
15p	1/15 (7)	—	[26]
15q	1/9 (11)	—	[32]
16p	7/21 (33)	—	[32]
16q	11/30 (37), 6/22 (27), 2/24 (8)	—	[32], [39], [23]
17p	6/8 (75), 16/20 (80), 5/19 (26), 13/28 (46), 14/20 (70), 34/63 (54), 15/27 (56), 27/41 (66), 7/34 (21), 18/23 (78), 15/28 (54), 25/28 (89)	17p13.3-13.1, 17p12-11.1 [44, 48], 17p13.3, [32, 46, 48]	[33], [30], [35], [32], [44], [24], [45], [28], [38], [46], [23], [48]
17q	5/16 (31), 12/31 (29), 45/64 (70), 11/30 (37), 21/28 (75), 64/120 (53), 23/30 (77)	17q21 [48], 17q22-23 [47, 48] 17q25-qter [48]	[33], [32], [24], [38], [46], [47], [48]
18p	0/6 (0), 3/9 (33)	—	[32], [28]
18q	0/8 (0), 31/52 (60)	18q23 [28]	[32], [28]
19p	11/32 (34)	—	[32]
19q	1/7 (14), 4/16 (25)	—	[33], [32]
20p&q	4/32 (13)	—	[32]
21p&q	0/6 (0), 0/12 (0), 0/12 (0)	—	[34], [35], [32]
22p&q	0/6 (0), 1/5 (20), 2/10 (20)	—	[29], [33], [32]
Xp	18/40 (45)	Xp21.1-11.4 [38]	[38]
Xq	—	—	

* If data from original paper cannot be extracted, largest number of tumours studied with highest frequency of LOH taken. Some data are combined from earlier papers covering the same samples: only the later publications are included here

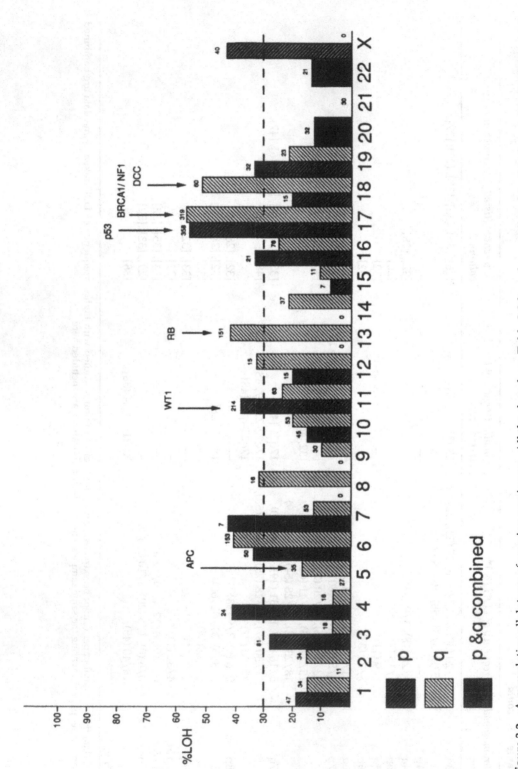

Figure 3.2 A cumulative allelotype of ovarian carcinoma. All the data from Table 3.2 have been collated in this figure. The LOH for each arm is represented by histrograms. X axis: chromosomal arms. Y axis: percentage loss of heterozygosity. The dashed line is placed at 30% LOH, a percentages thought to imply significance for the presence of a TSG within the region showing LOH. The numbers above each of the columns refers to the total number of tumour/blood pairs studied for each arm.

familial form of the disease is highly likely to be causal in the pathogenesis of a carcinoma, LOH elsewhere is more problematic. As genes such as p53, which control the cell cycle, become mutated, there is increasing likelihood of errors in DNA replication [21]. This can lead to non-disjunction, mitotic recombination and deletion. If, at one cell division, a large number of events occur together, then they may be selected for on the basis of only one such event being advantageous to tumour growth. The events on other chromosomes are thus merely neutral bystanders which do not have any disadvantage or advantage to the cancer cell.

Non-disjunction is probably the commonest mechanism by which tumours show LOH. This does not provide useful information for fine mapping of regions thought to contain TSGs and it has become apparent that large numbers of sporadic tumours will have to be studied in order to build up a convincing deletion map in ovarian carcinoma. Nevertheless, there is now a considerable amount of data and it is worthwhile to draw attention to some specific results shown in Table 3.2 and Figure 3.2 and to comment on possible future directions.

1. LOH is very frequent on chromosome 17. BRCA1, the unknown gene implicated in familial breast and ovarian carcinoma, is located at 17q12-21, but there are numerous genes (e.g. p53, NME1, NF1, prohibitin) on chromosome 17 which could account for the LOH. Two groups have reported LOH on 17q outside the BRCA1 region [47, 48].
2. Chromosome 6q appears to show frequent LOH, around 50% overall. Recent studies suggest that part of 6q27 may be the smallest region of LOH.
3. LOH involving 11p is common and may involve more than one region. Mutation analysis of WT1 has been negative [50].
4. One study has suggested that LOH on 18q may involve regions which are more telomeric than the putative TSG DCC. As DCC is a large gene, it will take a long time to eliminate mutations in DCC as a contributory factor to LOH on 18q.
5. The X chromosome shows LOH. X inactivation is non-random, implying a clonal origin for ovarian carcinoma. Since X inactivation normally occurs *in utero*, LOH of specific regions subject to inactivation may suggest that two hits are not necessary for the disabling of putative TSGs mapping to the X chromosome.
6. On the basis of this 'cumulative allelotype', other regions of the genome that may contain TSGs include 3p (several regions of 3p are implicated in small cell lung cancer, renal cell carcinoma and gynaecological cancers. The inherited cancer syndrome, von Hippel–Lindau, maps to 3p25), 13q (RB is at 13q14) and 16q (a site of frequent LOH in breast carcinoma). Although moderately frequent LOH is seen on 4p, 7p, 8q, 12q and 16p, the number of tumours studied for each arm is less than 25 and therefore the siting of TSGs on these arms must remain highly speculative.
7. From data accumulated from numerous LOH studies of other cancers, it seems unlikely that there are chromosomal arms where LOH is limited to ovarian carcinoma. It may be that groups of tumours (such as breast and ovarian carcinoma) show broadly similar patterns of LOH, but truly specific loci have not yet been uncovered. Generally speaking, inactivation of any one TSG is not restricted to a cell type. This may be especially true of TSGs such as p53 and RB which have a nuclear localization and are implicated in cell cycle control.

3.6 ACCUMULATION OF GENETIC HITS IN OVARIAN CARCINOMA

In the well-known genetic model of colorectal cancer [22] a particular order of genetic

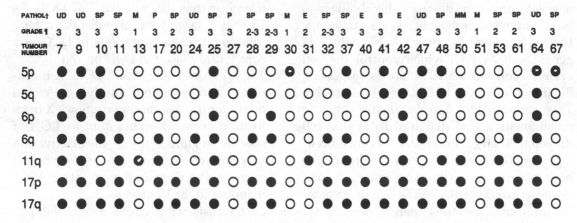

Figure 3.3 Loss of heterozygosity in 27 ovarian carcinomas on seven chromosomal arms: 5p, 5q, 6p, 6q, 11q, 17p and 17q. Shown here is the result of studying the same tumour/blood pairs with a number of markers on seven different chromosomes. ●, LOH with at least one marker on the denoted arm; ○, no LOH with any marker on the denoted arm; ◑; no information.

† Histopathological classification: UD, undifferentiated adenocarcinoma; SP, serous papillary carcinoma; P, papillary carcinoma; SPAC, serous papillary adenocarcinoma; M, mucinous adenocarcinoma; E, endometrioid adenocarcinoma; MM, mixed Müllerian tumour; S, serous carcinoma.

¶ Pathological grade based on criteria described previously [39].

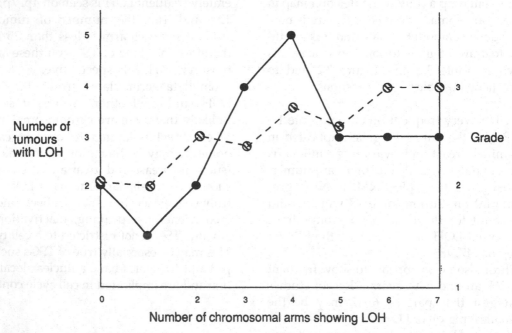

Figure 3.4 LOH: number of arms showing LOH per tumour and comparison with grade. The relationship between LOH and tumour grade in our series of tumours is demonstrated. X-axis: the number of chromosomal arms showing LOH (out of a maximum of seven; see Figure 3.3). Y-axis: (left) number of tumours with LOH, (right) grade. ●, LOH per arm; ◍, grade (see Figure 3.3). Mean number of arms lost per tumour is 4.3, mean grade is 2.5.

Table 3.3 Frequency of LOH on chromosomes 3p, 6q, 11p, 13q, 17 and 18q: correlations with tumour grade and stage

Locus or arm	Tumour type				Reference
	benign	borderline	low grade #	high grade #	
3p	NT	NT	2/20 (10)	4/5 (80)	[35]
6q	NT	NT	4/18 (22)	3/5 (60)	[35]
11p	NT	NT	5/22 (23)	3/4 (75)	[35]
11p	NT	0/2 (0)	0/6 (0)	5/9 (56) *	[43]
11p	0/4 (0)	0/2 (0)	5/11 (45)	5/8 (63)	[23]
13q	NT	NT	1/14 (7)	0/3 (0)	[35]
13q	1/4 (25)	2/5 (40)	11/15 (73)	4/7 (57)	[23]
17p	3/4 (75)	1/5 (20)	9/15 (60)	7/9 (78)	[23]
17p	NT	NT	4/17 (24)	1/2 (50)	[35]
17p at TP53	1/13 (8)	1/7 (14)	5/15 (33)	17/32 (53)	[24]
p53	NT	NT	3/13 (23)	6/18 (33)	[30]
17q	3/23 (13)	2/16 (13)	11/20 (55)	34/44 (77)	[24]
18q	NT	NT	3/7 (43)	28/45 (62)	[29]

NT = not tested

Where information available, low grade is stage I–II or grade 1–2, high grade is any score greater than this

* LOH at an adjacent locus is much less (<20%)

events was suggested, although it was made clear that it is the accumulation and not the order of genetic hits that is important for tumourigenesis. As mentioned above, it has been difficult to apply the same sort of analysis in the ovary. However, some data point in the same direction as that described for colorectal cancer. We have studied seven chromosomal arms in some detail. Figure 3.3 shows the results of our analysis. LOH is common on all the arms studied, but is particularly frequent on chromosome 17. Some tumours (e.g. tumour 7) show LOH on all arms studied, whereas in others (e.g. tumour 27) there is no LOH at any site. We also studied 12 benign tumours, but did not find any cases with LOH. Our work has also demonstrated that, unsurprisingly, higher grade ovarian carcinomas show a greater frequency of LOH than lower grade tumours (Figure 3.4). Whilst it is likely that at least some tumours can be explained by a stepwise progression model [22], in others the LOH–grade association might be due to an early mutation in a gene which predisposes to genomic instability and LOH, which might render a tumour grade 3 *de novo*. In this model, tumours do not move readily between grades and the LOH seen is largely secondary to other events.

There is preliminary evidence that particular patterns of LOH are associated with different grades of ovarian carcinomas. Some of these studies are summarized in Table 3.3. Insofar as the data can be compared, it seems that, compared with high grade tumours, in benign/borderline tumours or in the early stages (defined as grade 1–2 or stage I–II) of ovarian carcinoma, LOH is not especially frequent at any locus on chromosomes 3, 6, 11 and 18. There is some evidence that 13q and 17p LOH occurs at an earlier stage than other losses [23], but the 17p findings are not supported by other data [24], which hint at 17q LOH occurring before 17p. However, all this work is preliminary and mutation analysis of known TSGs in benign and borderline tumours and in different grades of ovarian carcinoma will be required for confirmation.

3.7 CONCLUSIONS

In this chapter we have outlined the way in which TSGs can be identified, described some of the work carried out toward this goal and reviewed the published literature on LOH in ovarian carcinoma. This field is moving very fast and it is likely that a number of new TSGs will be described within the next few years or so. Some of these may be implicated in inherited cancer syndromes. Although primary ultrasound screening looks helpful for those at high risk, automated DNA and gene product based tests are likely to prove more cost-effective, particularly when BRCA1 and other ovarian cancer susceptibility genes have been cloned. An understanding of the molecular pathogenesis of this disease should also result in more effective therapy, although significant improvement in the survival data resulting from this approach is very unlikely this century. However, a collaborative approach to the management of ovarian carcinoma offers the best hope for patients and those at risk. The addition of laboratory scientists to those already caring for these women will announce the arrival of molecular genetics as a clinical reality for cancer patients.

ACKNOWLEDGEMENTS

We would like to thank all the hospitals who have provided clinical material for our work. Ms S. Cottrell and Drs G.J. Allan, D.M. Black, I.G. Campbell, J. Ragoussis, E. Solomon and G.W.H. Stamp all contributed to the experiments carried out in the Human Immunogenetics Laboratory. This chapter is dedicated by W.F. to Dr J.D. Francis.

REFERENCES

1. Slevin, M.L. (1986) Ovarian cancer, in *Randomised Trials in Cancer – A Critical Review by Sites*, (eds M.L. Slevin and J. Staquet), Raven Press, New York, pp. 385–416.

2. Harris, H., Miller, O.J., Klein, G. *et al.* (1969) Suppression of malignancy by cell fusion. *Nature*, **223**, 363–8.

3. Saxon, P.J., Srivatsan, E.S. and Stanbridge, E.J. (1986) Introduction of human chromosome 11 via microcell transfer controls tumorigenic expression in HeLa cells. *EMBO J*, **5**, 3461–6.

4. Gelehrter, T.D. and Collins, F.S. (1990) *Principles of Medical Genetics*, Williams and Wilkins, Baltimore.

5. Yunis, J.J. and Ramsay, N. (1978) Retinoblastoma and a subband deletion of chromosome 13. *Am. J. Dis. Child.*, **132**, 161–3.

6. Strong, L.C., Riccardi, V.M., Ferrell, R.E. and Sparkes, R.S. (1981) Familial retinoblastoma and chromosomal deletion transmitted via an insertional translocation. *Science*, **213**, 1501–3.

7. Benedict, W.F., Murphree, A.L., Banerjee, A. *et al.* (1983) Patient with chromosome 13 deletion: evidence that the retinoblastoma gene is a recessive cancer gene. *Science*, **289**, 973–5.

8. DeMars, R. (1970) In 23rd Annual Symposium, Fundamental cancer research 1969. Williams and Wilkins, Baltimore, pp. 105–6.

9. Knudson, A.G. (1971) Mutation and cancer: statistical study of retinoblastoma. *Proc. Natl. Acad. Sci. USA*, **68**, 820–3.

10. Comings, D. (1973) A general theory of carcinogenesis. *Proc. Natl. Acad. Sci. USA*, **70**, 3324–8.

11. Knudson, A.G. (1978) Retinoblastoma: a prototypic hereditary neoplasm. *Semin. Oncol.*, **5**, 57–60.

12. Sparkes, R.S., Murphree, A.L., Lingua, R.W. *et al.* (1983) Gene for hereditary retinoblastoma assigned to human chromosome 13 by linkage to Esterase D. *Science*, **289**, 971–3.

13. Kan, Y.W. and Dozy, A.M. (1978) Polymorphism of DNA sequence adjacent to human β haemoglobin structural gene: relationship to sickle mutation. *Proc. Natl. Acad. Sci. USA*, **75**, 5631–5.

14. Solomon, E. and Bodmer, W.F. (1979) Evolution of a sickle variant gene. *Lancet*, **i**, 923.

15. Cavenee, W.B., Dryja, T.P., Phillips, R.A. *et al.* (1983) Expression of recessive alleles by chromosomal mechanism in retinoblastoma. *Nature*, **305**, 779–84.

16. Friend, S.H., Bernards, R., Rogelj, S. *et al.* (1986) A human DNA segment with properties of a gene that predisposes to retinoblastoma and osteosarcoma. *Nature*, **323**, 643–6.

17. Vogelstein, B., Fearon, E.R., Hamilton, S.R. *et al.* (1988) Genetic alterations during colorectal tumor development. *N. Engl. J. Med.*, **319**, 525–32.

18. Powell, D.E., Puls, L. and van Nagell, J. (1992) Current concepts in epithelial ovarian tumours: does benign to malignant transformation occur? *Hum. Pathol.*, **23**, 846–7.

19. Ballabio, A. (1993) The rise and fall of positional cloning? *Nature Genet.*, **3**, 277–9.

20. Dryja, T.P., McGee, T.L., Reichel, E. *et al.* (1990) A point mutation of the rhodopsin gene in one form of retinitis pigmentosa. *Nature*, **343**, 364–6.

21. Hartwell, L. (1992) Defects in a cell cycle checkpoint may be responsible for the genomic instability of cancer cells. *Cell*, **71**, 543–6.

22. Fearon, E.R. and Vogelstein, B. (1990) A genetic model for colorectal tumourigenesis. *Cell*, **61**, 759–67.

23. Gallion, H.H., Powell, D.E., Morrow, J.K. *et al.* (1992) Molecular genetic changes in human epithelial ovarian malignancies. *Gynecol. Oncol.*, **47**, 137–42.

24. Eccles, D.M., Russell, S.E.H., Haites, N.E and the ABE Ovarian Cancer Genetics Group (1992) Early loss of heterozygosity in ovarian cancer. *Oncogene*, **7**, 2069–72.

25. Sasano, H., Comerford, J., Silverberg, S.G. and Garrett, C.T. (1990) An analysis of abnormalities of the retinoblastoma gene in human ovarian and endometrial carcinoma. *Cancer*, **66**, 2150–4.

26. Li S-B., Schwartz, P.E., Lee, W-H. and Yang-Feng, T.L. (1991) Allele loss at the retinoblastoma locus in human ovarian cancer. *J. Natl. Cancer Inst.*, **83**, 637–40.

27. Jacobs, I.J., Kohler, M.F., Wiseman, R.W. *et al.* (1992) Clonal origin of epithelial ovarian carcinoma: analysis by loss of heterozygosity, p53 mutation and X-chromosome inactivation. *J. Natl. Cancer Inst.*, **84**, 1793–8.

28. Chenevix-Trench, G., Leary, J., Kerr, J. *et al.* (1992) Frequent loss of heterozygosity on chromosome 18 in ovarian adenocarcinoma which does not always include the DCC locus. *Oncogene*, **7**, 1059–65.

29. Lee, J.H., Kavanagh, J.J., Wharton, J.T. *et al.* (1989) Allele loss at the c-Ha-ras1 locus in human ovarian cancer. *Cancer Res.*, **49**, 1220–2.

30. Okamoto, A., Sameshima, Y., Yokoyama, S. *et al.* (1991) Frequent allelic losses and mutations of the p53 gene in human ovarian cancer. *Cancer Res.*, **51**, 5171–6.

31. Marks, J.R., Davidoff, A.M., Kerns, B.J. *et al.* (1991) Overexpression and mutation of p53 in epithelial ovarian cancer. *Cancer Res.*, **61**, 2979–84.

32. Sato, T., Saito, H., Morita, R. *et al.* (1991) Allelotype of human ovarian cancer. *Cancer Res.*, **51**, 5118–22.

33. Lee, J.H., Kavanagh, J.J., Wildrick, D.M. *et al.* (1990) Frequent loss of heterozygosity on chromosomes 6q, 11 and 17 in human ovarian carcinomas. *Cancer Res.*, **50**, 2724–8.

34. Ehlen, T. and Dubeau, L. (1990) Loss of heterozygosity on chromosomal segments 3p, 6q and 11p in human ovarian cancer. *Oncogene*, **5**, 219–23.

35. Zheng, J., Robinson, W.R., Ehlen, T. *et al.* (1991) Distinction of low grade from high grade human ovarian carcinomas on the basis of losses of heterozygosity on chromosomes 3, 6 and 11 and HER-2/*neu* gene amplification. *Cancer Res.*, **51**, 4045–51.

36. Jones, M.H. and Nakamura, Y. (1992) Deletion mapping of chromosome 3p in female genital tract malignancies using microsatellite polymorphisms. *Oncogene*, **7**, 1631–4.

37. Saito, S., Saito, H., Koi, S. *et al.* (1992) Fine scale deletion mapping of the distal long arm of chromosome 6 in 70 human ovarian cancers. *Cancer Res.*, **52**, 5815–17.

38. Yang-Feng, T.L., Li, S-B., Han, H. and Schwartz, P.E. (1992) Frequent loss of heterozygosity on chromosome Xp and 13q in human ovarian cancer. *Int. J. Cancer*, **52**, 575–80.

39. Foulkes, W.D., Ragoussis, J., Stamp, G.W.H. *et al.* (1993) Frequent loss of heterozygosity on chromosome 6 in human ovarian carcinoma. *Br. J. Cancer*, **67**, 551–9.

40. Vandamme, B., Lissens, W., Amfo, K. *et al.* (1992) Deletion of chromosome 11p13-11p15.5 sequences in invasive human ovarian cancer is a subclonal progression factor. *Cancer Res.*, **52**, 6646–52.

41. Viel, A., Giannini, F., Tumiotti, L. *et al.* (1992) Chromosomal localisation of two putative oncosuppressor genes involved in human ovarian tumours. *Br. J. Cancer*, **66**, 1030–6.

42. Foulkes, W.D., Campbell, I.G., Stamp, G.W.H. and Trowsdale, J. (1993) Loss of heterozygosity and amplification of chromosome 11 in human ovarian cancer. *Br. J. Cancer*, **67**, 268–73.

43. Eccles, D.M., Gruber, L., Stewart, M. *et al.* (1992) Allele loss on chromosome 11p is associated with poor survival in ovarian carcinoma. *Dis. Markers*, **10**, 95–9.

44. Tsao, S.W., Mok, C-H., Oike, K. *et al.* (1991) Involvement of p53 gene in the allelic deletion of chromosome 17p in human ovarian tumours. *Anticancer Res.*, **11**, 1975-82.

45. Eccles, D.M., Brett, L., Lessells, A. *et al.* (1992) Overexpression of the p53 protein and allele loss at 17p13 in ovarian carcinoma. *Br. J. Cancer*, **65**, 40–4.

46. Foulkes, W.D., Black, D.M., Stamp, G.W.H. *et al.* (1993) Very frequent loss of heterozygosity throughout chromosome 17 in sporadic ovarian carcinoma. *Int. J. Cancer*, **54**, 220–6.

47. Jacobs, I.J., Smith, S.A., Wiseman, R.W. *et al* (1993) A deletion unit on chromosome 17q in epithelial ovarian tumors distal to the familial breast/ovarian cancer locus. *Cancer Res.*, **53**, 1218–21.

48. Phillips, N., Ziegler, M., Saha, B. and Xynos, F. (1993) Allelic loss on chromosome 17 in human ovarian carcinoma. *Int. J. Cancer*, **54**, 85–91.

49. Allan, G.J., Cottrell, S., Trowsdale, J. and Foulkes, W.D. (1994) Loss of heterozygosity on chromosome 5 is a late event and is not associated with mutations in APC at 5q21–22. *Hum. Mutation*, **3**, 283–92.

50. Bruening, W., Gross, P., Sato, T. *et al.* (1993) Analysis of the 11p13 Wilms' tumour suppressor gene (WT1) in ovarian tumours. *Cancer Invest.*, **11**, 393–9.

Chapter 4

The BRCA1 gene in sporadic breast and ovarian cancer

D.M. BLACK and E. SOLOMON

4.1 INTRODUCTION

The majority of cases of breast and ovarian cancer appear to be sporadic; that is, they arise without a clear genetic susceptibility because the cases lack an obvious inherited component. However, there are some families in which there are several affected individuals, indicating either a clustering of sporadic cases or an inherited genetic effect. In other, rarer families, there is a clear inherited susceptibility to either breast or ovarian cancer which can be traced through consecutive generations. In these families the disease usually occurs at an early age and often bilaterally. Interestingly, the risk of ovarian cancer is increased in relatives of women with breast cancer and vice versa. This observation suggests the existence of one or more genes which predispose to both breast and ovarian cancer [1].

The transmission of the disease has been investigated in such familial cases and it has been shown that at least a proportion of breast cancer can be explained by inherited mutations in one or more autosomal dominant genes [1–4]. The contribution these autosomal dominant genes make to total breast cancer cases is age dependent and over one-third of the cases diagnosed before the age of 30 are estimated to be due to inheritance of a susceptibility allele. This contribution is reduced to about 1% of cases diagnosed after the age of

80. There does not seem to be such an age effect in ovarian cancer.

4.2 GENETICS

In late 1990 Mary-Claire King and her colleagues at the University of California (Berkeley) succeeded in showing the first convincing linkage data in breast cancer families with a polymorphic locus, CMM86 (D17S74), which mapped to the long arm of human chromosome 17 [15]. This discovery instigated the search for the predisposing gene on 17q which has been called BRCA1 (*breast cancer 1*). Linkage to this region of 17q was clearly confirmed in three large pedigrees with an inherited predisposition to both breast and ovarian cancers [6]. Subsequently, the combined data from many different groups in a worldwide familial breast–ovarian cancer consortium have demonstrated that in almost all families with breast and ovarian cancer, and about half of those with only breast cancer, the disease is linked to the BRCA1 gene [7]. This gene may be responsible for over 90% of the inherited susceptibility to ovarian cancer.

Over the last few years we and others have isolated a large number of highly polymorphic markers from 17q in an effort to build genetic and physical maps of the region

39

around the BRCA1 locus. These markers have been predominantly microsatellites of the (CA)n repeat type. (CA)n repeats are short runs of poly(CA)n/(GT)n which occur frequently in mammalian DNA. By analysing several such markers on 17q, the BRCA1 gene has been shown to lie in a less than 4 cM interval, which is flanked by two (CA)n repeats: one in the THRA1 gene and the second at the locus D17S183 [8,9]. It may be possible to further reduce the size of the BRCA1 region by typing further markers on additional families and identifying recombinants (Chapter 2). Critical recombinants in this region have to be scrutinized in these families either for evidence against linkage to BRCA1 or the removal of sporadic cases, which are always going to be complications in such a common disease. It is unlikely that the BRCA1 region will be reduced substantially by a genetic mapping approach due to the genetic heterogeneity and the high frequency of sporadic breast cancer. The best that can realistically be hoped for is a 2 cM interval with the BRCA1 gene somewhere therein. Other strategies to pinpoint the BRCA1 gene are therefore in progress.

4.3 LOSS OF HETEROZYGOSITY IN BREAST AND OVARIAN TUMOURS

With very few exceptions, the genes which lead to dominantly inherited cancer susceptibility, such as the APC gene in familial polyposis coli (a type of colon cancer) or the RB gene in retinoblastoma, actually operate recessively at the cellular level. That is, both copies of the gene are mutated or inactivated in the target cell giving rise to the tumour. In the case of an inherited susceptibility, one mutation is inherited in the germ line, followed by a second mutational event in a cell of the target tissue. Similarly, when the same gene is involved in sporadic cancers of the same type, two mutations must occur at the somatic level

within the same target cell. Genes that behave in this manner have been called **tumour suppressor genes** (as opposed to dominantly acting oncogenes) and are believed, in their normal function, to be involved in growth control or differentiation. The hallmark of tumour suppressor gene inactivation is the loss of genetic material, often known as loss of heterozygosity (LOH) in the region of the chromosome in which it resides [10].

If familial breast and ovarian cancer develops due to inactivation of a tumour suppressor gene, the disease would occur in individuals who inherit one mutant allele in the germ line and suffer a second mutational event in the target tissue (e.g. breast ductal or ovarian epithelium), thereby removing the remaining dominant wild type allele. Sporadic cancer would arise when both events occur somatically in either a breast ductal epithelial cell or an ovarian epithelial cell. The search for loss of heterozygosity is currently underway on both familial and sporadic breast and ovarian tumours for two reasons. First, if LOH is seen in the region of BRCA1 it suggests that the gene is a tumour suppressor, which in turn has implications for the types of biological experiments which might be done towards its isolation. Second, LOH has proved a powerful method for narrowing the region within which a tumour suppressor gene is located, particularly in colon cancer [11].

To date, LOH studies have provided conflicting evidence as to whether or not BRCA1 is a tumour suppressor gene. Chromosome 17q markers are lost at significant frequencies in sporadic breast [12,13] and ovarian cancer [14,15]. Sato *et al.* found LOH in over 30% (29 out of 93) of sporadic breast tumours, using D17S74, the probe which provided the original linkage to chromosome 17q. More recently, Futreal *et al.* have used (CA)n repeats around the BRCA1 locus to look at LOH in 20 sporadic breast tumours [13]. They have made the remarkable finding that with a (CA)n repeat at the THRA1 locus at 17q12,

LOH was seen in almost 80% (11 out of 14) of their breast tumours. If this result can be confirmed it would indicate that BRCA1 is probably a tumour suppressor gene. It would also suggest that BRCA1 is involved in the majority of sporadic as well as familial breast cancers. We have used this marker, together with others which span the BRCA1 region, to look for LOH (Figure 4.1). In 100 patients with sporadic breast tumours, of which 50 were premenopausal (age of diagnosis less than 40 years) and 50 were postmenopausal (age of diagnosis greater than 60 years), we detected LOH on chromosome 17q in 34 tumour samples as shown in Figure 4.2. Almost all the tumours which showed loss did so with multiple markers in the region, indicating that the LOH could be due to loss of either the

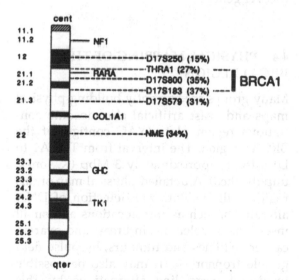

Figure 4.1 Idiogram of the long arm of human chromosome 17. The NFI gene at 17q11.2, the RARA gene at 17q21.1, the COL1A1 gene at 17q21.4, the GHC gene cluster at 17q23.2 and the TK1 gene at 17q24.3 are shown as reference markers. The polymorphic markers used in the LOH study are also shown, together with the percentage loss seen at each marker. The BRCA1 region, which is flanked by THRA1 and D17S183, is also indicated.

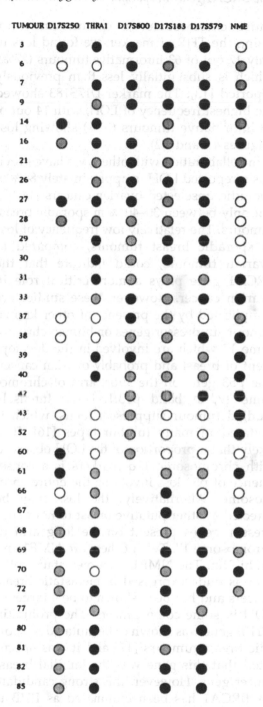

Figure 4.2 A list of the 34 tumours which showed LOH with chromosome 17q markers. The tumour ID numbers are also shown. ●, loss; ○ no loss; ◉ not informative; blank, not determined.

41

entire chromosome or chromosome arm. Using the THRA1 marker, we found loss in only 17 out of 63 informative tumours (27%), which is substantially less than previously reported [13]. The marker D17S183 showed the highest frequency of LOH, with 14 out of 38 informative tumours (37%) showing loss (Figures 4.1 and 4.2).

In collaboration with others, we have previously reported LOH in approximately 80% of sporadic unselected ovarian cancers [14,15], but only between 30–40 % in sporadic breast tumours. The relatively low frequency of loss in sporadic breast tumours, compared to ovarian tumours, could indicate that the BRCA1 gene plays a more critical role in ovarian cancer. However, these studies are complicated by the presence of other known tumour suppressor genes on human chromosome 17 which are involved in the development of breast and probably ovarian cancer. The p53 gene on the short arm of chromosome 17, at band p13.1, is an intensely studied tumour suppressor locus, which is mutated in many tumour types [16]. It is likely that a proportion of the LOH observed with chromosome 17q markers is a consequence of p53 loss involving the entire chromosome. Alternatively, the loss may be directed at other putative breast tumour suppressor genes present on the long arm of chromosome 17. Two of these are NME1 and prohibitin. The NME1 (non-metastatic cells) gene is underexpressed in metastatic breast cancers and has been shown to be a target of LOH in some colon cancers. The prohibitin (PHB) gene was shown to be mutated in sporadic breast tumours [17] and it was speculated that this gene was the familial breast cancer gene. However, this strong candidate for BRCA1 has been eliminated as PHB is distal to GIP on chromosome 17q and is therefore not within the flanking markers for BRCA1 (Figure 4.1). Studies on breast and ovarian tumours from BRCA1 linked families also show LOH with chromosome 17q

markers [18]. As expected, the alleles which are linked to the disease in these families are retained in the tumours and the wild type alleles are lost, causing homozygosity or hemizygosity for the BRCA1 mutation. Such observations indicate that the BRCA1 gene may be identified by LOH studies on breast and ovarian tumours, especially those which are of early onset. Other tumour suppressor genes have been identified by this approach. Most notably, the DCC (deleted in colon cancer) gene on chromosome 18q was localized solely on the basis of LOH studies [19]. Therefore, if enough tumours are analysed with probes from the BRCA1 region it should be possible to identify small deletions around this locus. Isolation and characterization of the genes present in these deletions could eventually lead to the identification of the BRCA1 gene.

4.4 PHYSICAL MAPPING OF THE BRCA1 REGION

Many groups are currently building physical maps and yeast artificial chromosome contiguous region plots (YAC contigs) of the BRCA1 region. The interval from THRA1 to D17S183 is approximately 3 Mbp (K. Jones, unpublished). A detailed physical map of this region will facilitate the detection of DNA alterations, such as translocations and small insertions or deletions, in breast and ovarian cancer cell lines and tumours, by pulse field gel electrophoresis. It may also be possible to detect germ line alternations by this approach, as was the case for the NF1 gene, another tumour suppressor gene on chromosome 17q [20,21]. A YAC contig of the BRCA1 region is being constructed by many groups. This resource will facilitate both the construction of a physical map and the generation of further genetic markers and probes. These can be used for the screening of cDNA libraries and 'zoo blots' for the detection of evolutionary conserved sequences, which may indicate the location of exons [22].

4.5 FUTURE DEVELOPMENTS

The intense efforts which are currently ongoing will lead to the isolation of the BRCA1 gene in the near future. Once this gene is identified it will immediately open up opportunities for screening women from high risk families to determine if they have inherited the disease susceptibility allele. It may also give an opportunity for the detection of mutant cells shed into the blood from presymptomatic breast and ovarian tumours. The role of the BRCA1 gene in other cancers can also be addressed. It has recently been reported that male relatives of women with breast cancer have an increased risk of prostate cancer, so the BRCA1 gene may also be important in this disease [23].

REFERENCES

1. Lynch, H.T., Watson, P., Conway, T.A. and Lynch, J.F. (1992) Natural history and age at onset of hereditary breast cancer. *Cancer*, **69**, 1404–7.

2. Newman, B., Austin, M.A., Lee, M. and King, M-C. (1988) Inheritance of human breast cancer: evidence for autosomal dominant transmission in high-risk families *Proc. Natl. Acad. Sci. USA*, **85**, 3044–8.

3. Claus, E.B., Risch, N.J. and Thompson, W.D. (1990) Age at onset as an indicator of familial risk of breast cancer. *Am. J. Epidemiol.*, **131**, 961–72.

4. Claus, E.B., Risch, N.J. and Thompson, W.D. (1991) Genetic analysis of breast cancer in the cancer and steroid hormone study. *Am. J. Hum. Genet.*, **48**, 232–42.

5. Hall, J.M., Lee, M.K., Newman, B. *et al.* (1990) Linkage of early-onset familial breast cancer to chromosome 17q21. *Science*, **250**, 1684–9.

6. Narod, S.A., Feunteun, J., Lynch, H.T. *et al.* (1991) Familial breast–ovarian cancer locus on chromosome 17q12-q23. *Lancet*, **338**, 82–3.

7. Easton, D.F., Bishop, D.T., Ford, D. and Cockford, G.P. (1993) Genetic linkage analysis in familial breast and ovarian cancer. Results from 214 families. *Am. J. Hum. Genet.*, **52**, 678–701.

8. Bowcock, A.M., Anderson, L.A., Black, D.M. *et al.* (1993) THRA1 and D17S183 flank an interval of <4 cM for the breast–ovarian cancer gene (BRCA1) on chromosome 17q21. *Am. J. Hum. Genet.*, **52**, 718–21.

9. Goldgar, D.E., Cannon-Albright, L.A., Oliphant, A. *et al.* (1993) Chromosome 17q linkage studies of 18 Utah breast cancer kindreds. *Am. J. Hum. Genet.*, **52**, 743–8.

10. Knudson, A.G. and Strong, L.C. (1972) Mutation and cancer: a model for Wilms' tumor of the kidney. *J. Natl. Cancer Inst.*, **48**, 313–24.

11. Ponder, B.A.J. (1990) Inherited predisposition to cancer. *Trends Genet.*, **6**, 213–18.

12. Sato, T., Tanigami, A., Yamakawa, K. *et al.* (1990) Allelotype of breast cancer: cumulative allele losses promote tumor progression in primary breast cancer. *Cancer Res.*, **50**, 7184–9.

13. Futreal, P.A., Soderkvist, P., Marks, J.R. *et al.* (1992) Detection of frequent allelic loss on proximal chromosome 17q in sporadic breast carcinoma using microsatellite length polymorphisms. *Cancer Res.*, **52**, 2624–7.

14. Foulkes, W.D., Black, D.M., Stamp, G.W.H. *et al.* (1993) Very frequent loss of heterozygosity throughout chromosome 17 in sporadic ovarian carcinoma. *Int. J. Cancer*, **54**, 220–5.

15. Foulkes, W.D., Black, D.M., Solomon, E., and Trowsdale, J. (1991) Allele loss on chromosome 17q in sporadic ovarian cancer. *Lancet*, **338**, 444–5.

16. Marshall, C.J. (1991) Tumor suppressor genes. *Cell*, **64**, 313–26.

17. Sato, T., Saito, H., Swenson, H. *et al.* (1992) The human prohibitin gene located on chromosome 17q21 is mutated in sporadic breast cancer. *Cancer Res.*, **52**, 1643–6.

18. Smith, S.A., Easton, D.F., Evans, D.G.R. and Ponder, B.A.J. (1992) Chromosome 17 allele loss in familial ovarian cancer. *Nature Genet.*, **2**, 128–31.

19. Fearon, E.R., Cho, K.R., Nigro, J.M. *et al.* (1990) Identification of a chromosome 18q gene that is altered in colorectal cancers. *Science*, **247**, 49–56.

20. Cawthon, R.M., Weiss, R., Xu, G.F. *et al.* (1990) A major segment of the neurofibromatosis type 1 gene: cDNA sequence, genomic structure and point mutations. *Cell*, **62**, 193–201.

21. Wallace, M.R., Marchuk, D.A., Anderson, L.B. *et al.* (1990) Type 1 neurofibromatosis gene: identification of a large transcript disrupted in three NF1 patients. *Science*, **249**, 181–6.

22. Wicking, C. and Williamson, B. (1991) From linked marker to gene. *Trends Genet.*, **7**, 288–92.

23. Tulinius, H., Egilsson, V., Olafsdottir, G. and Sigvaldson, H. (1992) Risk of prostate, ovarian and endometrial cancer among relatives of women with breast cancer. *Lancet*, **305**, 855–7.

Chapter 5

Allele losses on chromosome 17 in ovarian tumours

C.M. STEEL, D.M. ECCLES, L. GRUBER, M. WALLACE, A. LESSELS, J.M. MORSMAN, H. GABRA, R.C.F. LEONARD and B.B. COHEN

5.1 INTRODUCTION

Analysis of tumours for localized loss of heterozygosity (LOH) or 'allele imbalance' is a well-recognized approach to the detection and mapping of tumour suppressor genes [1]. Studies in ovarian cancer have identified regional LOH on chromosomes 3p, 6q, 11p, 17p and 17q [2–9]. Much of the work in this field has concentrated on chromosome 17, where high rates of allele imbalance have been recorded on both arms. Attention has also been drawn to this chromosome by the recent assignment of a breast–ovarian cancer gene to 17q12-21 through linkage analysis in affected families [10].

Using 11 polymorphic loci mapping to different regions of chromosome 17 (Figure 5.1), we have compared peripheral blood and tumour derived DNA from a consecutive series of patients undergoing surgery for primary ovarian neoplasms [3,6,7]. Data are presented here on the first 45 patients for whom complete results are available.

5.2 PATIENTS, MATERIALS AND METHODS

5.2.1 CLINICAL SAMPLES

Ovarian tumour tissue obtained at surgery was transferred directly to dry ice or liquid nitrogen and then stored at −70°C until processed. Heparinized peripheral blood was collected in the postoperative period. The purpose of the research (which had received local ethical committee approval) was explained and informed consent for DNA analysis was obtained from all patients.

5.2.2 HISTOLOGY

A portion of each tumour was fixed in formalin (without prior freezing) and processed by paraffin wax embedding, sectioning and staining with haematoxylin and eosin. Tumours were staged on the basis of findings at surgery, together with histological examination of biopsies from the omentum and from any other tissues that appeared to be involved macroscopically.

5.2.3 DNA EXTRACTIONS

High MW DNA was obtained from blood and from finely chopped frozen tumour tissue by lysis in buffered SDS, digestion with RNAase and proteinase K, followed by phenol:chloroform extraction and ethanol precipitation [3].

5.2.4 SOUTHERN BLOTTING AND PROBING

Restriction enzyme digestion and probing with YNZ22, MCT35.1 and THH59 (D17S5,

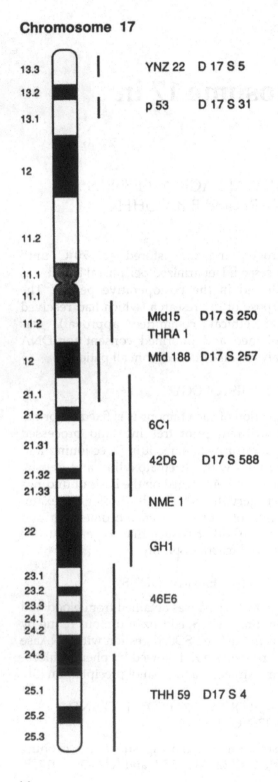

Chromosome 17

D17S31 and D17S4) to detect the corresponding VNTR or biallelic polymorphisms have been described previously [3].

5.2.5 PCR AND DETECTION OF MICROSATELLITE POLYMORPHISMS

DNA samples were amplified using the primer pairs and conditions specified for the eight microsatellite containing sequences in the international collaborative breast–ovarian cancer family linkage study [10]. Products of the PCR reactions were separated by electrophoresis in 12½% polyacrylamide denaturing gels, electrotransferred to Hybond® nylon membrane and hybridized to ^{32}P labelled poly-CA probe or to $(AAAG)_6$ in the case of the GH1 sequence which has a tetranucleotide repeat. The alleles of the microsatellite sequences were then visualized by autoradiography. This indirect probing procedure tends to reduce the laddering effect that often complicates the identification of oligonucleotide repeat alleles [12].

By sequential loading of gels four loci can be analysed in each track (Figure 5.2). Three autoradiographs, with different exposure times, were made from each membrane since the sensitivity of detection of allele imbalance can vary with the intensity of signal. Most PCR reactions and gel separations were repeated at least twice for every sample and more often, if required, until an unequivocal result was obtained.

5.3 RESULTS AND DISCUSSION

With the exception of the biallelic markers D17S31 (40% heterozygous) all of the sequences probed were informative in at least half the patients (range 50–72%) and every patient was heterozygous for at least four of

Figure 5.1 Idiogram of chromosome 17 with the current regional and subregional assignment of 11 polymorphic loci examined in this study. Data from refs 9, 10 and 11.

46

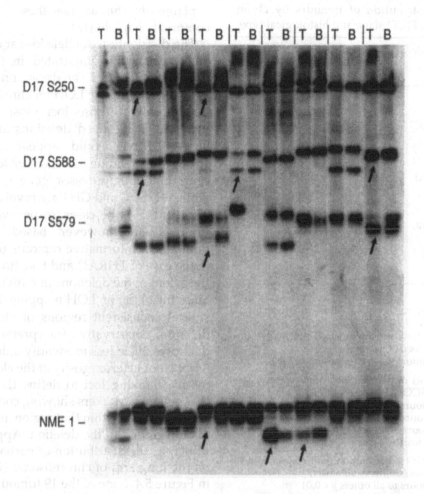

Figure 5.2 One complete autoradiograph showing comparisons of eight tumour (T) and blood (B) paired DNA samples in adjacent tracks. Four polymorphic markers are present in each track and examples of allele imbalance in the tumour, when compared with the corresponding blood DNA, are indicated by arrows.

the 11 loci (range 4–10, mean 6.7). Fourteen of the 45 tumours showed loss of heterozygosity at every informative chromosome 17 locus while a further 12 showed no allele imbalance at any locus. Nineteen tumours had lost an allele at one or more loci but retained heterozygosity elsewhere on the chromosome. While recognizing the dangers of oversimplification, these three categories are taken, for

the purposes of the present analysis, to represent loss of one complete copy of chromosome 17, retention of two intact copies and partial loss of one chromosome 17 respectively. The distribution of histological types and stages of tumour among these three categories is shown in Table 5.1. There is a highly significant association between chromosome 17 loss and advancing tumour stage. Whole

47

Table 5.1 Distribution of tumours by chromosome 17 status, FIGO stage and histological type

Histological type	Benign/ borderline	FIGO stage I/II	III/IV
Endometrioid		1H	
		4D	1L
Mucinous	4H	3H	1H
		1D	1D
Serous/ undifferentiated	1D	1D	2H
			8D
			12L
Other (teratoma, granulosa cell, adenofibroma)	2D	1D	1H
		1L	

Key:

H = Retained heterozygosity at all informative chromosome 17 loci

D = Retained heterozygosity at some informative chromosome 17 loci, LOH at others

L = LOH at all informative chromosome 17 loci

Statistical analysis of distribution with respect to stage (≤ FIGO II *vs* ≥ FIGO III)
  For 12 'H' tumours *vs* all others $p < 0.05$
  For 19 'D' tumours *vs* all others $p = 0.18$ NS
  For 14 'L' tumours *vs* all others $p < 0.002$
  (Fisher's exact test)

Statistical analysis of distribution with respect to histological type (serous/undiff *vs* all others)
  For 12 'H' tumours *vs* all others $p < 0.01$
  For 19 'D' tumours *vs* all others $p = 0.9$ NS
  For 14 'L' tumours *vs* all others $p < 0.005$
  (Fisher's exact test)

chromosome loss is also strongly correlated with aggressive histological appearances. Twelve of the 14 tumours in this category were of serous or undifferentiated type. The only case with complete loss of heterozygosity which was not FIGO stage III or IV was a teratoma and the apparent anomaly is readily

explained by the fact that these tumours are commonly haploid [13].

The distribution of allele loss at each of the loci examined is illustrated in Figure 5.3. Concentrating the analysis on tumours showing incomplete LOH on chromosome 17 may highlight those loci most frequently included in localized deletions and on this basis THRA1 would appear to be the strongest candidate as a marker for an adjacent tumour suppressor gene (71% LOH), while D17S250 and GH1 are involved in only 25% and 23% of cases respectively. These findings are however based on small numbers of informative tumours (only seven in the case of THRA1) and take no account of the extent of the deletions in individual cases. Since the object of 'LOH mapping' is to define shortest consistent regions of chromosome deletion, conservative interpretation of the data uses allele loss to identify a deletion but *retention* of heterozygosity at the closest informative flanking loci to define the extent of that deletion. Markers showing constitutional homozygosity within that region are assumed to be included in the deletion. Applying that principle, the distribution of partial deletions on the long arm of chromosome 17 is shown in Figure 5.4. Nine of the 19 tumours had two non-contiguous regions of deletion on chromosome 17 and one tumour had three such regions. No tumour had a deletion confined to the short arm while eight had deletions involving the long arm only.

Previous studies on a series of ovarian cancers that includes the present set have demonstrated only a single common region of deletion on 17p, which is probably identified with the p53 gene [3,6]. The findings reported here suggest that there may be two

Figure 5.3 Distribution of allele loss at each of the 11 polymorphic loci examined. The left hand column represents the percentage of all informative samples (i.e. those for which the blood DNA was heterozygous) in which allele imbalance was recorded. The right hand column represents the same data derived only from the 19 tumours showing an incomplete pattern of allele loss on chromosome 17.

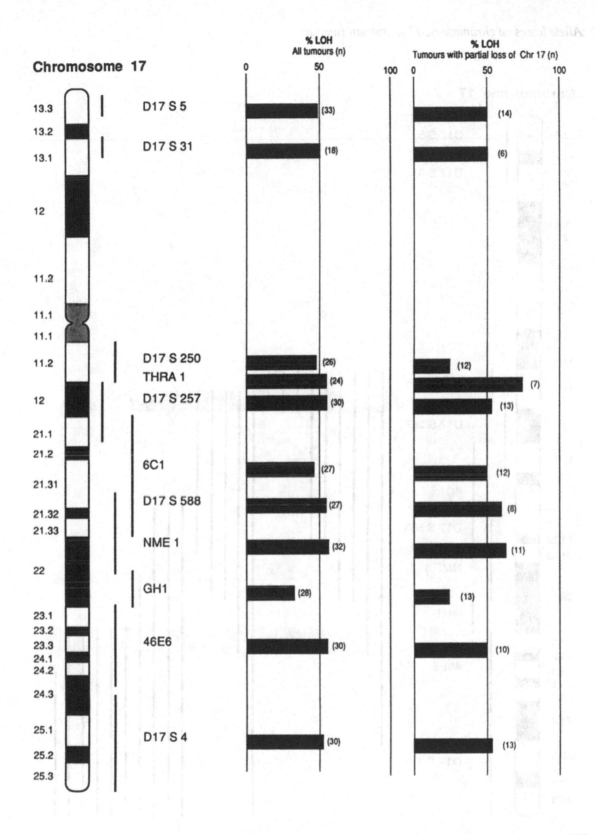

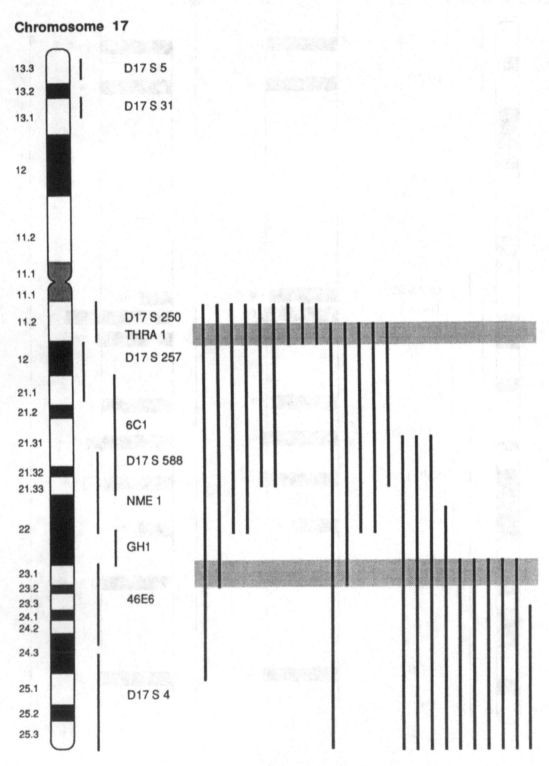

'shortest regions of overlap' (SROs) defined by deletions on the long arm. These are indicated by hatching in Figure 5.4. The proximal site, flanked by D17S250 and D17S579, includes the THRA1 locus and possibly also the postulated BRCA1 tumour suppressor gene [10]. The distal site appears to be flanked by GH1 and 46E6 but could be anywhere distal to GH1. Only one mapped long arm deletion covers neither of the shaded regions and that was found in a tumour which also carried deletions of the short arm and the proximal long arm SRO. Ten long arm deletions cover the proximal site only, nine the distal one only and four encompass both. Neither of these 17q SROs corresponds to the deletion unit recently identified by Jacobs and colleagues in a similar study [9]. Their series of tumours evidently included a very much lower proportion of cases with partial deletion of chromosome 17. Our data do not exclude the possibility of one or more additional SROs within 17q21-22; however, no 17q deletion that we have mapped includes that region without extending into either the proximal or the distal common deletion site or both. We therefore interpret the high frequency of deletions in 17q21-22 as a reflection of the overlap of deletions primarily involving a proximal or a distal SRO. The two studies concur on the association between chromosome 17 loss and serous or undifferentiated carcinoma of advanced FIGO stage.

We have examined the distribution of partial chromosome 17 deletion in relation to histological type and FIGO stage for the 19 informative tumours and find that, in the absence of a 17p deletion, tumours with loss of the proximal or the distal 17q SRO, or both, belong mainly to the benign, borderline or FIGO stage I–II categories and are distributed among all histological types. Only one out of eight is a serous adenocarcinoma of FIGO stage III–IV. Conversely, deletion of the short arm plus either or both of the long arm SROs tends to be found among advanced stage tumours and predominantly in serous adenocarcinomas (Table 5.2).

This strongly reinforces the conclusion from our previous studies that 17q lesions are early events in ovarian carcinogenesis while

Table 5.2 Distribution of 'D' tumours by site of chromosome 17 deletion, FIGO stage and histological type

Histological type	Benign/ borderline	FIGO stage	
		I/II	III/IV
Endometrioid		2q	
		1p+q	
Mucinous		1q	1p+q
Serous/ undifferentiated	1q		1q
			1p+q 6p+q
Other	2q	1q	
		1p+q	

Key

q = Tumours with deletions confined to long arm (either or both SRO sites)

p+q = Tumours with deletions including short and long arms

No tumour had a deletion on the short arm only. One tumour with partial deletion of the long arm was uninformative for short arm loci

Statistical analysis of distribution with respect to stage (≤ FIGO II *vs* ≥ FIGO III)
For 8 'q' tumours *vs* 10 'p+q' tumours $p < 0.025$ (Fisher's exact test)

Statistical analysis of distribution with respect to histological type (serous/undifferentiated *vs* all others)
For 8 'q' tumours *vs* 10 'p+q' tumours $p < 0.08$ (Fisher's exact test)

Figure 5.4 Estimated extent of 24 hemizygous segments on the long arm in the subset of tumours showing incomplete deletions of chromosome 17. Each deletion is assumed to be limited by the closest flanking markers demonstrated to have retained heterozygosity in the tumour. Several tumours carried multiple deletions separated by regions of retained heterozygosity. A minimum of two 'shortest regions of overlap', indicated by the hatched bands, can be deduced from this data set.

deletion of a region on 17p (probably reflecting loss of wild type p53) is associated with more advanced disease. The new findings reported here suggest that two separate genes on the long arm of chromosome 17, one at q11-12 (which may correspond to BRCA1) and the other at q23-25, are involved in the aetiology of ovarian cancer.

ACKNOWLEDGMENTS

The authors are grateful to all gynaecologists in Lothian and Fife for their cooperation in this study, to Mrs I McKenzie and Miss A Gallacher for expert assistance and to Messrs Norman Davidson, Sandy Bruce and Douglas Stuart for artwork. The study was supported by a grant from the Scottish Hospitals Endowment Research Trust.

REFERENCES

1. Ponder, B.A.J. (1988) Gene losses in human tumours. *Nature*, **335**, 400–2.
2. Lee, J.H., Kavanagh, J.J., Wildrick, D. M. *et al.* (1990) Frequent loss of heterozygosity on chromosome 6q, 11 and 17 in human ovarian carcinomas. *Cancer Res.*, **50**, 2724–8.
3. Eccles, D.M., Cranston, G., Steel, C.M. *et al.* (1990) Allele loss on chromosome 17 in human epithelial ovarian cancer. *Oncogene*, **5**, 1599–601.
4. Russell, S.E.H., Hickey, G.I., Lowry, W.S. *et al.* (1990) Allele loss from chromosome 17 in ovarian cancer. *Oncogene*, **5**, 1581–3.
5. Foulkes, W., Black, D., Solomon, E. and Trowsdale, J. (1991) Allele loss on chromosome 17 in sporadic ovarian cancer. *Lancet*, **338**, 444–5.
6. Eccles, D.M., Brett, L., Lessells, A. *et al.* (1992) Overexpression of the p53 protein and allele loss at 17p13 in ovarian carcinoma. *Br. J. Cancer*, **65**, 40–4.
7. Eccles, D.M., Russell, S.E.H., Haites, N.E. *et al.* (1992) Early loss of heterozygosity on 17q in ovarian cancer. *Oncogene*, **7**, 2069–72.
8. Eccles, D.M., Gruber, L., Stewart, M. *et al.* (1992) Allele loss on chromosome 11p is associated with poor survival in ovarian cancer. *Dis. Markers*, **10**, 95–9.
9. Jacobs, I.J., Smith, S.A., Wiseman, R.W. *et al.* (1993) A deletion unit on chromosome 17q in epithelial ovarian tumours distal to the familial breast/ovarian cancer locus. *Cancer Res.*, **53**, 1218–21.
10. Easton, D.F., Bishop, D.T., Ford, D. and Cockford, G.P. (1993) Genetic linkage analysis in familial breast and ovarian cancer – results from 214 families. *Am. J. Hum. Genet.*, **52**, 678–701.
11. Solomon, E. and Ledbetter, D.H. (1991) Report of the committee on genetic constitution of chromosome 17. Eleventh International Workshop on Human Gene Mapping. *Cytogenet. Cell Genet.*, **58**, 686–738.
12. Cohen, B.B., Wallace, M.R. and Crichton, D.N. (1992) A comparison of procedures for analysing microsatellite (CA)-repeat polymorphisms. *Mol. Cell Probes*, **6**, 439–42.
13. Kaiser-McCaw, B. and Latt, S.A. (1977) X-chromosome replication in parthenogenic benign ovarian teratomas. *Hum. Genet.*, **38**, 163–8.

Chapter 6

Cloning and molecular characterization of monoclonal antibody-defined ovarian tumour antigens

I.G. CAMPBELL, W.D. FOULKES, T.A. JONES, L.G. POELS and J. TROWSDALE

6.1 INTRODUCTION

In an effort to develop additional treatments and improved methods for early detection of ovarian cancers a number of monoclonal antibodies (MAbs) have been generated against cell surface antigens of epithelial ovarian cancer (EOC). Therapies using these reagents to target ovarian cancers have so far been disappointing. Identifying the antigens recognized by the antibody may be important for improving the targeting of antibody based therapy. For example, detailed molecular analysis of the polymorphic epithelial mucin gene, MUC1, has shown that differential glycosylation of a tandem repeat unit is responsible for the appearance of novel epitopes in breast, ovarian and other adenocarcinomas [1]. This information has opened up new possibilities for immunotherapy with mucins since these structures are highly immunogenic and are relatively tumour specific. The encouraging results of such studies prompted us to undertake the cloning of the genes for other MAb defined tumour antigens based on an expression cloning technique [2]. In this chapter we briefly summarize the important characteristics of the genes cloned so far and discuss their possible function in ovarian cancer.

6.2 CLONING STRATEGY AND RESULTS

All the cDNAs were cloned using an expression cloning system described in detail previously [3,4] and the overall strategy is outlined in Figure 6.1. After each MAb specific clone was isolated, its identity as the *in vivo* target was confirmed either by comparison of the size of products produced by transfectants with that derived from cell lines and/or by correlation of cell surface reactivity with the presence of corresponding levels of mRNA. To ascertain if mutation was the basis for tumour specific reactivity of the MAb the sequences of cDNAs from carcinoma cell lines were then compared with those derived from normal tissues. The deduced amino acid sequence was used to search for homologous proteins in EMBL and Swiss protein databases and to analyse the protein for any distinctive structural motifs. Finally, the chromosomal localization of the gene was determined using fluorescence *in situ* hybridization and by molecular techniques. The involvement of the region in chromosomal aberrations such as allele loss, amplification or rearrangement was investigated in tumour and normal DNA from a collection of 30 ovarian tumours. By combining these techniques we hoped to be

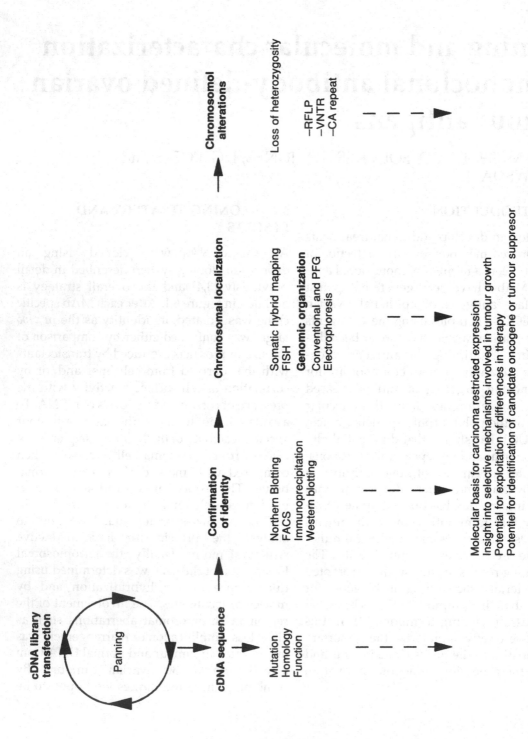

Figure 6.1 Project strategy. Abbreviations: YAC, yeast artificial chromosome; PFG, pulse field gel; RFLP, restriction fragment length polymorphism; VNTR, variable number tandem repeat.

Table 6.1 Cloned ovarian tumour antigens

MAb	% EOC +ve	Size	Homology	Function	Chromosome	References
MOV18 LK26	90	38 kd	FOLR-1	Folate receptor 1	11q13.3-13.5	[4,6,22,23]
OVTL-3	90	40 kd	Ig superfamily	Channel/receptor?	3q13.3-13.31	[7,9]
OVTL-30	85	90 kd	Ig superfamily ICAM-1	Adhesion	19p13.3-13.2	[13]
G253	85	90 kd	Ig superfamily	Adhesion	19q13.1-13.3	[19,20]

able to explain fully the molecular basis for the tumour specific expression of these antigens. Table 6.1 summarizes the details of the MAbs used and the possible function of the antigen based on homology with proteins of known function or similarities in structural features.

6.2.1 MOV18/LK26

In earlier studies we described the cloning of the cDNA encoding the antigen detected by MAb MOV18 [4]. Its identification as the adult folate receptor (FOLR1) and the finding that expression is greatly elevated in EOC suggested that either folate is limiting in this environment or that other defects in the tumour cells affect their ability to utilize the folate that is available. In either case this information should provide an impetus for the re-evaluation of antifolate therapy in EOC. In particular the high affinity of the receptor for folate, in the order of 10^{-9} M [5], and its massive overexpression relative to normal tissues suggest that perhaps low levels of antifolates may be more effective and obviously less toxic than the usual maximum tolerable dose regimens. Recently we demonstrated that another MAb, designated LK26 and raised against a choriocarcinoma cell line, also recognizes FOLR1 [6].

6.2.2 OVTL-3

The MAb OVTL-3 has a highly restricted reactivity with EOC and defines a surface glycoprotein, OA3, which has been used for immunotargeting [7,8]. cDNAs expressing OA3 encoded a 323 amino acid protein with five putative transmembrane spanning domains (Figure 6.2), which was reminiscent of a membrane receptor or channel but of a new type having no similarity with any of the known families [9]. In addition, the extracellular domain revealed significant homology to V regions of the immunoglobulin superfamily, particularly to those of the IgV related sequence from cartilage link proteins and poliovirus receptor.

OA3 is the first example of an immunoglobulin domain related protein associated with multiple transmembrane domains. Many members of the immunoglobulin superfamily participate in cell-to-cell recognition and signalling [10] and elucidation of the natural ligand for OA3 could have important therapeutic implications. Interestingly, a protein data bank search found 28% homology between OA3 and a protein from vaccinia virus, VA38. Hydrophobicity analysis clearly shows them to be structurally related. No functional information is currently available for VA38 but it has been suggested that it may be involved in the membrane permeability changes induced following virus infection [11]. What role OA3 plays in EOC and indeed normal cells is unknown but its presence on vaccinia virus should facilitate determination of its function.

The basis for the tumour specificity of OVTL-3 was investigated by examining the

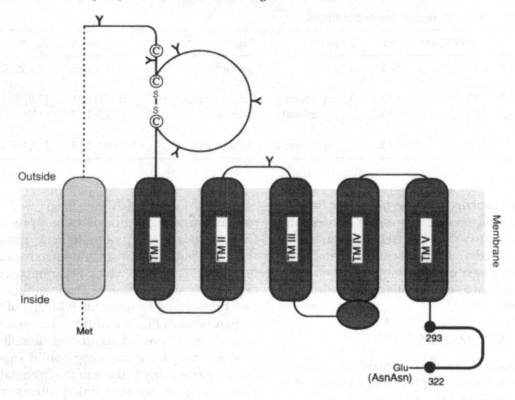

Figure 6.2 Structural model for OA3. Cylinders (dark shading) indicate transmembrane domains TM I-V and a possible NH₂ terminus TM region is indicated (light shading). Putative sites of N-glycosylation (Y) and extracellular cysteine residues Ⓒ are indicated. A cysteine pair is shown (S-S) based on homology with the immunoglobulin superfamily. The domain is most likely of the V-type based on the longer distance (74 amino acids) between cysteine residues and homology with human cartilage link protein and poliovirus receptor. The thick line at the COOH terminus region is deleted in shorter splice variants of OA3.

expression of OA3 in normal tissues and carcinoma cell lines at the mRNA level and by surface reactivity with the antibody. We were surprised to find that in all the normal tissues examined, significant levels of OA3 message were detected, certainly as high as the most strongly reactive carcinoma cell lines (Figure 6.3). Paradoxically, the *in vivo* reactivity of OVTL-3 is highly restricted to ovarian carcinoma although the epithelia of normal endometrium, fallopian tube, endocervix and lymphocytes show weak reactivity [7,12]. None of the eight tissues examined – heart, brain, placenta, lung, liver, skeletal muscle, kidney or pancreas – have been reported to show OVTL-3 reactivity. These data suggest that the epitope recognized by OVTL-3 is associated with differences in post-translational modification in normal versus tumour cells or may be the result of altered associations with other membrane proteins. Glycosylation differences are unlikely to be responsible inasmuch as treatment of cells with O-linked and N-linked sugar inhibitors has no quantitative or qualitative effect on OVTL-3 binding to carcinoma cell lines. Alternatively, it

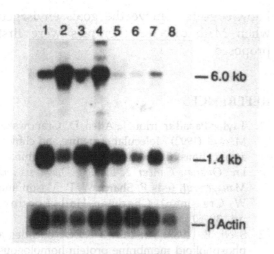

Figure 6.3 Expression of OA3 mRNA on a Northern blot of normal human tissue. The blot was probed and washed under stringent conditions and exposed for 24 hrs at –70°C with an intensifying screen. Each track contained approximately 2 mg of poly(A)+ RNA from either heart (track 1), brain (track 2), placenta (track 3), lung (track 4), liver (track 5), skeletal muscle (track 6), kidney (track 7) or pancreas (track 8). The bottom panel is the result with a β-actin probe. The sizes of the transcripts in kilobases are indicated on the right of the figure.

is conceivable that expression is post-transcriptionally controlled with no protein being translated despite the abundance of OA3 message in normal cells. We have not as yet been able to test this due to the lack of a suitable antibody for immunoprecipitations or Western blots.

6.2.3 OVTL-30

This antibody is reactive with approximately 85% of EOC [13]. cDNA sequences expressing the antigen OA30 were identified as being similar to the gene coding for the inter-

cellular adhesion molecule 1 (ICAM-1), a 90 kd inducible surface glycoprotein that promotes adhesion in immunological and inflammatory reactions [14]. ICAM-1 is a ligand of lymphocyte function associated antigen 1 (LFA-1), a member of the integrin family of cell-to-cell and cell-to-matrix receptors. Cell adhesion molecules of the immunoglobulin superfamily may play important roles in tumourigenesis and the development of metastatic disease [15]. In a variety of human malignancies tumour progression has been observed to be associated with changes in cell adhesion molecule expression. In particular, ICAM-1 has been associated with more advanced forms of disease and the development of melanoma with metastatic potential [16] although in neuroblastoma the expression was restricted to low grade tumours with favourable outcome [17]. Clearly ICAM-1 expression and its role in malignant behaviour is tissue specific and may reflect local secretions of cytokines. It is difficult to determine if ICAM-1 is a positive or negative prognostic factor in EOC since the majority of cases present as late stage tumours, but in a limited number of benign tumours OVTL-30 reactivity was infrequent and weak [13]. Soluble ICAM-1 has been used as a serum marker in liver metastasis [18] and may also be a useful serum marker to monitor tumour burden in EOC patients.

6.2.4 G253

The MAb G253 is an IgG_{2a} antibody raised against an astrocytoma cell line [19,20] but subsequently found to be overexpressed in the majority of ovarian carcinomas. The G253 cDNA encodes a novel 90 kd protein and, as with OA3 and ICAM-1, is a member of the immunoglobulin superfamily (manuscript in preparation). It shares sequence and structural homology with proteins associated with tumour metastasis and it is most likely that its normal function is to direct cell-to-cell adhesion. G253 does not appear to participate in homophilic binding and identification of the natural ligand will be of some importance.

6.3 CONCLUSIONS

The preponderance of immunoglobulin superfamily proteins is a striking feature of the tumour antigens cloned so far and may be a measure of their importance in the development of the malignant phenotype. In no case have these antigens been found to be unique molecules. They are normal proteins that are either overexpressed, inappropriately expressed or post-translationally altered in cancer cells. We have found no evidence that mutation of these genes is the basis for the production of novel epitopes. With the exception of FOLR1 no significant allele loss or amplification has been detected and in this case it is likely that FGF-3 (previously INT-2) and/or the *bcl*-1 gene are driving these genomic alterations and in any event do not influence FOLR1 expression [21].

The identification of the immunoglobulin superfamily genes ICAM-1, G253 and OA3 as ovarian carcinoma antigens highlights the importance of cell adhesion in the development of EOC. However, these molecules represent only half of the adhesion process since each requires a ligand to complete its function. It will be important to determine the ligands for G253 and OA3 as these may give clues to their function in the same way that the identification of folate as the ligand for FOLR1 is providing insight into selective pressures faced by EOC.

The great hopes of MAb directed therapy have largely remained unfulfilled which is particularly disappointing as it initially presented itself as an ideal tumour targeting strategy. Our understanding of tumour antigens is gradually expanding and the challenge for the future is to harness this knowledge to achieve the goals envisaged when MAb directed therapies were first proposed.

REFERENCES

1. Taylor-Papadimitriou, J., Allen, D., Granowska, M. *et al.* (1992) Molecular structure and clinical applications of a cancer-associated mucin. In *Ovarian Cancer 2, Biology, Diagnosis and Management*, (eds F. Sharp, W. P. Mason and W. Creasman), Chapman Hall, London, pp. 39–50.

2. Seed, B. (1987) An LFA-3 cDNA encodes a phospholipid membrane protein homologous to its receptor CD2. *Nature*, **329**, 840–2.

3. Campbell, I.G., Foulkes, W.D., Jones, T.A. *et al.* (1992) Cloning of genes encoding ovarian carcinoma-specific antigens. In *Ovarian Cancer 2, Biology, Diagnosis and Management*, (eds F. Sharp, W.P. Mason and W. Creasman), Chapman & Hall, London, pp. 73–86.

4. Campbell, I.G., Jones, T.A., Foulkes, W.D. *et al.* (1991) Folate binding protein is a marker for ovarian cancer. *Cancer Res.*, **51**, 5329–38.

5. Henderson, G.B. (1990) Folate binding proteins. *Ann. Rev. Nutr.*, **10**, 319–35.

6. Garin-Chesa, P., Campbell, I., Saigo, P. E. *et al.* (1993) Trophoblast and ovarian cancer antigen LK26. *Am. J. Pathol.*, **142**, 557–67.

7. Poels, L.G., Peters, D., van Megen, Y. *et al.* (1986) Monoclonal antibody against human ovarian tumor associated antigens. *J. Natl. Cancer Inst.*, **76**, 781–91.

8. Buist, M.R., Kenemans, P., Vermorken, J.B. *et al.* (1992) Radioimmunotargeting in ovarian carcinoma patients with indium-111 labelled monoclonal antibody OV-TL3 F(ab')2: pharmacokinetics, tissue distribution, tumour imaging. *Int. J. Gynecol. Cancer*, **2**, 23–34.

9. Campbell, I.G., Freemont. P.S., Foulkes, W.D. *et al.* (1992) An ovarian tumour marker with homology to vaccinia virus contains an IgV-like region and multiple transmembrane domains. *Cancer Res.*, **52**, 5416–20.

10. Williams, A.F. and Barclay, A.N. (1988) The immunoglobulin superfamily – domains for cell surface recognition. *Ann. Rev. Immunol.*, **6**, 318–405.

11. Smith, G.L., Chan, Y.S. and Howard, S.T. (1991) Nucleotide sequence of 42 kbp of vaccinia virus strain WR from near the right inverted terminal repeat. *J. Gen. Virol.*, **72**, 1349–76.

12. Massuger, L.F.A., Kenemans, P., Claessens, R.A.M.J. *et al.* (1991) Detection and localization of ovarian cancer with radiolabeled monoclonal antibodies. *Eur. J. Obstet. Gynecol. Reprod. Biol.*, **41**, 47–63.

13. Boerman, O.C., Makkink, W.K., Thomas, C.M.G. *et al.* (1990) Monoclonal antibodies that discriminate between human ovarian carcinomas and benign ovarian tumours. *Eur. J. Cancer*, **26**, 117–27.

14. Simmonds, D., Makgoba, M.W. and Seed, B. (1988) ICAM, an adhesion ligand of LFA-1, is homologous to the neural-cell adhesion molecule NCAM. *Nature*, **331**, 624–7.

15. Johnson, J.P. (1991) Cell adhesion molecules of the immunoglobulin supergene family and their role in malignant transformation and progression to metastatic disease. *Cancer Metastasis Rev.*, **10**, 11–12.

16. Holzmann, B., Brocker, E.B., Lehmann, J.M. *et al.* (1987) Tumor progression in human malignant melanoma: five stages defined by their antigenic phenotypes. *Int. J. Cancer*, **39**, 466–71.

17. Favrot, M.C., Combaret, V., Goillot, E. *et al.* (1991) Expression of leucocyte adhesion molecules on 66 clinical neuroblastoma specimens. *Int. J. Cancer*, **48**, 502–10.

18. Tsujisaki, M., Imai, K., Hirata, H. *et al.* (1991) Detection of circulating intercellular adhesion molecule-1 antigen in malignant diseases. *Clin. Exp. Immunol.*, **85**, 3–8.

19. Rettig, W.J., Chesa, P.G., Beresford, H.R. *et al.* (1986) Differential expression of cell surface antigens and glial fibrillary acidic protein in human astrocytoma subsets. *Cancer Res.*, **46**, 6406–12.

20. Rettig, W.J., Garin-Chesa, P., Beresford, H.R. *et al.* (1988) Cell-surface glycoproteins of human sarcomas: differential expression in normal and malignant tissues and cultured cells. *Immunology*, **85**, 3110–14.

21. Foulkes, W.D., Campbell, I.G. Stamp, G.W.H. *et al.* (1993) Loss of heterozygosity and amplification on chromosome 11q in human ovarian cancer. *Br. J. Cancer*, **67**, 268–73.

22. Miotti, S., Canevari, S., Menard, S. *et al.* (1987) Characterization of human ovarian carcinoma-associated antigens defined by monoclonal antibodies with tumor-restricted specificity. *Int. J. Cancer*, **39**, 297–303.

23. Ragoussis, J., Senger, G., Trowsdale, J. *et al.* (1992) Genomic organisation of the human folate receptor genes on chromosome 11q13. *Genomics*, **14**, 423–30.

Chapter 7

New insights into the genetics of human ovarian epithelial tumor development

S. ZWEIZIG, J. ZHENG, M. WAN, T.M. KIM, M. VELICESCU, J. GOSEWEHR
and L. DUBEAU

7.1 INTRODUCTION

Much progress was made during the last decade toward the identification and characterization of several of the genetic determinants of carcinogenesis. The actual mechanisms of tumorigenesis remain largely unknown in spite of these advances. Much of the difficulty comes from the complexity of the neoplastic phenotype itself. Indeed, this phenotype is not characterized by single, but by multiple abnormalities which can each vary in importance in individual tumors. Examples of different manifestations of the neoplastic phenotype include uncontrolled growth, ability to destructively infiltrate neighboring tissues, ability to metastasize to distant organs, aberrant cell differentiation, etc. It is likely that these properties are independent of each other and are therefore under separate genetic controls, as not all are present at the same time in individual tumors. The complexity of the problem is further increased by the fact that according to the concept of tumor progression first advanced by Foulds [1] and Nowell [2], neoplastic cells are not stable but in constant evolution, resulting in high degrees of heterogeneity within a given tumor mass.

The ovarian epithelial tumor model is an attractive one in which to study the mechanisms of tumorigenesis, in the light of the above mentioned difficulties. Firstly, it allows the isolation of some of the components of the malignant phenotype. The constituents of this model include cystadenomas and tumors of low malignant potential (LMPs) in addition to carcinomas. The first two entities are distinguished from the carcinomas by their lack of invasive and metastatic abilities. Thus, clonal molecular abnormalities associated with their development may be associated with uncontrolled cell proliferation but not with invasion or metastasis. We have used the criteria recommended by the Federation of Gynecologic Oncologists (FIGO) to further subdivide the carcinomas according to their histologic grades, as this approach allows further separation of specific phenotypic properties. Low grade carcinomas according to these criteria have retained their abilities to form specialized structures such as glands or papillae, whereas high grade carcinomas form amorphous solid tumor blocks.

The other reason for the attractiveness of the ovarian model is the relatively high stability of the different tumor entities that compose this model. We favor the view that cystadenomas, LMPs and even different grades of carcinomas are stable and independent from each other as opposed to representing different stages of tumor progression. Although some carcinomas may possibly develop from pre-existing cystadenomas or LMPs, our working hypothesis is that most of them arise *de novo* and that cystadenomas or LMPs do not show gradual and inevitable progression toward carcinomas. Indeed, large cystadenomas several cm in diameter are histologically indistinguishable from small ones except for their size. LMPs or low grade carcinomas that recur several months or even years after initial surgery are usually histologically similar to the original tumors. On the other hand, small incidental carcinomas are sometimes seen with no histological evidence of an adjacent pre-existing cystadenoma. There is certainly very little evidence for a gradual progression toward histologically more complex and biologically more aggressive lesions.

Much of the recent work done in our laboratory has been based on the reasoning that this relative stability of the different constituents of the ovarian model, especially the cystadenomas and LMPs, may result in reduced heterogeneity and thus facilitate identification of their determinants. We have therefore examined the frequencies of genetic abnormalities in ovarian cystadenomas, LMPs and in carcinomas of low or high histologic grade to determine if certain genetic lesions are associated with specific disease states. We anticipated that qualitative molecular differences would be found between such entities in addition to purely quantitative ones. We were particularly interested in comparing LMPs or cystadenomas to carcinomas because, as mentioned above, such studies may lead to the distinction of the molecular determinants of tumor proliferation from those of invasion or metastasis. Although these studies are still ongoing, we have almost completed an allelotype of ovarian epithelial tumors subdivided into LMPs and low and high grade carcinomas and have also examined the frequencies of loss of heterozygosity

on selected chromosomes in cystadenomas. The frequencies of mutation in the p53 gene were also examined in the same tumors. The results of these studies and our conclusions regarding the mechanisms of ovarian tumorigenesis are summarized in this chapter.

7.2 MATERIALS AND METHODS

7.2.1 SOURCE OF TUMOR AND BLOOD SPECIMENS

Fresh specimens of tumor tissues used for allelotype studies were obtained from the surgical pathology departments of either the Women's Hospital of the Los Angeles County Medical Center or the Kenneth Norris Jr. Comprehensive Cancer Center. Frozen histologic sections of all tumors were first examined to verify the presence of neoplastic cells and to ensure that the specimens did not contain unacceptable amounts of non-neoplastic cells such as in stromal tissues. The entire tumor specimens were also reviewed to verify that the lesions were primary ovarian tumors of epithelial origin. Non-epithelial ovarian tumors as well as mixed epithelial/mesenchymal tumors were not used. We also elected not to use Müllerian-like primary peritoneal tumors. Tumors were discarded if the possibility of a primary endometrial or tubal origin could not be ruled out. In addition, we have discarded any tumor where the possibility of a metastasis to the ovary from a non-ovarian source could not be ruled out with high degrees of confidence.

High molecular weight DNA was extracted from each selected specimen as described [3]. Fresh blood samples were drawn from each patient and processed for extraction of high molecular weight DNA as described [3]. Archival tissue sections were obtained from pathology departments at the above two hospitals in the few experiments where such tissues were used.

7.2.2 ALLELOTYPE ANALYSES

A few genetic loci were examined by conventional Southern blotting analysis as previously described [3]. However, most loci were examined by enzymatically amplifying 50 ng of high molecular weight DNA obtained from blood and tumor samples of each patient using primers for microsatellite polymorphisms. PCR mixes were of 25 μl and contained 1 μCi of ^{32}P-dCTP. The radiolabelled PCR products were electrophoresed on denaturing polyacrylamide gels and the position of the alleles for each locus was determined by autoradiography. One of the difficulties with this PCR based approach is that the relative amounts of the two parental alleles of a given locus are not always maintained during enzymatic amplification, resulting in random preferential amplification of one of the alleles. This problem was encountered almost exclusively when using archival tissue sections as the PCR template. We have therefore elected not to use archival specimens for allelotype studies in order to minimize the possibility of this artefact. In addition, we have taken further precautions by repeating all experiments showing the presence of allelic losses several times in order to verify the authenticity of the losses. Experiments done on cystadenomas or those aimed at selectively amplifying specific areas of a tumor using the SURF technique (see below), which were done on archival specimens, were repeated approximately 10 times each.

Genetic loci examined by PCR or probes used for Southern blotting analysis were as follows.

- Chromosome 1p: DIS116 [4], pMUC-10 *
- Chromosome 1q: D1S117 [5], D1S103 [6]
- Chromosome 2q: glucagon [7], interleukin-1 [8], gamma-B-crystallin [9]
- Chromosome 3p: pBH302 [3], pH3H2 [3]
- Chromosome 3q: D3S196 [10]
- Chromosome 4q: FABP2 [11]
- Chromosome 5p: D5S117 [12]
- Chromosome 5q: D5S134 [13], CSF-1 receptor [14]
- Chromosome 6p: pHHH156˙, pZFD6 ˙
- Chromosome 6q: Arg-1 [15], D6S87 [15], D6S255 [15], D6S2⁺, D6S37⁺, c-myb⁺, estrogen receptor [16]
- Chromosome 9q: D9S63 [17]
- Chromosome 11p: TH [18], H-*ras* [3], insulin [3]
- Chromosome 13q: FTL-1 [19], D13S128 [20], D13S133 [20]
- Chromosome 14q: D14S45 [21], T cell receptor delta [22]
- Chromosome 15q: IGFR [23], CYP19 [24]
- Chromosome 16p: D16S319 [25]
- Chromosome 16q: D16S289 [25]
- Chromosome 17p: p53, D17S513 [26], pYNZ22 [3]
- Chromosome 17q: GH [27], D17S250 [28], G3PA [29]
- Chromosome 18p: D18S37 [30]
- Chromosome 18q: MBP [31]
- Chromosome 19p: D19S76 [32]
- Chromosome 19p: apoliprotein CII [33]
- Chromosome 20p: CSTP1 [34], D20S27 [35]
- Chromosome 20q: SRC [36]
- Chromosome 21q: APP [37], D21S167 [38]
- Chromosome 22q: CYP2D [39]
- Chromosome Xp: DMD [40], Kallman [41]
- Chromosome Xq: AR [42], Alport [43].

7.2.3 SELECTIVE AMPLIFICATION OF INDIVIDUAL TUMOR AREAS BY SURF

Selected tumor cells were amplified separately from archival tissue sections using the SURF technique as described by Shibata *et al.* [44]. Briefly, 4 micron thick tissue sections were stained with hematoxylin and eosin but not cover-slipped. Selected cells were painted

---

* Probe obtained from Dr S.J. Gendler, Imperial Cancer Research Fund Laboratories, London.
˙ Probe obtained from American Type Culture Collection, Rockvillie, MD.

manually with water-insoluble black ink using a Sharpie® permanent marker pen (Sanford Corp., Bellwood, IL) and UV-irradiated for two hours with a trans-illuminator (UVP Inc., San Gabriel, CA) resulting in degradation of all DNAs except in the areas protected by black ink. Tissue sections were transferred to microcentrifuge tubes, incubated overnight at 56°C in 100 µl/ml proteinase K, heated in boiling water for 10 minutes and used directly in PCR mixes for allelic loss studies or for determination of p53 mutations.

7.2.4 DETERMINATION OF THE PRESENCE OF p53 MUTATIONS BY RNA-SSCP AND DOUBLE STRANDED DNA SEQUENCING

The presence of p53 mutations was examined in either high molecular weight DNA from LMPs and carcinomas or in archival tissue sections of cystadenomas. Enrichment for neoplastic cells in cystadenomas was achieved using the SURF technique (see above). Exons 5–6 and 7–8 of the p53 gene were first amplified enzymatically. The products were then reamplified using primers for approximately 125 base pair fragments from the above exons. One of the PCR primers used for each reamplification reaction contained the T7 RNA polymerase promoter sequence at its 5'-end as described by Danenberg *et al.* [45]. The reaction products were then used as templates for RNA synthesis using this polymerase [45]. The radiolabelled RNA fragments were electrophoresed on 6% polyacrylamide gels under non-denaturing conditions. The presence of mutations resulted in shifts in electrophoretic mobilities of the RNA fragments. All cases where the presence of mutation was supected based on this initial screening were then reexamined by double stranded DNA sequencing using a dsDNA Cycle Sequencing System kit (Bethesda Research Laboratories, Gaithersburg, MD).

7.3 RESULTS

7.3.1 ALLELOTYPE OF HUMAN OVARIAN CARCINOMAS

Several laboratories have reported studies on losses of heterozygosity at various chromosomal loci in human ovarian carcinomas [3,46–60]. One of these studies [59] was comprehensive, showing data on every somatic chromosomal arm (allelotype). There was only partial agreement between the different studies, perhaps reflecting the fact that ovarian tumors include several different histologic types which may have different etiologies and mechanisms. Evidence that such differences exist was indeed reported [59]. In addition, our earlier work suggested that marked differences in frequencies of specific molecular abnormalities may exist between tumors of different histologic grades [3]. We have initiated our own allelotype study which included only primary Müllerian-derived ovarian epithelial tumors. The tumors were of the three most common histologic types (serous, endometrioid and mucinous), although a few tumors with clear cell differentiation were also used. They were subdivided into LMPs and into carcinomas of low or high histologic grades in order to examine the molecular differences between these subgroups.

Although the above studies are still ongoing, they are almost complete and current results are shown in Figure 7.1. The figure shows frequencies of allelic losses for carcinomas of high histologic grade only, as available evidence suggests that some chromosomal arms are more frequently involved in such losses in high grade lesions [3]. Results for 12 different chromosomal arms are currently pending, as indicated. Chromosomes showing high frequencies of allelic loss in this tumor population included 6q (55%), 11p (39%), 13q (63%), 17p (60%) and 17q (66%). Other studies have also shown similar losses at these loci in ovarian carcino-

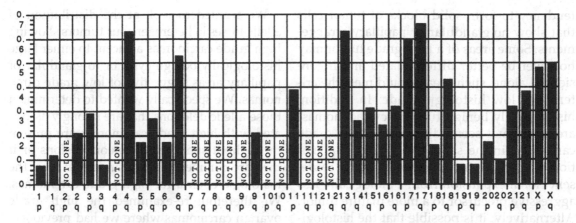

Figure 7.1 Allelotype of human ovarian carcinomas of high histologic grades.

mas [46,47,50,52–56,58–60]. Chromosome 17q is of particular interest because it is thought to be associated with familial predisposition to breast and ovarian carcinomas [61,62]. Two of the chromosomes showing high frequencies of loss of heterozygosity in our population of high grade carcinomas have not previously been associated with these tumors to our knowledge. They are the long arm of chromosome 4 and the long arm of chromosome X. Twelve of 20 tumors examined from patients heterozygous for a microsatellite repeat polymorphism at the FABP2 locus on chromosome 4q28-q31 showed reduction to homozygosity at this locus. We are currently attempting to further define the role of this genetic region in ovarian tumorigenesis. With regard to the long arm of chromosome X, the potential significance of allelic losses on this chromosome in ovarian tumors is discussed later.

7.3.2 ALLELIC DELETIONS THAT DISTINGUISH LOW GRADE FROM HIGH GRADE CARCINOMAS

We next compared the above frequencies of allelic deletions to those present in carcinomas of low histologic grades as our earlier

work suggested that some genetic loci may be specifically associated with the high grade phenotype [3]. Chromosomes where such an association was strongest were 11p, 13q and Xq. Allelic deletions on other frequently affected chromosomes such as 6q, 17p and 17q were also more frequent in high grade tumors but the differences were not as marked as for the above chromosomes and were not statistically significant.

We conclude that inactivation of one or several genes on chromosomes 11p, 13q or Xq plays an important role during ovarian tumorigenesis. However, these genetic abnormalities may be specifically associated with the acquisition of phenotypic properties that distinguish tumors of high histologic grade from low grade carcinomas and may possibly not be directly involved in the acquisition of invasive and metastatic abilities.

7.3.3 ALLELIC DELETIONS IN HISTOLOGICALLY BENIGN OR LOW GRADE MALIGNANT TUMORS ADJACENT TO HIGH GRADE CARCINOMAS

Ovarian tumors are often heterogeneous with regard to histologic grade or malignant behavior. High grade carcinomas have a tendency to form solid blocks of tumor cells that show no glandular or papillary arrangements. Some areas of a high grade tumor may however be better differentiated and if considered alone, such areas would meet the criteria for low histologic grade. In addition, histologically benign tumors (cystadenomas) are sometimes seen adjacent to a high grade carcinoma in the same ovary. One explanation is that such heterogeneous lesions represent clonal expansion from a biologically less aggressive precursor to a more mature tumor. Alternatively, it is possible that the histologically less aggressive areas in such lesions are not pre-existing precursors but are merely manifestations of tumor heterogeneity or that the different histologic areas represent collisions between unrelated neoplasms.

We took advantage of the observations of molecular differences between carcinomas of low and high histologic grades to address these questions, which are central to our understanding of ovarian tumor development. The results shown in Table 7.1 suggested that allelic deletions on chromosomes 11p, 13q or Xq may distinguish high grade from low grade ovarian carcinomas. We have also examined 11 different cystadenomas for allelic deletions on chromosome 11p and did not observe any (results not shown).

We wanted to look at the distribution of allelic losses in heterogeneous tumors showing high grade carcinomas adjacent to either large histologically benign cysts or to glandular or papillary areas suggestive of low grade carcinomas. We specifically wanted to determine if those allelic deletions that are strongly associated with high grade carcinomas are present throughout such heterogeneous lesions or if they are confined to those areas that meet the histologic criteria for high grade carcinomas. We therefore re-examined the high grade ovarian carcinomas where we had previously demonstrated the presence of allelic deletions on chromosome 11p and identified several tumors showing phenotypic heterogeneity. We enzymatically amplified the different histologic areas individually from archival tissue sections using the SURF technique (see above) and examined the presence or absence of allelic losses on chromosome 11p in all neoplastic areas separately. The results (Zheng *et al.*, in preparation) clearly showed that allelic deletions on this chromosome, although found only in tumors containing poorly differentiated solid areas characteristic of high histologic grades, were not confined to such areas in phenotypically heterogeneous lesions and were even present in adjacent histologically benign neoplastic cysts. These results rule out

Table 7.1 Association between allelic losses on chromosomes 11p, 13q and Xq and grade of ovarian carcinomas

Chromosome	*Number of tumors with allelic losses/number of cases examined from heterozygous patients*		*Double-sided p values (Fisher's exact test)*
	Low grade carcinomas	*High grade carcinomas*	
11p	0/14	12/31	0.009
13q	0/13	19/22	0.0004
Xq	0/10	12/25	0.007

the possibility that the different histologic areas represent collisions between independent tumors. We interpret these data as supportive of a model where the histologically less aggressive areas in the above tumors are not typical cystadenomas or low grade carcinomas and may be manifestations of phenotypic heterogeneity rather than representing pre-existing precursor lesions.

7.3.4 POINT MUTATIONS IN THE p53 GENE IN LOW AND HIGH GRADE OVARIAN CARCINOMAS

The p53 gene has been the subject of extensive investigations following the initial reports that it can function as a tumor suppressor gene. These studies have demonstrated that point mutations concentrated in specific exons of this gene are found frequently in a large variety of different tumor types. Several authors have also reported the presence of such mutations in ovarian carcinomas [55,56,63–65]. We have examined the frequencies of such mutations in our tumor population as we wanted to determine if molecular abnormalities involving this locus would distinguish high grade ovarian carcinomas from low grade carcinomas, LMPs and cystadenomas.

The tumors were first screened for the presence of mutations in exons 5–8 using the method of RNA-SSCP as described by Danenberg *et al.* [45]. Those tumors showing evidence of mutation were then further examined by DNA sequencing. The results (Table 7.2) showed the presence of mutations in 15

of 31 high grade carcinomas. The fact that such mutations were also seen in a significant proportion of low grade carcinomas suggests that abnormalities at this locus are compatible with the low grade phenotype and are not directly involved in controlling the phenotypic changes that distinguish high from low grade carcinomas. However, the fact that no p53 mutations were detected in either cystadenomas or LMPs suggests that such mutations are rare in the latter lesions, which lack invasive and metastatic abilities. The results are suggestive of a direct role for the p53 protein in controlling invasive and metastatic abilities.

7.3.5 ALLELIC LOSSES IN LMPs

The results shown in Figure 7.1 demonstrated that several chromosomal arms are affected frequently by allelic deletions in high grade ovarian carcinomas and further studies suggested that allelic deletions on certain chromosomes may distinguish such high grade lesions from carcinomas of low histologic grades. We were therefore interested to determine which if any of the chromosomal arms examined were affected frequently in LMPs. All chromosomal arms studied in Figure 7.1 were therefore also examined for the presence or absence of loss of heterozygosity in 10 LMPs from which high molecular DNA was available to us. We have elected not to increase our tumor population with archival specimens because of such specimens showing false-positive losses of

Table 7.2 Frequencies of mutations in exons 5–8 of the p53 gene in different types of ovarian epithelial tumors

Cystadenomas	LMPs	Low grade carcinomas	High grade carcinomas
0/10	0/10	3/12	13/31

p (cystadenomas and LMPs *vs* carcinomas) = 0.001
p (low grade *vs* high grade carcinomas) = 0.48

heterozygosity due to preferential allelic amplification. The results showed that allelic losses were rare in LMPs and that several such tumors contained no detectable losses. Of all the chromosomes examined, only one was found to be frequently associated with allelic losses in our population of LMPs. This was the long arm of chromosome X. Allelic deletions on this chromosome, more specifically those involving the androgen receptor locus in the pericentrometric region, were seen in three of six (50%) LMPs informative for the locus. Autoradiographs demonstrating loss of heterozygosity on this chromosome in two of these tumors are shown in Figure 7.2. Interestingly, the same locus is among those found to be infrequently involved by allelic losses in carcinomas of low histologic grade, although it was affected by such losses in 50% of high grade carcinomas (Table 7.1). Differences in frequencies of allelic loss at this

locus in LMPs compared to those seen in low grade carcinomas (3/6 *vs.* 0/10) were significant by Fisher's exact test (2-sided $p = 0.04$).

7.3.6 A MODEL FOR OVARIAN EPITHELIAL TUMOR DEVELOPMENT

Our conclusions from the above studies are summarized in Figure 7.3, which is our current working model for the development of ovarian epithelial tumors. We suggest that inactivation of one or several genes on the long arm of chromosome X plays an important role in ovarian tumorigenesis. Such abnormalities, however, are probably not directly involved in the control of invasive or metastatic abilities as they occur frequently in LMPs. Instead, they may be important for the control of neoplastic cell proliferation. Other abnormalities, which are frequent in carcinomas of all grades but infrequent or absent in

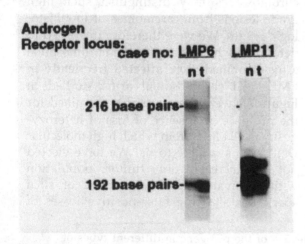

Figure 7.2 Losses of heterozygosity on chromosome Xq in LMPs. DNAs from patient's normal blood cells (n) or tumor (t) were amplified enzymatically using primers for the androgen receptor locus. The radiolabeled PCR products were electrophoresed on denaturing polyacrylamide gels and autoradiographed. The results show loss of one of the two parental alleles in both tumor samples.

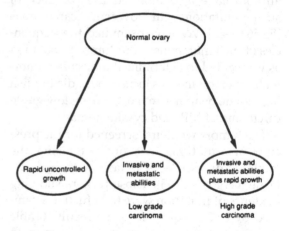

Figure 7.3 A model for the development of human ovarian epithelial tumors. We suggest that the genetic determinants of LMPs, which lead to uncontrolled growth, are different from those of carcinoma, which lead to invasive and metastatic abilities. The presence of both types of determinants in a given tumor leads to carcinomas of higher histologic grade. (Reproduced from Genetics of ovarian carcinoma development, In *Current Perspectives on Molecular and Cellular Oncology*, Volume 2, JAI Press Ltd., London.)

LMPs, are probably more directly involved in invasive or metastatic behavior. Such abnormalities include inactivation of genes on chromosomes 6q, 17p and 17q as well as mutations in the p53 gene. When present in carcinomas, allelic deletions on chromosome Xq lead to tumors of high histologic grades.

7.4 DISCUSSION

We have presented preliminary data from an allelotype of primary ovarian epithelial tumors subdivided into LMPs, low grade carcinomas and high grade carcinomas. Chromosome regions affected frequently by losses of constitutional heterozygosity in this study are for the most part similar to those reported in other studies. Exceptions are the long arm of chromosome 4, which to our knowledge has not previously been associated with ovarian tumorigenesis, and the pericentromeric region of the long arm of chromosome X.

The results of our experiments also provided evidence that LMPs, low grade ovarian carcinomas and high grade carcinomas may be distinguished from each other by qualitative molecular differences in addition to purely quantitative ones. These conclusions may provide clues about the nature of the genetic determinants of individual components of the neoplastic phenotype in general. We suggest that chromosomal abnormalities strongly associated with high grade but not with low grade carcinomas, although impotant for ovarian tumorigenesis, may not be directly involved in the control of invasive and metastatic abilities. Instead, they may be specific determinants of those properties that distinguish high grade from low grade tumors. Morphologically, these properties are manifested as solid poorly differentiated blocks of tumor cells. Although the reasons for these morphologic changes are not fully understood, they could be at least partly due to increased rates of proliferation. This hypothesis is supported by the fact that the only clonal molecular abnormality which we have so far observed in a significant proportion of LMPs – allelic losses on chromosome Xq – is also among those that most clearly distinguish high grade from low grade carcinomas. We suggest that inactivation of one or several genes on this chromosome probably leads to increased cell proliferation but not to invasive and metastatic abilities, with allelic losses at this locus being frequent in LMPs. The rarity of such losses in low grade carcinomas is explained by the idea that when present in carcinomas, the superimposition of these abnormalities onto determinants of the invasive and metastatic phenotype results in tumors of high histologic grades. Direct verification of this model awaits isolation and further characterization of the genetic target of the allelic deletions on chromosome Xq. Activation of the k-*ras* proto-oncogene may be another example of a molecular abnormality frequently present in LMPs [66]. This abnormality may also lead to increased cell proliferation as opposed to invasive or metastatic abilities based on the above reasoning. However, its distribution among carcinomas of different histologic grades has not to our knowledge been examined.

Our data also provide evidence against stepwise progression of ovarian tumors from cystadenomas to LMPs and carcinomas of increasing histologic grade. The presence of large histologically benign cysts adjacent to ovarian carcinomas has been regarded as evidence for clonal expansion of carcinomas from pre-existing cystadenomas. However, results reported in this chapter demonstrate that the histologically benign portions of such heterogeneous tumors contain genetic abnormalities that are usually not seen in typical cystadenomas. It is possible that such heterogeneous tumors start out as histologically benign and that manifestations of malignancy only develop later. However, our molecular analyses suggest that such histologically benign cysts contain molecular changes characteristic of carcinomas and may therefore be best regarded as carcinomas in spite of their histologic appearances. Likewise, areas of a high grade tumor that would meet the criteria for low grade carcinoma if considered alone, contained genetic abnormalities associated with high grade lesions. The finding of molecular abnormalities such as allelic deletions on chromosome Xq, which are more frequent in LMPs than in low grade carcinomas, also provides evidence against progression of low grade ovarian carcinomas from pre-existing LMPs.

The finding that histologically benign cysts adjacent to carcinomas are genetically different from pure cystadenomas also suggests a potential approach, based on molecular analyses, to identify those histologically benign tumors more likely to develop manifestations of malignancy or more likely to contain microscopic carcinomas. Such approaches may eventually complement histologic examination of cystadenomas by surgical pathologists.

The finding of qualitative molecular differences between ovarian cystadenomas, LMPs and carcinomas of low and high histologic grades supports the notion that they constitute separate entities as opposed to different points in a single disease spectrum. The data also emphasize the possibility of using the ovarian epithelial tumor model to isolate different components of the neoplastic phenotype and study their determinants separately. The suggestion of an association between ovarian tumor cell proliferation and allelic losses on chromosome Xq is particularly interesting. Additional support for a role of this chromosome in regulation of cell proliferation comes from the evidence that it plays a role in the control of *in vitro* cell senescence [67,68]. Further evidence for a direct role in ovarian cell proliferation specifically is suggested by the observation that patients with Turner syndrome, who are born with a single X chromosome, have undeveloped ovaries (gonadal dysgenesis). Thus, both alleles of this chromosome are necessary for ovarian development. It is presently not clear if the above deletions involve active or inactive X chromosomes. The genetic target of those deletions must escape X inactivation if the deletions are on the inactive chromosome. The importance of this chromosome for the control of proliferation of other tumor cell types is currently unclear.

ACKNOWLEDGMENTS

This work was supported by grant number R29 CA51167 from the US National Cancer Institute and by grant number EDT-11B from the American Cancer Society.

REFERENCES

1. Foulds, L. (1956) The histologic analysis of mammary tumors in mice II. The histology of responsiveness and progression. *J. Natl. Cancer Inst.*, **17**, 713–52.
2. Nowell, P.C. (1976) The clonal evolution of tumor cell populations. *Science*, **194**, 23–8.
3. Zheng, J.P., Robinson, W.R., Ehlen, T. *et al.* (1991) Distinction of low grade from high grade human ovarian carcinomas on the basis of losses of heterozygosity on chromosomes 3, 6, and 11 and HER-2/*neu* gene amplification. *Cancer Res.*, **51**, 4045–51.
4. Sharma, V., Allen, L., Magenis, R.E. and Litt, M. (1991) A dinucleotide repeat polymorphism at the D1S116 locus. *Nucleic Acids Res.*, **19**, 1169.
5. Sharma, V. and Litt, M. (1991) Dinucleotide repeat polymorphism at the D1S117 locus. *Nucleic Acids Res.*, **19**, 1168.
6. Weber, J.L., Kwitek, A.E. and May, P.E. (1990) Dinucleotide repeat polymorphism at the D1S103 locus. *Nucleic Acids Res.*, **18**, 2199.
7. Wu, S., Xiang, K. and Bell, G.I. (1991) Dinucleotide repeat polymorphism in the human glucagon gene (GCG). *Nucleic Acids Res.*, **19**, 1163.

8. Todd, S. and Naylor, S.L. (1991) Dinucleotide repeat polymorphism in the human interleukin 1,alpha gene (IL1A). *Nucleic Acids Res.*, **19**, 3756.

9. Polymeropoulos, M.H., Xiao, H., Rath, D.S. and Merril, C.R. (1991) Trinucleotide repeat polymorphism at the human gamma-B-crystallin gene. *Nucleic Acids Res.*, **19**, 4571.

10. Weber, J.L., May, P.E., Patterson, D. *et al.* (1990) Dinucleotide repeat polymorphism at the D3S196 locus. *Nucleic Acids Res.*, **18**, 4635.

11. Polymeropoulos. M.H., Rath, D.S., Xiao, H. and Merril, C.R. (1990) Trinucleotide repeat polymorphism at the human intestinal fatty acid binding protein gene (FABP2). *Nucleic Acids Res.*, **18**, 7198.

12. Weber, J.L., Kwitek, A.E. and May, P.E. (1990) Dinucleotide repeat polymorphisms at the D5S107, D5S108, D5S111, D5S117 and D5S118 loci. *Nucleic Acids Res.*, **18**, 4035.

13. Koorey, D.J., McCaughan, G.W., Trent, R.J. and Gallagher, N.D. (1992) Dinucleotide repeat polymorphism at the D5S134 locus linked to the adenomatous polyposis coli (APC) gene. *Hum. Mol. Genet.*, **1**, 655.

14. Polymeropoulos, M.H., Xiao, H., Rath, D.S. and Merril, C.R. (1991) Dinucleotide repeat polymorphism at the human c-fms protooncogene for the CFS-1 receptor (CFS1R). *Nucleic Acids Res.*, **19**, 1160.

15. Wilkie, P.J., Polymeropoulos, M.H., Trent, J.M. *et al.* (1993) Genetic and physical map of 11 short tandem repeat polymorphisms on human chromosome 6. *Genomics*, **15**, 225–7.

16. Del Senno, L., Aguiari, G.L. and Piva, R. (1992) Dinucleotide repeat polymorphism in the human estrogen receptor (ESR) gene. *Hum. Mol. Genet.*, **1**, 354.

17. Kwiatkowski, D.J., Henske, E.P., Weimer, K. *et al.* (1992) Construction of a GT polymorphism map of human 9q. *Genomics*, **12**, 229–40.

18. Polymeropolous, M.H., Xiao, H. and Merril, C.R. (1991) Tetranucleotide repeat polymorphism at the human tyrosine hydroxylase gene (TH). *Nucleic Acids Res.*, **19**, 3753

19. Polymeropoulos, M.H., Rath, D.S., Xiao, H. and Merril, C.R. (1991) Dinculeotide repeat polymorphism at the human fms-related tyrosine kinase gene (FLT1). *Nucleic Acids Res.*, **19**, 2803.

20. Petrukhin, K.E., Speer, M.C., Cayanis, E. *et al.* (1993) A microsatellite genetic linkage map of human chromosome 13. *Genomics*, **15**, 76–85.

21. Luty, J.A. and Litt, M. (1991) Dinucleotide repeat polymorphism at the D14S45 locus. *Nucleic Acids Res.*, **19**, 4308.

22. Jordan, S.A., McWilliam, P., O'Brian, D.S. and Humphries, P. (1991) Dinucleotide repeat polymorphism at the T cell receptor delta locus (TCRD). *Nucleic Acids Res.*, **19**, 1959.

23. Polymeropoulos, M.H., Rath, D.S., Xiao, H. and Merril, C.R. (1991) Dinucleotide repeat polymorphism at the human gene for insulin-like growth factor I (IFGI). *Nucleic Acids Res.*, **19**, 5797.

24. Polymeropoulos, M.H., Xiao, H., Rath, D.S. and Merril, C.R. (1991) Tetranucleotide repeat polymorphism at the human aromatase cytochrome P-450 gene (CYP19). *Nucleic Acids Res.*, **19**, 195.

25. Shen, Y., Thompson, A.T., Holman, K. *et al.* (1991) Four dinucleotide repeat polymorphisms on human chromosome 16 at D16S289, D16S318, D16S319 and D16S320. *Hum. Mol. Genet.*, **1**, 773.

26. Oliphant, A.R., Wright, E.C., Swensen, J. *et al.* (1991) Dinucleotide repeat polymorphism at the D17S513 locus. *Nucleic Acids Res.*, **19**, 4794.

27. Polymeropoulos, M.H., Rath, D.S., Xiao, H. and Merril, C.R. (1991) A simple sequence repeat polymorphism at the human growth hormone locus. *Nucleic Acids Res.*, **19**, 689.

28. Weber, J.L., Kwitek, A.E., May, P.E. *et al.* (1990) Dinucleotide repeat polymorphisms at the D17S250 and D17S261 loci. *Nucleic Acids Res.*, **18**, 4640.

29. Stoffel, M. and Bell, G.I. (1992) Microsatellite polymorphism in the human platelet glycoprotein IIIa gene (GP3A) on chromosome 17. *Nucleic Acids Res.*, **20**, 1172.

30. Sharma, V., Guo, Z. and Litt, M. (1992) Dinucleotide repeat polymorphism at the D18S37 locus. *Hum. Mol. Genet.*, **1**, 289.

31. Polymeropoulos, M.H., Xiao, H. and Merril, C.R. (1991) Tetranucleotide repeat polymorphism at the human myelin basic protein (MBP). *Hum. Mol. Genet.*, **1**, 658.

32. Weber, J.L. and May, P.E. (1990) Dinucleotide repeat polymorphism at the D19S76 locus. *Nucleic Acids Res.*, **18**, 2835.

33. Hegele, R.A. and Tu, L.L. (1991) Variation within intron 3 of the apoliprotein CII gene. *Nucleic Acids Res.*, **19**, 3162.

34. Polymeropoulos. M.H., Xiao, H., Rath, D.S. and Merril, C.R. (1991) Dinucleotide repeat polymorphism at the human cysteine–proteinase inhibitor pseudogene (CSTP1). *Nucleic Acids Res.*, **19**, 1164.

35. Weber, J.L. and May, P.E. (1990) Dinucleotide repeat polymorphism at the D20S27 locus. *Nucleic Acids Res.*, **18**, 2202.

36. Xiang, K., Philippe, G., Seino, M. *et al.* (1991) Dinucleotide repeat polymorphism in the human SRC gene on chromosome 20. *Nucleic Acids Res.*, **19**, 6967.

37. Mant, R., Parfitt, E., Hardy, J. and Owen, M. (1991) Mononucleotide repeat polymorphism in the APP gene. *Nucleic Acids Res.*, **19**, 4572.

38. Guo, Z., Sharma, V., Patterson, D. and Litt, M. (1990) TG repeat polymorphism at the D21S167 locus. *Nucleic Acids Res.*, **18**, 4967.

39. Polymeropoulos, M.H., Rath, D.S., Xiao, H. and Merril, C.R. (1991) Dinucleotide repeat polymorphism at the human debrisoquine 4-hydroxylase (CYP2D) locus. *Nucleic Acids Res.*, **19**, 1961.

40. Hugnot, J.P., Recan, D., Jeanpierre, M. *et al.* (1991) A highly informative CACA repeat polymorphism upstream of the human dystrophin gene (DMD). *Nucleic Acids Res.*, **19**, 3159.

41. Bouloux, P.M., Hardelin, J.P., Munroe, P. *et al.* (1991) A dinucleotide repeat polymorphism at the Kallmann locus (Xp22.3). *Nucleic Acids Res.*, **19**, 5453.

42. Sleddens, H.F., Osstra, B.A., Brinkmann, A.O. and Trapman, J. (1992) Trinucleotide repeat polymorphism in the androgen receptor gene (AR). *Nucleic Acids Res.*, **20**, 1427.

43. Barker, D.F., Cleverly, J. and Fain, P.R. (1992) Two CA-dinucleotide polymorphisms at the COL4A5 (Alport syndrome) gene in Xq22. *Nucleic Acids Res.*, **20**, 929.

44. Shibata, D., Hawes, D., Li, Z.H. *et al.* (1992) Specific genetic analysis of microscopic tissue after selective ultraviolet radiation fractionation and the polymerase chain reaction. *Am. J. Pathol.*, **141**, 539–43.

45. Danenberg, P.V., Horikoshi, T., Volkenandt, M. *et al.* (1992) Detection of point mutations in human DNA by analysis of RNA conformation polymorphism(s). *Nucleic Acids Res.*, **20**, 573–9.

46. Foulkes, W.D., Campbell, I.G., Stamp, G.W. and Trowsdale, J. (1993) Loss of heterozygosity and amplification on chromosome 11q in human ovarian cancer. *Br. J. Cancer*, **67**, 268–73.

47. Eccles. D.M., Russell, S.E., Hattes, N.E. *et al.* (1992) Early loss of heterozygosity on 17q in ovarian cancer. The ABE Ovarian Cancer Genetics Group. *Oncogene*, **7**, 2069–72.

48. Jones, M.H. and Nakamura, Y. (1992) Deletion mapping of chromosome 3p in female genital tract malignancies using microsatellite polymorphisms. *Oncogene*, **7**, 1631–4.

49. Chenevix Trench, G., Leary, J., Kerr, J. *et al.* (1992) Frequent loss of heterozygosity on chromosome 18 in ovarian adenocarcinoma which does not always include the DCC locus. *Oncogene*, **7**, 1059–65.

50. Eccles, D.M., Cranston, G., Steel, C.M. *et al.* (1990) Allele losses on chromosome 17 in human epithelial ovarian carcinoma. *Oncogene*, **5**, 1599–601.

51. Russell, S.E., Hickey, G.I., Lowry, W.S. *et al.* (1990) Allele loss from chromosome 17 in ovarian cancer. *Oncogene*, **5**, 1581–3.

52. Gallion, H.H., Powell, D.E., Smith, L.W. *et al.* (1990) Chromosome abnormalities in human epithelial ovarian malignancies. *Gynecol. Oncol.*, **38**, 473–7.

53. Ehlen, T. and Dubeau, L. (1990) Loss of heterozygosity on chromosomal segments 3p, 6q and 11p in human ovarian carcinomas. *Oncogene*, **5**, 219–23.

54. Jacobs, I.J., Kohler, M.F., Wiseman, R.W. *et al.* (1992) Clonal origin of epithelial ovarian carcinoma: analysis by loss of heterozygosity, p53 mutation and X-chromosome inactivation. *J. Natl. Cancer Inst.*, **84**, 1793–8.

55. Eccles, D.M., Brett, L., Lessells, A. *et al.* (1992) Overexpression of the p53 protein and allele loss at 17p13 in ovarian carcinoma. *Br. J. Cancer*, **65**, 40–4.

56. Tsao, S.W., Mok, C.H., Oike, K. *et al.* (1991) Involvement of p53 gene in the allelic deletion of chromosome 17p in human ovarian tumors. *Anticancer Res.*, **11**, 1975–82.

57. Eccles, D.M., Gruber, L., Stewart, M. *et al.* (1992) Allele loss on chromosome 11p is associated with poor survival in ovarian cancer. *Dis. Markers*, **10**, 95–9.

58. Saito, S., Saito, H., Koi, S. *et al.* (1992) Fine-scale deletion mapping of the distal long arm of chromosome 6 in 70 human ovarian cancers. *Cancer Res.*, **52**, 5815–17.

59. Sato, T., Saito, H., Morita, R. *et al.* (1991) Allelotype of human ovarian cancer. *Cancer Res.*, **51**, 5118–22.

60. Lee, J.H., Kavanagh, J.J., Wildrick, D.M. *et al.* (1990) Frequent loss of heterozygosity on chromosomes 6q, 11, and 17 in human ovarian carcinomas. *Cancer Res.*, **50**, 2724–8.

61. Narod, S.A., Feunteun, J., Lynch, H.T. *et al.* (1991) Familial breast–ovarian cancer locus on chromosome 17q12–q23. *Lancet*, **338**, 82–3.

62. Hall, J.M., Lee, M.K., Newman, B. *et al.* (1990) Linkage of early-onset familial breast cancer to chromosome 17q21. *Science*, **250**, 1684–9.

63. Mazars, R., Pujol, P., Maudelonde, T. *et al.* (1991) p53 mutations in ovarian cancer: a late event? *Oncogene*, **6**, 1685–90.

64. Kihana, T., Tsuda, H., Teshima, S. *et al.* (1992) High incidence of p53 gene mutation in human ovarian cancer and its association with nuclear accumulation of p53 protein and tumor DNA aneuploidy. *Jpn. J. Cancer Res.*, **83**, 978–84.

65. Yaginuma, Y. and Westphal, H. (1992) Abnormal structure and expression of the p53 gene ·in human ovarian carcinoma cell lines. *Cancer Res.*, **52**, 4196–9.

66. Mok, S.C.-H., Bell, D.A., Knapp, R.C. *et al.* (1993) Mutation of k-*ras* protooncogene in human ovarian epithelial tumors of borderline malignancy. *Cancer Res.*, **53**, 1489–92.

67. Klein, C.B., Conway, K., Wang, X.W. *et al.* (1991) Senescence of nickel-transformed cells by an X chromosome: possible epigenetic control. *Science*, **251**, 796–9.

68. Wang, X.W., Lin, X., Klein, C.B. *et al.* (1992) a conserved region in human and Chinese hamster X chromosomes can induce cellular senescence of nickel-transformed Chinese hamster cell lines. *Carcinogenesis*, **13**, 555–61.

Part Two
Tumour Biology

Chapter 8

Molecular and biological factors in the pathogenesis of ovarian cancer

J.S. BEREK and O. MARTÍNEZ-MAZA

8.1 INTRODUCTION

Ovarian cancer, which results in higher mortality than any other gynecologic malignancy, is the fourth leading cause of cancer deaths in women in the United States [1]. A major factor in this high mortality is that at the time of diagnosis most patients already have advanced disease. Early detection in ovarian cancer is hampered by the lack of appropriate tumor markers and clinically, most ovarian cancer patients fail to develop significant symptoms until they reach advanced stage disease. Ovarian cancer has a high frequency of metastasis, yet generally remains localized within the peritoneal cavity [2].

Tumor development has been associated with the aberrant, dysfunctional expression and/or mutation of various genes. This can include oncogene overexpression, amplification or mutation, aberrant tumor suppressor (antioncogene) expression or mutation and the inappropriate expression of cytokines and growth factors and/or the cellular receptors for these molecules. Also, subversion of host antitumor immune responses may play a role in the pathogenesis of cancer [3,4].

Most ovarian cancers appear to arise from the ovarian epithelium, a single layer of cells that is found on the surface of the ovary.

While several factors have been implicated in the genesis and growth of ovarian cancer, several studies have shown that the frequency of ovulation is associated with an increased risk for the development of ovarian cancer [1,5–7]. Because ovulation is associated with the disruption of the surface epithelium of the ovary, the ovarian epithelium must proliferate to heal this ovulation associated wound. Therefore, ovulation must be associated with the production of growth factors that enhance the growth and/or differentiation of ovarian epithelial cells. Certainly, various cytokines and growth factors, including transforming growth factor α (TGF-α) and IL-6, have been seen in ovarian follicular fluid [7–9]. Perhaps the repetitive proliferation of ovarian epithelial cells associated with ovulation contributes to the development of ovarian cancer by increasing the chance for a genetic accident (error in DNA replication) that could contribute to the activation of an oncogene or the inactivation of a tumor suppressor gene. Such event(s), combined with the inherent ability of ovarian epithelial cells to respond to and produce cytokines and growth factors, could explain, in part, the high frequency of ovarian cancer and its association with ovulation.

8.2 ONCOGENES

The aberrant expression of various oncogenes in ovarian cancer has been described. These include HER-2/*neu*, *ras*, *myc*, *fms*, *jun* and *myb* [10–17]. The many oncogenes that have been characterized can be divided into a few major groups, based on their biological role and cellular location [14,18]. For instance, several oncogenes, including HER-2/*neu* and *fms*, appear to encode for transmembrane receptor molecules involved in ligand binding. Other oncogenes, including *ras*, represent inner membrane proteins involved in signal transduction. Finally, oncogenes including *myc*, *myb* and *jun* represent nuclear transcriptional regulatory proteins. Therefore, proto-oncogenes represent various cellular proteins with normal physiologic roles in various cellular processes involved in the induction of cellular growth and differentiation. These activities are subverted by mutation or overexpression, resulting in part in the generation of the transformed phenotype.

Recently, the role of HER-2/*neu* in ovarian cancer has received much attention [11,19,20]. HER-2/*neu* is an oncogene product that was seen to be overexpressed in breast cancer; overexpression of HER-2/*neu* in breast cancer was seen to be associated with a poor prognosis [20]. Normal ovarian epithelium expresses low to moderate levels of HER-2/*neu* [11]. HER-2/*neu* is overexpressed in about 30% of ovarian malignancies and appears to be indicative of poor clinical prognosis and poor survival [11,19,20]. Therefore, HER-2/*neu* has the potential to be clinically useful as a marker for ovarian cancer.

Lichtenstein and coworkers have shown that HER-2/*neu* overexpressing ovarian tumor cell lines were more resistant to TNF or lymphokine activated killer (LAK) cell mediated lysis than cells that expressed lower levels of HER-2/*neu*, suggesting that overexpression of this oncogene might impart a biological advantage to tumor cells by enhancing their resistance to cytotoxicity [21].

The HER-2/*neu* oncogene [20] fits into the category of both oncogene and growth factor receptor, since the HER-2/*neu* gene is both a proto-oncogene and appears to code for an epidermal growth factor (EGF) receptor-like molecule [22]. Recently, a ligand (growth factor?) that binds to this putative growth factor receptor has been described and partially characterized [23]. Another oncogene that has been seen to be overexpressed in ovarian cancer is c-*fms* which also encodes for a growth factor receptor, in this case, for the receptor for M-CSF [24]. Interestingly, ovarian cancer cells also have been seen to produce M-CSF [24,25].

Since the HER-2/*neu* gene product appears to be a growth factor receptor, antibodies directed to the extracellular portion of this molecule might be able to downregulate its growth promoting activity. Bast and coworkers have found that anti-HER-2/*neu* monoclonal antibodies to cells that overexpress HER-2/*neu* can inhibit their growth [25,26].

8.3 ANTIONCOGENES

Another genetic lesion that has been implicated in the genesis and development of ovarian cancer involves the p53 tumor suppressor gene: the p53 gene has been seen to be overexpressed (and mutated) in about 30–50% of ovarian cancers [27–29]. The p53 gene, on chromosome 17p, is a tumor suppressor gene and mutations or loss of p53 have been seen in many human cancers. The product of the p53 gene is a nuclear phosphoprotein that can be expressed by normal cells and plays a role in the regulation of cellular growth and development, but which is overexpressed when mutated [27,30,31]. The loss of normal p53 function, due to mutation and overexpression or to deletion of the normal p53 gene, is often associated with a malignant phenotype.

Mutation of p53 results in the dominant transformed phenotype, since the expression of a mutant form of this tumor suppressor gene leads to the dysfunction of normal p53, by preventing the association of p53 to form a functional DNA-binding, regulatory complex.

In recent studies, we have seen that p53 tumor suppressor gene expression can be induced in an ovarian cancer cell line by TNF-α, together with the induction of cell death by apoptosis [32]. Therefore, a mechanism by which TNF induces tumor cell death may involve the upregulation of tumor cell p53 gene expression.

Another tumor suppressor gene that has been suggested to play a role in the development of ovarian cancer is the retinoblastoma (RB) locus: a significant high frequency of allelic deletion of RB has been seen in ovarian cancer tissue [33].

8.4 GROWTH FACTORS AND CYTOKINES

Cytokines and growth factors have been seen to play important roles in the development and growth of cancer [34,35], including ovarian cancer [6,7,36,37]. In fact, it has been proposed that epithelial ovarian cancer may be a cytokine propelled disease [6,7].

Among the several growth factors that have been examined in ovarian cancer are transforming growth factor β (TGF-β), and EGF and related factors, including TGF-α [7,11,38]. TGF-β is a 24 kd glycoprotein that can inhibit the growth of many epithelial cells [39]. EGF is a 6 kd glycoprotein with a structure similar to TGF-α that can stimulate the proliferation of normal ovarian epithelial cells; both EGF and TGF-α bind to the same receptor [10,38]. The response of ovarian cancer cell lines to EGF and TGF-α appears variable [7]. In fact, Bast and coworkers have seen that malignant epithelial ovarian cells are less responsive to EGF than their non-malignant counterparts

[38]. TGF-β, which can act as an autocrine growth inhibitory factor for normal ovarian epithelial cells, may act in a similar fashion for some ovarian cancer cells [38]. Therefore, the loss of the ability to produce active TGF-β or to respond to this factor may have occurred in some ovarian cancers.

Various cytokines, including TNF-α, interleukin 1 (IL-1), macrophage/monocyte colony stimulating factor (M-CSF) and interleukin 6 (IL-6) may also play impotant roles in ovarian cancer pathogenesis [6,37,38,40–42]. Cytokines including IL-1 and IL-6 have been seen to enhance the proliferation of some ovarian cancer cell lines [38,43] and various cytokines have been seen to be produced by ovarian cancer cells, including M-CSF, GM-CSF, IL-1, TNF-α and IL-6 [40–42].

Many ovarian cancer cells express both M-CSF and *fms*, the M-CSF receptor [24,25,38,41,42]. M-CSF is a homodimeric 90 kd glycoprotein. Levels of *fms* transcripts were seen to correlate strongly with ovarian tumors in high histological grade and advanced clinical stage and were associated with a poor clinical outcome [42]. Also, elevated plasma levels of M-CSF were seen in 70–80% of patients with ovarian cancer [24,38,42]. It has been postulated that M-CSF stimulated macrophages might produce other cytokines, such as IL-1 or IL-6, that can further stimulate tumor cell growth [42]. Therefore, M-CSF could potentially act as both an autocrine/paracrine tumor stimulatory factor and as a factor that can modify the tumor cell environment, resulting in enhanced tumor cell growth.

8.4.1 INTERLEUKIN 6

IL-6 is a growth and differentiation inducing factor that is potentially relevant to the development and/or progression of ovarian cancer. IL-6 has been shown to act as an autocrine/paracrine growth factor for several types of human tumors, including multiple myeloma cells [44,45] and renal cancer cells [46]. In our own recent work we found IL-6 to act as an autocrine growth factor for AIDS associated Kaposi's sarcoma [47]. Also, IL-6 has been shown to act as a programmed cell death preventing factor in B cell tumors [48]. Our studies indicate that many epithelial ovarian cancer cells produce IL-6 [49].

IL-6 is a pleiotropic cytokine with a wide range of biological effects [50,51]. The gene for IL-6 has been cloned and sequenced and the structure of the IL-6 gene described. IL-6 is a 26 kd glycoprotein, consisting of 212 amino acids based on a sequence deduced from cloned IL-6 cDNA, with some sequence homology with human G-CSF, as well as several recently described cytokines, including oncostatin M (OSM), ciliary neurotrophic growth factor (CNTF) and leukemia inhibitory factor (LIF). The gene for IL-6 in humans is on chromosome 7 and consists of five exons and four introns. The biological activities that have been described for IL-6 include: induction of differentiation of activated B cells, support of plasmacytoma and myeloma growth, induction of acute phase reactants and stimulation of hepatocytes, nerve growth factor-like activity, induction of cytotoxic T cells and support of hematopoietic differentiation [50]. Clearly, IL-6 is a pleiotropic factor with both growth and differentiation inducing properties. IL-6 can be produced by several types of cells, including T lymphocytes, monocyte/macrophages, fibroblasts, certain tumor cells, epithelial cells and endometrial cells.

The receptor for IL-6 (IL-6R) has been cloned [52]. It is composed of two polypeptides: an 80 kd IL-6 binding protein, which is associated on IL-6 binding to a dimer composed of a second, 130 kd signal transducing molecule. We have detected IL-6R (80 kd) expression in ovarian cancer cells [53]. Recently, the gene for NF-IL6, a nuclear transcription factor that binds to a cytokine responsive (IL-1) element in the IL-6 regula-

tory region, was cloned [54]. The NF-IL6 protein has some homology with the *fos* and *myc* oncogene products and interacts with the NF-IL-6 binding motif within the IL-6 gene regulatory region, inducing IL-6 gene expression. Normally, NF-IL-6 is not expressed, but its expression is induced by exposure of IL-6 producing cells to various inducers of IL-6 gene expression, including LPS or cytokines.

We have seen that ovarian cancer cells of epithelial origin (which constitute 90% of ovarian cancers) produce and secrete IL-6 [49]. Several epithelial ovarian cancer cell lines, including SKOV-3, OVCAR-3 and CAOV-3, produced substantial amounts of biologically active IL-6 [49]. Ovarian cancer cell lines of non-epithelial origin (PA-1 and 222) did not secrete IL-6, although cytoplasmic IL-6 was detected in PA-1 as well as in all epithelial ovarian cancer cell lines tested [49]. Primary ovarian tumor cell cultures also produced substantial levels of IL-6 [49] with primary isolates of ovarian tumor cells displaying intracellular IL-6 by immunoperoxidase staining. The IL-6 produced by ovarian cancer cells was examined by radioimmunoprecipitation and found to correspond in molecular weight to monocyte/lymphoid derived IL-6 [49]. Also, IL-6 mRNA expression indicated that most epithelial ovarian tumor cells lines display detectable levels of IL-6 gene expression [49]. Several cytokines (IFN-γ, IL-1 and TNF) were seen to upregulate IL-6 production by ovarian tumor cell lines [49]. Primary cultures of normal human ovarian epithelium were also seen to produce IL-6 [55]. These results indicate that ovarian cancer cells, including established ovarian cancer cell lines, primary tumor isolates and normal ovarian epithelial cells, produce biologically active IL-6 that is indistinguishable from the IL-6 produced by peripheral blood mononuclear cells.

Ovarian cancer cells also express the IL-6 receptor. In a recent study, we detected expression of the 80 kd subunit of the IL-6 receptor in most ovarian cancer cell lines tested by Northern blot analysis [53]. Naturally, if IL-6 is an autocrine positive or negative growth factor, ovarian cancer cells should be producing not only detectable quantities of secreted IL-6 and IL-6 mRNA, but also should express detectable quantities of IL-6 receptor. Therefore, the observation that ovarian cancer cells express the IL-6 receptor allows the possibility that IL-6 might play a role as a growth/differentiation/viability factor for these cells.

Elevated levels of IL-6 were detected in the ascitic fluid [49] and serum [56] of women with ovarian cancer. Ascitic fluids isolated from patients with ovarian cancer had very high (3.2–42 ng ml^{-1}) levels of IL-6, while those from control, non-cancer patients were much lower (1.8–2.6 ng ml^{-1}) [49]. Elevated serum IL-6 levels were seen to correlate with the presence of more extensive disease: elevated (>0.2 units ml^{-1}) levels of IL-6 were seen in 16/21 (76%) of ovarian cancer patients with macroscopic disease, but only in 13% of patients with microscopic disease or in 17% of healthy control donors [56]. The mean serum IL-6 concentration in the group of ovarian cancer patients with macroscopic disease (n=21) was 0.26 ± 0.04 (sem); serum levels of IL-6 in healthy adult donors were 0.12 ± 0.03 units ml^{-1} (max. <0.020) [56]. Serum IL-6 reached very elevated levels (>1 unit ml^{-1}) in some patients.

Recently, we examined the *in vivo* biological effects of IL-6, by correlating levels of IL-6, acute phase proteins (C'-reactive protein – CRP, haptoglobin and α_2 macroglobulin) and lgM/A/G in ovarian cancer patients' ascitic fluid or serum (unpublished observations). Significantly elevated levels of IL-6, CRP, haptoglobin and IgA and decreased levels of lgM were seen in ovarian cancer ascites (n=36), when compared to peritoneal fluids from a control group (donors with non-malignant gynecologic conditions; n=20). Again, in this study elevated serum IL-6

levels (6.5 ± 5.2 *vs.* 0.2 ± 0.02 U/ml) were seen in ovarian cancer (n=7), as well as increased serum CRP, when compared to controls (n=7). Ascites CRP correlated with IL-6 in both ovarian cancer (*p*<0.01) and in controls (*p*<0.001). These results suggest that the increased levels of IL-6, present *in vivo* in patients with ovarian cancer, are associated with increased levels of acute phase proteins and IgA. This is particularly interesting, since IL-6 can act both as a B cell stimulating factor, inducing the differentiation of activated B cells to lg secreting cells, and as a potent inducer for the production of acute phase reactants [50,57–59].

Another recent observation suggests that IL-6 can play a role as a growth factor for ovarian cancer cells: activated monocytes produce factors that enhance ovarian tumor cell growth. Working with Dr Robert Bast and colleagues at Duke University, we have seen that culture supernatants from activated human monocytes, which support ovarian tumor growth, contained significant amounts of IL-6 [43]. Furthermore, anti-IL-6 serum inhibited part of this monocyte produced growth supporting activity. Therefore, IL-6 has the potential to act as a paracrine growth factor for ovarian cancer cells. Also, we have seen that ovarian cancer cells cultured in serum-free conditions, which result in greatly decreased endogenous IL-6 production, require exogenous IL-6 for optimal proliferation (unpublished observation).

While it is clear that IL-6 can act as an autocrine/paracrine growth factor for human tumors, the complete role of IL-6 in the host response to cancer or as a tumor growth promoting or suppressing factor is not clear [37]. Certainly, IL-6 has the potential to modulate antitumor immune responses and may thereby act as an inhibitory factor for tumor cell growth.

Recently, we have examined the possibility that IL-6 acts as an autocrine growth factor for ovarian cancer cells by inhibiting

IL-6 gene expression by exposure to IL-6 antisense oligonucleotides. This was seen to result in greatly decreased cellular proliferation: exposure of ovarian cancer cell lines (CAOV-3, OVCAR-3 and OC-436) to various concentrations of a single-stranded antisense IL-6 oligodeoxynucleotide, specific for a sequence in the second coding exon of the IL-6 gene, resulted in decreased IL-6 production and a >80–85% inhibition of cellular proliferation [53]. However, the addition of exogenous IL-6 failed to restore the proliferation of the antisense-treated cells. Also, antibodies to IL-6 did not consistently inhibit cell growth nor did rIL-6 enhance growth at low cell concentrations. These results suggest that exogenous IL-6 does not directly induce the proliferation of ovarian cancer cells, although endogenous IL-6 production is needed for optimal cell growth. As the majority of epithelial ovarian cancers produce IL-6, the direct specific inhibition of IL-6 gene expression may be of potential therapeutic value.

Preliminary studies indicate that various tumor cells can be protected from NK cell mediated killing by IL-6 (unpublished observations). Cells (CAOV-3 ovarian cancer cells) treated with dexamethasone, which results in greatly decreased IL-6 production [60], showed greatly increased sensitivity to NK cell mediated lysis [61]. Addition of exogenous recombinant IL-6 to dexamethasone treated cells restored resistance to NK lysis. These preliminary results suggest that IL-6 (endogenously produced or exogenous) can protect tumor cells from NK mediated killing.

8.4.2 INTERLEUKIN 10

Epithelial malignancies of the ovary remain confined to the peritoneal cavity even in advanced stages of the disease. It has been suggested that the growth of ovarian cancer intraperitoneally (IP) could be related to the local deficiency of antitumor immune effector mechanisms, allowing tumor growth within the peritoneal cavity [62]. The presence of immunosuppressive factors in the ascites from ovarian epithelial tumor-bearing patients has previously been described [63,64]. In recent studies, we observed that ascitic fluid from patients with ovarian cancer contains significantly elevated levels of IL-10 [65], a cytokine with various immunosuppressive activities.

IL-10 was originally identified as cytokine synthesis inhibitory factor (CSIF) because of its activity as an inhibitor of cytokine production [66]. The gene for IL-10 has been cloned [67]. This 35–40 kd cytokine is produced by the 'type 2' CD4 positive helper T cell clones (TH2) and inhibits the cytokine production of the 'type 1' subset (TH1) in murine systems. TH1 and TH2 are two subpopulations of T helper cells, initially defined in the mice, that control the nature of an immune response by secreting characteristic and mutually antagonistic sets of cytokines [68]: TH1 clones specifically produce IL-2 and IFN-γ, whereas TH2 clones produce IL-4, IL-5, IL-6 and IL-10. IL-10 inhibits the production of IL-2 and IFN-γ by TH1 cells [69]. While T cells corresponding strictly to TH1 and TH2 subsets have not been described in humans, increasing evidence points to the existence of TH1 and TH2 type responses in humans; a similar dichotomy between TH1 and TH2 type responses has recently been reported in the human [70,71]. Human IL-10 also inhibits the synthesis of IFN-γ and other cytokines by human peripheral blood mononuclear cells [72]. Furthermore, IL-10 is exceedingly potent at suppressing the release of cytokines such as IL-1, IL-6, IL-8 and TNF-α by activated monocytes [73–75]. IL-10 further downregulates class II MHC (major histocompatibility complex molecule) expression on monocytes, resulting in a strong reduction in antigen presenting capacity of these cells [74]. Together, these observations support the concept that

IL-10 plays an important role not only in the regulation of T cell responses, but also as an anti-inflammatory mediator. IL-10 is produced by T cells, B cells and monocytes [72]. Among T cells, CD4 positive cells appear to be the main producers of IL-10, whereas CD8 positive cells appear to be poor producers of this cytokine.

Very recently, we measured levels of various cytokines in ascites obtained from women with ovarian cancer, in collaboration with Dr John Abrams of DNAX Inc, and found that levels of various cytokines, measured by ELISA, were significantly elevated when compared to levels in peritoneal fluid from women who did not have ovarian cancer. In particular, levels of IL-10 and, as expected, IL-6 were seen to be particularly elevated in ovarian cancer ascites [65]. Our preliminary results indicate that ovarian cancer cells do not produce IL-10: ovarian cancer cell lines and primary tumor cells cultured *in vitro* did not produce detectable levels of IL-10, while several of these lines did produce IL-6. Elevated levels of IL-10 were seen in nearly all ascites samples from women with ovarian cancer. Because peritoneal immunosuppression is characteristically seen in this disease, we are currently examining the role of IL-10 as a potential peritoneal immunosuppressive factor in ovarian cancer.

8.4.3 PERITONEAL CYTOKINES IN OVARIAN CANCER

Since the development of ovarian cancer may involve cytokine dysregulation, we recently determined the levels of various cytokines in ascites collected from women with ovarian cancer, in collaboration with Dr John Abrams at DNAX. As already mentioned, high levels of ascites IL-6 and IL-10 are seen in the great majority of ovarian cancer cases. Approximately 50–60% of cases were seen also to contain significant ascites levels of IL-2, TNF-α, IFN-γ, G-CSF and GM-CSF [76]. Levels of various cytokines, including IL-6, IL-10, TNF-α, G-CSF and GM-CSF, were seen to be significantly elevated compared to levels of these same cytokines seen in peritoneal fluids from non-cancer patients. A similar pattern was seen in sera from women with ovarian cancer, with IL-6 and IL-10 being the most frequently detected serum cytokines. A significant correlation was seen between IL-6 (and IL-10) and acute phase proteins and immunoglobulins, as well as the immunosuppressive activity of ascitic fluids and tumor histological stage. Studies to determine whether a specific cytokine/tumor marker/acute phase reactant pattern could be useful in monitoring the progress of patients with ovarian cancer are underway.

Certainly, it is possible that certain cytokine patterns, in particular high levels of IL-10, could result in a peritoneal environment characterized by immune unresponsiveness and promotion of tumor growth.

8.5 CONCLUSIONS

The dysregulation of various biological and molecular factors may play important roles in the development and progression of ovarian cancer. These include oncogene overexpression, mutation or loss of antioncogenes, growth factor and cytokine stimulation and modification of the host environment and host antitumor immune response. Understanding the specific mechanisms involved in ovarian cancer development and growth will allow opportunities for the rational design of effective antitumor treatment modalities.

ACKNOWLEDGMENTS

The authors express their gratitude for the laboratory work and assistance of Cathy Casey, Walter Gotlieb, Michael Johnson, Klara Kaldi, Reba Knox, Robert Stenson and

Joanna Watson and for the generous provision of reagents by John Abrams and Tadamitsu Kishimoto.

REFERENCES

1. Silverberg, E., Boring, C.C. and Squires, T.S. (1990). Cancer statistics 1990. *Ca - A Cancer J. Clin.*, **40**, 9.

2. Berek, J.S. (1994) Epithelial ovarian cancer. In *Practical Gynecologic Oncology 2nd edn.*, (eds J.S. Berek and N.F. Hacker), Williams and Wilkins, Baltimore, p. 327.

3. Bookman, M.A. and Bast, R.C. Jr. (1991) Immunobiology and immunotherapy of ovarian cancer. *Semin. Oncol.*, **18**, 270.

4. Bookman, M.A. and Berek, J.S. (1992) Biologic and immunologic therapy of ovarian cancer. *Hematol. Oncol. Clin. North Am.*, **6**, 941.

5. Piver, M.S. (1987) Epidemiology of ovarian cancer. In *Ovarian Malignancies: Diagnosis and Therapeutic Advances*, (ed. M.S. Piver), Churchill Livingstone, Edinburgh, pp. 1–10.

6. Malik, S. and Balkwill, F. (1991) Epithelial ovarian cancer: a cytokine propelled disease? *Br. J. Cancer*, **64**, 617.

7. Mills, G.B., Hashimoto, S., Hurteau, J. *et al.* (1992) Regulation of growth of human ovarian cancer cells. In *Ovarian Cancer 2: Biology, Diagnosis and W. Management*, (eds F. Sharp, W.P. Mason and W. Creasman), Chapman & Hall, London, pp. 127– 45.

8. Motro, B., Itin, A., Sachs, L. and Keshet, E. (1990) Pattern of interleukin 6 gene expression *in vivo* suggests a role for this cytokine in angiogenesis. *PNAS*, **87**, 3092.

9. Buyalos, R.P., Watson, J.M. and Martínez-Maza, O. (1992) Detection of interleukin-6 in human follicular fluid. *Fertil. Steril.*, **57**, 1230.

10. Berchuck, A., Kohler, M.F. and Bast, R.C. Jr. (1992) Oncogenes in ovarian cancer. *Hematol. Oncol. Clin. N. Am.*, **6**, 813.

11. Berchuck, A., Marks, J.R. and Bast, R.C. Jr. (1992) Expression of the epidermal growth factor receptor, HER-2/*neu* and p53 in ovarian cancer. In *Ovarian Cancer 2: Biology, Diagnosis and Management*, (eds F. Sharp, W.P. Mason and W. Creasman), Chapman & Hall, London, pp. 53–9.

12. Kommoss, F., Bauknecht, T., Birmelin, G. *et al.* (1992) Oncogene and growth factor expression in ovarian cancer. *Acta Obstet. Gynecol. Scand.*, (Suppl.), **155**, 19.

13. Barletta, C., Lazzaro, D., Prosperi Porta, R. *et al.* (1992) *c-myb* activation and the pathogenesis of ovarian cancer. *Eur. J. Gynaecol. Oncol.*, **13**, 53.

14. Baker, V.V., Borst, M.P., Dixon, D. *et al.* (1990) *c-myc* amplification in ovarian cancer. *Gynecol. Oncol.*, **38**, 340.

15. Boltz, E.M., Kefford, R.F., Leary, J.A. *et al.* (1989) Amplification of *c-ras-Ki* oncogene in human ovarian tumours. *Int. J. Cancer*, **43**, 428.

16. Zhou, D.J., Gonzalez-Cadavid, N., Ahuja, H. *et al.* (1988) A unique pattern of proto-oncogene abnormalities in ovarian adenocarcinomas. *Cancer*, **62**, 1573.

17. Rodenburg, C.J., Koelma, I.A., Nap, M. and Fleuren, G.J. (1988) Immunohistochemical detection of the *ras* oncogene product p21 in advanced ovarian cancer. Lack of correlation with clinical outcome. *Arch. Pathol. Lab. Med.*, **112**, 151.

18. Bishop, J.M. (1991) Molecular themes in oncogenesis. *Cell*, **64**, 235.

19. Berchuck, A., Kamel, A., Whitaker, R. *et al.* (1990) Overexpression of HER-2/*neu* is associated with poor survival in advanced epithelial ovarian cancer. *Cancer Res.*, **50**, 4087.

20. Slamon, D.J., Godolphin, W., Jones, L.A. *et al.* (1989) Studies of HER-2/*neu* proto-oncogene in human breast and ovarian cancer. *Science*, **244**, 707.

21. Lichtenstein, A., Berenson, J., Gera, J.F. *et al.* (1990) Resistance of human ovarian cancer cells to tumor necrosis factor and lymphokine-activated killer cells: correlation with expression of HER/*neu* oncogenes. *Cancer Res.*, **50**, 7364.

22. Kokai, Y., Dobashi, K., Weiner, D.B. *et al.* (1988) Phosphorylation process induced by epidermal growth factor alters the oncogenic and cellular *neu* (NGL) gene products. *PNAS*, **85**, 5389.

23. Peles, E., Bacus, S.S., Koshi, R.A. *et al.* (1992) Isolation of the *neu*/HER-2 stimulatory ligand: a 44 kd glycoprotein that induces differentiation of mammary tumor cells. *Cell*, **69**, 205.

24. Kacinsky, B.M., Carter, D., Mittal, K. *et al.* (1990) Ovarian adenocarcinomas express *fms-*

complementary transcripts and *fms* antigen, often with co-expression of CSF-1. *Am. J. Pathol.*, **137**, 135.

25. Ramakrishnan, S., Xu, F.J., Brandt, S.J. *et al.* (1989) Constitutive production of macrophage colony-stimulating factor by human ovarian and breast cancer cell lines. *J. Clin. Invest.*, **83**, 921.

26. Bast, R.C. Xu, F.J., Rodriguez, G.C. *et al.* (1992) Inhibition of breast and ovarian tumour cell growth by antibodies and immunotoxins reactive with distinct epitopes on the extracellular domain of HER-2/*neu* (c-erbB2). In *Ovarian Cancer 2: Biology, Diagnosis and Management*, (eds F. Sharp, W. Mason and W. Creasman), Chapman & Hall, London, pp. 67–71.

27. Marks, J.R., Davidoff, A.M., Kerns, B.J. *et al.* (1991) Overexpression and mutation of p53 in epithelial ovarian cancer. *Cancer Res.*, **51**, 2979.

28. Mazars, R., Pujol, P., Maudelonde, T. *et al.* (1991) p53 mutations in ovarian cancer: a late event? *Oncogene*, **6**, 1685.

29. Okamoto, A., Sameshima, Y., Yokoyama, S. *et al.* (1991) Frequent allelic losses and mutations of the p53 gene in human ovarian cancer. *Cancer Res.*, **51**, 5171.

30. Hollstein, M., Sidransky, D., Vogelstein, B. and Harris, C.C. (1991) p53 mutations in human cancers. *Science*, **253**, 49.

31. Levine, A.J., Momand, J. and Finlay, C.A. (1991) The p53 tumour suppressor gene. *Nature*, **351**, 453.

32. Gotlieb, W.H., Watson, J.M., Rezai, A. *et al.* (1994) Upregulation of p53 tumor suppressor gene expression by tumor necrosis factor-alpha: relation to the production of apoptosis in an ovarian cancer cell line. *Am. J. Obstet. Gynecol.*, **170**, 1121–30.

33. Li, S.B., Schwartz, P.E., Lee, W.H., Yang-Feng, T.L. (1991) Allele loss at the retinoblastoma locus in human ovarian cancer. *J. Natl Cancer Inst.*, **83**, 637.

34. Aaronson, S.A. (1991) Growth factors and cancer. *Science*, **254**, 1146.

35. Cross, M. and Dexter, T.M. (1991) Growth factors in development, transformation, and tumorigenesis. *Cell*, **64**, 271.

36. Malik, S., Naylor, M.S. and Balkwill, F.R. (1992) Cytokines and ovarian cancer. In *Ovarian Cancer 2: Biology, Diagnosis and Management*, (eds F. Sharp, W.P. Mason and W. Creasman), Chapman & Hall, London, pp. 87–92.

37. Martínez-Maza, O. and Berek, J.S. (1991). Interleukin 6 and cancer therapy. *In Vivo*, **5**, 583.

38. Bast, R.C., Xu, F.J., Rodriguez, G.C. *et al.* (1992) Factors regulating the growth of normal and malignant ovarian epithelium. In *Ovarian Cancer 2: Biology, Diagnosis and Management*, (eds F. Sharp, W.P. Mason and W. Creasman), Chapman & Hall, London, pp. 61–6.

39. Wakefield, L.M. and Sporn, M.B. (1990). Suppression of carcinogenesis: a role for TGF-β and related molecules in prevention of cancer. In *Tumor Suppressor Genes*, (ed. G. Klein), Marcel Dekker, New York, pp. 217–43.

40. Berek, J.S., Watson, J.M. and Martínez-Maza, O. (1992) Role of interleukin-6 in ovarian cancer. In *Ovarian Cancer 2: Biology, Diagnosis and Management*, (eds F. Sharp, W.P. Mason and W. Creasman), Chapman & Hall, London, pp. 101–13.

41. Carson, L.F., Moradi, M.M., Li, B.Y. *et al.* (1992) Characterization of cytokines produced by ovarian cancer cells. In *Ovarian Cancer 2: Biology, Diagnosis and Management*, (eds F. Sharp, W.P. Mason and W. Creasman), Chapman & Hall, London, pp. 93–9.

42. Kacinsky, B.M. (1992) CSF-1 and its receptor on ovarian and other gynaecological neoplasms. In *Ovarian Cancer 2: Biology, Diagnosis and Management*, (eds F. Sharp, W.P. Mason and W. Creasman), Chapman & Hall, London, pp. 115–25.

43. Wu, S., Rodabaugh, K., Watson, J.M. *et al.* (1992) Stimulation of ovarian tumor cell proliferation with monocyte products including IL-1-alpha, IL-6 and tumor necrosis factor-alpha. *Am. J. Obstet. Gynecol.*, **166**, 997.

44. Kawano, M., Hirano, T., Matsuda, T. *et al.* (1988) Autocrine generation and requirement of BSF-2/IL-6 for human multiple myelomas. *Nature*, **332**, 83.

45. Klein, B., Zhang, X.G., Jourdan, M. *et al.* (1989). Paracrine rather than autocrine regulation of myeloma-cell growth and differentiation by interleukin-6. *Blood*, **73**, 517.

46. Miki, S., Iwano, M., Miki, Y. *et al.* (1989) Interleukin-6 (IL-6) functions as an *in vitro* autocrine growth factor in renal cell carcinomas. *FEBS Lett.*, **250**, 607.

47. Miles, S.A., Rezai, A.R., Salazar-Gonzalez, J.F. *et al.* (1990) AIDS Kaposi's sarcoma-derived cells produce and respond to interleukin-6. *PNAS*, **87**, 4068.

48. Sabourin, L.A. and Hawley, R.G. (1990) Suppression of programmed death and G1 arrest in B-cell hybridomas by interleukin-6 is not accompanied by altered expression of immediate early response genes. *J. Cell Physiol.*, **145**, 564.

49. Watson, J., Sensintaffar, J. L., Berek, J.S. and Martínez-Maza, O. (1990) Constitutive production of interleukin 6 by ovarian cell lines and by primary ovarian tumor cultures. *Cancer Res.*, **50**, 6959.

50. Hirano, T., Akira, S. and Kishimoto, T. (1990) Biological and clinical aspects of interleukin 6. *Immunol. Today*, **11**, 443.

51. Kishimoto, T. and Hirano, T. (1988) Molecular regulation of B lymphocyte response. *Ann. Rev. Immunol.*, **6**, 485.

52. Yamasaki, K., Taga, T., Hirata, Y. *et al.* (1988) Cloning and expression of human interleukin-6 (BSF-2/IFNb$_2$) receptor. *Science*, **241**, 825.

53. Watson, J.M., Berek, J.S. and Martínez-Mara, O. (1993) Growth inhibition of ovarian cancer cells induced by antisense IL-6 oligonucleotides. *Gynecol. Oncol.*, **49**, 8–15.

54. Akira, S., Isshiki, H., Sugita, T. *et al.* (1990) A nuclear factor for IL-6 expression (NF-IL6) is a member of a C/EBP family. *EMBO J.*, **9**, 1897.

55. Lidor, Y.J., Xu, F.I., Martínez-Maza, O. *et al.* (1993) Constitutive production of macrophage colony stimulating factor and IL-6 by human ovarian surface epithelial cells. *Exp. Cell Res.*, **207**, 332–9.

56. Berek, J.S., Chung, C., Kaldi, K. *et al.* (1991) Serum IL-6 levels correlate with disease status in epithelial ovarian cancer patients. *Am. J. Obstet. Gynecol.*, **164**, 1038.

57. Marinkovic, S., Jahreis, G.P., Wong, G.G. and Baumann, H. (1989) IL-6 modulates the synthesis of a specific set of acute phase plasma proteins *in vivo. J. Immunol.*, **142**, 808.

58. Stenson, R., Watson, J.M., Korzeniowski, P.A. *et al.* (1991) Generation, characterization and growth in nude mice of two ovarian tumor cell lines. Abstract, Society of Gynecological Investigation meeting.

59. Tosato, G., Seamon, K.B., Goldman, N.D. *et al.* (1988) Identification of a monocyte-derived human B cell growth factor as interferon-b$_2$ (BSF-2, IL-6). *Science*, **239**, 502.

60. Ray, A., Tatter, S.B., Santhanam, U. *et al.* (1989) Regulation of expression of interleukin-6: molecular and clinical studies. *Ann. NY Acad. Sci.*, **557**, 353.

61. Johnson, M.T., Watson, J.M., Berek, J.S. and Martínez-Maza, O. (1992) Interleukin-6 induces resistance of ovarian tumors to natural killer cell-mediated cytotoxicity. *Proc. Soc. Gynecol. Invest.*, Abstract.

62. Berek, J.S. Bast, R.C., Lichtenstein, A. *et al.* (1984) Lymphocyte cytotoxicity in the peritoneal cavity and blood of patients with ovarian cancer. *Obstet. Gynecol.*, **64**, 708.

63. Badger, A., Oh, S. and Moolten, F. (1981) Differential effects of an immunosuppressive fraction from ascites fluid of patients with ovarian cancer on spontaneous and antibody dependent cytotoxicity. *Cancer Res.*, **41**, 1133.

64. Johnson, M.T., Sensintaffar, J.L., Watson, J.M. *et al.* (1991) Detection and preliminary characterization of an immune suppressive factor in ascites from women with ovarian cancer. *Proc. Soc. Gynecol. Invest.*, Abstract.

65. Gotlieb, W.H., Abrams, J.S., Watson, J.M. *et al.* (1992) Presence of IL-10 in the ascites of patients with ovarian and other intra-abdominal cancers. *Cytokine*, **4**, 385–90.

66. Fiorentino, D.F., Bond, M.W. and Mosmann, T.R. (1989) Two types of mouse helper T cell. IV. Th2 clones secrete a factor that inhibits cytokine production by Th1 clones. *J. Exp. Med.*, **170**, 2081.

67. Moore, K.W., Vieira, P., Fiorentino, D.F. *et al.* (1990) Homology of cytokine synthesis inhibitory factor (IL-10) to the Epstein–Barr virus gene BCRFI. *Science*, **248**, 1230.

68. Mosmann, T.R. and Moore, K.W. (1991) The role of IL-10 in crossregulation of TH1 and TH2 responses. *Immunol. Today*, **12**, A49.

69. Fiorentino, D.F., Zlotnik, A., Vieira, P. *et al.* (1991) IL-10 acts on the antigen-presenting cell

to inhibit cytokine production by Th1 cells. *J. Immunol.*, **146**, 3444.

70. Del Prete, G.F., de Carli, M., Ricci, M. and Romagnani, S. (1991) Helper activity for immunoglobulin synthesis of T helper type 1 (Th 1) and Th2 human T cell clones: the help of Th1 clones is limited by their cytolytic capacity. *J. Exp. Med.*, **174**, 809.

71. Romagnani, S. (1991) Human TH1 and TH2 subsets: doubt no more. *Immunol. Today*, **12**, 256.

72. Zlotnik, A. and Moore, K.W. (1991) Interleukin 10. *Cytokine*, **3**, 366.

73. Bogdan, C, Vodovotz, Y. and Nathan, C. (1991) Macrophage deactivation by IL-10. *J. Exp. Med.*, **174**, 1549.

74. De Waal Malefyt, R., Abrams, J., Bennett, B. *et al.* (1991) IL-10 inhibits cytokine synthesis by human monocytes: an autoregulatory role of IL-10 produced by monocytes. *J. Exp. Med.*, **174**, 1209–20.

75. Fiorentino, D.F., Zlotnik, A., Mosmann, T.R. *et al.* (1991) IL-10 inhibits cytokine production by activated macrophages. *J. Immunol.*, **147**, 3815.

76. Watson, J.M., Gotlieb, W.H., Abrams, J.H. *et al.* (1993) Immune analysis of ascitic fluid from patients with ovarian cancer: relationship between cytokines, acute phase proteins, immunoglobulins, immunosuppression and tumor classification. *Proc. Soc. Gynecol. Invest.*, **186** (abstract), 8.

Chapter 9

Cytokines and ovarian cancer

M.S. NAYLOR, F. BURKE and F.R. BALKWILL

9.1 INTRODUCTION

Cytokines can influence the growth and spread of a tumour in both positive and negative ways. Endogenous cytokines or those used as therapy may act as direct cytostatic agents preventing cell proliferation and encouraging differentiation. In some microenvironments, particularly when nutritional conditions are suboptimal, cytokines may also be cytotoxic, initiating apoptosis of the tumour cells. Therapeutic administration, local endogenous cytokines or genetically engineered local cytokine production may stimulate host immune responses to the tumour leading to cell and cytokine mediated destruction of the malignant cells. Under certain circumstances cytokines can also mediate destruction of the tumour neovasculature or deplete the tumour environment of essential nutrients.

Conversely, these regulatory molecules may promote tumour growth and spread. For example, cytokines may act as growth factors. They can also be viability factors that prevent programmed cell death and may inhibit response to cytotoxic chemotherapy. The influence of cytokines on tumour vasculature is very dependent on the local microenvironment. Although the vessels can be destroyed in some instances, cytokines can also stimulate angiogenesis, as well as promote the

development of other elements of the tumour stroma. Genes for cytokines that act as growth suppressors may be altered or deleted in tumour cells. Finally, certain cytokines can promote bone and extracellular matrix destruction, thus encouraging tumour spread.

In this chapter we detail the production of the cytokine tumour necrosis factor, TNF, which may act as a growth/viability factor in human ovarian cancer and be involved in tumour spread, and describe the therapeutic action of interferon-γ, a cytokine that can be cytostatic or cytotoxic in human ovarian cancer.

9.2 TUMOUR NECROSIS FACTOR AND OVARIAN CANCER

The cytokine tumour necrosis factor, TNF, was originally identified as an agent that was selectively cytotoxic for some tumour cell lines [1] and caused necrosis of certain murine tumours [2] and human tumour xenografts [3]. However, this cytokine has a number of biological activities that could promote the growth and invasive capacity of tumours [4]. For example, TNF may act directly as a growth factor for fibroblasts [5], thus contributing to the generation of tumour stroma [6]. TNF also has wide ranging effects

89

on endothelial cells including promotion of chemotaxis and stimulation of angiogenesis [7,8]. TNF modulates certain metalloproteinase genes [9,10] that are associated with high invasive activity and metastatic potential [11].

We have demonstrated previously that TNF can promote tumour progression *in vivo*. In xenograft models, intraperitoneal injection of recombinant human TNF (rhuTNF) causes ascitic human ovarian cancer cells to clump and form multiple solid tumours on the peritoneal surface [12]. Other groups have shown that certain human tumour cell lines express TNF *in vitro* and that prolonged exposure to TNF leads to the development of resistance to

the cytotoxic effects of TNF and constitutive secretion of TNF by these cells [13].

Here we describe TNF cytokine and receptor distribution in 81 ovarian neoplasms and 12 samples of normal ovary. We have studied expression of TNF mRNA and of the p55/p75 TNF receptors by *in situ* hybridization techniques and related this to histologic grading of the tumour. Using immunohistochemistry we have assayed for the presence of TNF and TNF receptor protein. We have also assessed the interaction of macrophages and tumour cells in the tumour microenvironment.

TNF gene expression was found in 45 of 63 cases of ovarian cancer and localized to epithelial tumour areas (Figure 9.1). These

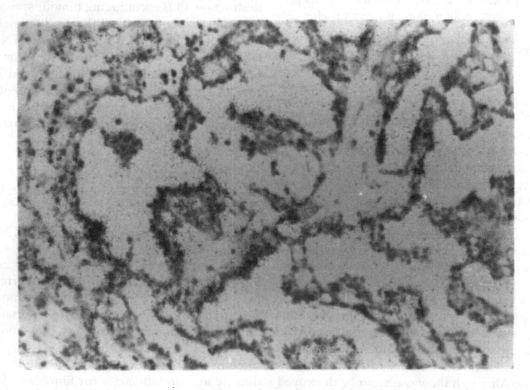

Figure 9.1 Relative distribution of TNF gene expression and macrophages. *In situ* hybridization with a ^{35}S-labeled antisense TNF riboprobe demonstrates that expression is confined to malignant epithelial cells as determined by silver grain deposition following autoradiography for 10 days (×200)

Table 9.1 Frequency and extent of TNF expression in ovarian neoplasms

Tumor type	No. of cases	Total no. +ve	+	++	+++
Serous	40	29	17	11	1
Undifferentiated adenocarcinoma	3	2	1	1	–
Mucinous	14	3	2	1	–
Endometrioid	5	2	1	1	–
Clear cell	1	0	–	–	–
Miscellaneous	18	1	1	–	–

+++ = >20 cells/hpf; ++ = 2–20 cells/hpf; + = 0.2–2 cells/hpf; +/− = <0.2 cells/hpf where hpf = high power field. The different neoplasias studied were representative of their relative frequency in the general population

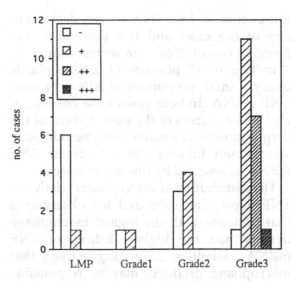

Figure 9.2 Relationship of serous ovarian tumour grade with frequency of TNF gene expression. +++ = mean >20 cells/hpf; ++ = mean <2–20 cells/hpf; + = mean <2 cells/hpf, where hpf=high power field. Poorly differentiated (grade III) carcinomas show significantly higher quantitative and qualitative levels of TNF expression ($p<0.005$ Fisher's exact test). LMP=low malignant potential.

data are summarized in Table 9.1. The pattern and extent of TNF expression was unlike that found in other cancers studied, including breast, cervical and colorectal cancers, where less than 0.1% of cells in the stroma containing TNF mRNA. In ovarian cancer biopsies, as many as 65% of cells in a maximal high power field were found to express TNF. The level and frequency of TNF expression increases with progression from borderline tumours (low malignant potential) to poorly differentiated tumours (grade 3) (Fisher's exact test, significance $p<0.005$) (Figure 9.2).

The distribution of immunoreactive TNF protein appeared to be different from that of TNF mRNA. In some cases the epithelial areas contained a number of tumour cells and macrophages that stained with the anti-TNF monoclonal antibody. However, the majority of immunoreactive TNF protein was detected in the stroma and at the epithelial/stromal borders, also reflecting the distribution of macrophages. Such disparities between mRNA and protein have been seen previously with TNF [14]. This disparity may be usual for rapidly secreted proteins, where the immunoreactivity reflects slower release

and/or greater stability of protein or even uptake by other cells.

TNF p55 receptor expression was detected in all cases studied (n = 12). While p55 was confined to the epithelial tumour areas, its distribution was more homogeneous than that of TNF mRNA expression. In contrast, p75 TNF receptor expression was found at the tumour–stromal interface and over cells in the malignant gland lumina. The distribution appears to relate to the macrophage distribution. Immunohistochemistry for the receptors reflected the *in situ* hybridization results.

Expression of TNF induced cytokines was investigated in relation to TNF expression. IL-1β expression was found in 23 of 68 cases assessed. The distribution and extent of IL-1β mRNA was unlike that of TNF. IL-1β gene expression was scattered, found at lower levels (generally <0.1% of the population) in a similar distribution to that of the macrophage population. IL-1α mRNA was not detected in any of the cases and IL-6 expression was found in two of 12 cases in stromal areas.

In two of 12 biopsies of non-neoplastic ovary a small proportion of cells expressed TNF mRNA. In both cases these cells localized to focal areas of the externa theca of the corpus luteum. Normal ovarian mesothelium, stroma and follicles did not contain TNF mRNA as assessed by this methodology.

The distribution of macrophages relative to TNF expressing cells and the observation that tumours with the highest macrophage density had the highest indices of TNF mRNA labelling are suggestive that macrophage products may be responsible for this induction. It is widely known that activated macrophages secrete a number of factors, including TNF itself, that can induce TNF expression in adjacent cells [13,15]. Recent studies by Wu *et al.* (personal communication, R. Bast) have provided *in vitro* evidence that this may be what is occurring in ovarian cancer. Studies in our laboratory have shown that *in vivo* treatment of ovarian cancer xenografts with TNF results in TNF expression in the epithelial tumour cells. There is also evidence that tumours themselves secrete chemotactic factors that attract macrophages into the tumour [16,17].

Soluble TNF receptors have been found at high levels in a number of disease states including ovarian cancer [18]. While the cellular source of these TNF binding proteins has not been determined, our *in situ* results may provide the answer. Coexpression by the tumour cells of both TNF and its receptor suggests the existence of both autocrine and paracrine mechanisms of action.

Our current knowledge of TNF and the observations recorded in our study lend support to the following hypothesis:

1. Ovarian tumours produce a range of chemotactic factors that attract macro-phages into the tumour microenvironment. These may include members of the CSF family, e.g. M-CSF, and the chemokine family, e.g. MCP-1.

2. Macrophages are activated by soluble factors in the local microenvironment, perhaps elicited as part of the host response to the tumour, resulting in the production of TNF.

3. Production of TNF by macrophages within the stromal areas of the tumour induces TNF expression in adjacent tumour epithelial cells. Tumour cells have acquired the ability to express TNF as part of the transformation event either by derepression through genetic mutation or through acquisition of the ability to encode a dominant transcription factor. TNF mRNA encoded by the tumour epithelial cells has a longer half-life than that of the macrophages which is reflected in the distribution of expressing cells.

4. Acquisition of TNF expression renders epithelial cells refractile to the cytotoxic effects of TNF and also has further effects on the process of tumourigenesis, e.g. angiogenesis, adhesion, invasion and tissue remodelling.

Production of TNF by ovarian cancer cells could result in resistance to the cytotoxic action of host derived TNF [13] or exogenous rhuTNF administered in the therapeutic setting. TNF has been used in several clinical trials but no significant improvements in survival have been reported. Local production by tumour cells and their consequent resistance may in part explain these disappointing results.

The aberrant expression of this potent cytokine and its actions in promoting tumour spread may indicate that TNF therapy would be inappropriate for some ovarian cancers and that TNF antagonists may have therapeutic potential.

9.3 THE THERAPEUTIC POTENTIAL OF INTERFERON-γ IN OVARIAN CANCER

There have been several clinical trials over the past few years administering recombinant human IFN-γ (rhIFN-γ) to patients with ovarian cancer. In two studies no responses were observed in patients with advanced ovarian cancer receiving interperitoneal (IP) IFN-γ [19,20]. Out of 58 evaluable patients with residual epithelial ovarian cancer, Pujade-Lauraine *et al.* [21] found that an IP dose of 20×10^6 U/m^2 twice per week for three to four months resulted in 15 complete and two partial responses in those patients with limited tumour burden. Further details of this trial are reported in Chapter 24.

In our laboratory, we have established three xenograft models of human ovarian cancer [22]. The tumours grow as ascites in the peritoneum, but if they are treated for seven days with human TNF, they develop multiple solid tumour deposits over the peritoneal surface. The histological appearance of these TNF pretreated tumours resembles stage III ovarian cancer. Malik *et al.* [23] demonstrated that human IFN-γ at doses equivalent to those given in humans has direct antitumour activity on free floating ascitic tumour cells and solid intraperitoneal tumours. There was evidence for a cytotoxic action of IFN-γ against the free floating tumour cell clumps in the peritoneum with cure of peritoneal disease in two of the models. Histological analysis of solid tumours following treatment with human IFN-γ showed evidence of increased cell death and during treatment the architecture of the tumour was gradually lost. Large areas of hypocellular epithelial mucin were evident in the treated tumours and an overall reduction in the number of epithelial cells was observed. However, these tumours were not cured and did eventually progress. We have begun to investigate optimal dose and schedule of IFN-γ in these models and to look for markers predictive of response.

Earlier scheduling experiments showed that daily therapy with rhIFN-γ at a dose of 1.5×10^5 U proved to be effective at prolonging survival [23]. Further experiments were undertaken to see whether shorter treatment periods and and/or higher doses were as effective as daily therapy in one of the xenografts HU, which was the most sensitive to the antiproliferative effects of IFN-γ. These are shown in Figure 9.3. Survival times in all treatment groups were statistically better than control injected groups. Using the log rank test, daily therapy was shown to be the most effective in terms of survival. The mice in this group also received considerably less rhIFN-γ (8.4×10^6 U) compared with the mice receiving the dose of 7.5×10^5 U/day in four 5-day treatment cycles (15×10^6 U). Thus it appears that daily treatment is the most effective and that IFN-γ needs to be continually present to give optimal results. Earlier studies [23] have indicated that daily injections in the murine model are equivalent to three times weekly regimens in humans because the IFN-γ is cleared more rapidly in mice. The best route may be an IP depot preparation of IFN-γ for treatment of ovarian cancer.

To study the mechanisms of antitumour activity of IFN-γ, we investigated the role of the IFN-γ induced enzyme indoleamine dioxygenase, IDO, which converts tryptophan to kynurenine. Depletion of tryptophan induced by this enzyme has been implicated in the cell growth inhibitory effects of IFN-γ *in vitro* [24,25]. The antitumour activity of IFN-γ in the ascitic and solid tumour form of the xenografts was preceded by a fall in tumour tryptophan and a corresponding rise in tumour kynurenine. The extent to which tryptophan alteration occurred in the models varied but did not appear to be related to IFN-γ response in terms of ultimate survival. There was a significant depletion in tryptophan and a corresponding increase in kynurenine in the solid tumour models. HU, the xenograft which was most responsive to

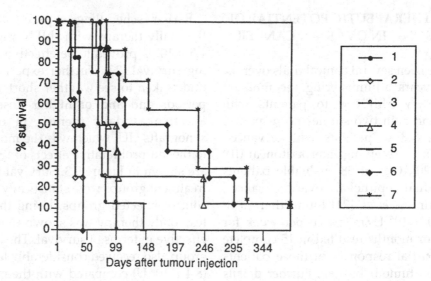

Figure 9.3 Effects of various doses and schedules of IFN-γ on the survival of mice bearing the HU xenograft. 1. Control injection for 3 days, rest 7 days × 4; 2. Control injection for 5 days, rest 7 days × 4; 3. Hu IFN-γ 1.5 × 10⁵ U for 3 days rest for 7 days × 4; 4. Hu IFN-γ 1.5 × 10⁵ U for 5 days rest for 7 days × 4; 5. Hu IFN-γ 7.5 × 10⁵ U for 3 days rest for 7 days × 4; 6. Hu IFN-γ 7.5 × 10⁵ U for 5 days rest for 7 days × 4; 7. Hu IFN-γ 1.5 × 10⁵ U daily for 56 days.

IFN-γ therapy, showed changes in tryptophan and kynurenine that were maximal at 24 hours, less dramatic at days 2 and 4 and had returned to normal values by day 7. This is shown in Figure 9.4. In another of the xenografts, LA, IFN-γ treatment also resulted in tryptophan depletion which, unlike the HU xenograft, was maintained throughout the treatment period (data not shown).

Northern analysis demonstrated that mRNA for IDO was detectable six hours post-treatment in the HU xenograft and continued to be present after seven days of daily therapy (data not shown). *In situ* hybridization studies confirmed these findings and revealed the presence of IDO mRNA in the human tumour cells from eight hours through to seven days. RNA analysis by both Northern blot and *in situ* hybridization did not reflect the tryptophan data. It may be that the cells are using alternative mechanisms to recover from tryptophan depletion or that the IDO gene is regulated post-transcriptionally.

Studies to further understand these findings are underway.

We have begun to look at other markers which may lead to changes predictive of response to IFN-γ and may also be involved in changes in tryptophan. One such marker is tryptophanyl tRNA synthetase. Northern analysis and *in situ* hybridization in two of the xenografts showed significant induction of mRNA for this marker after IFN-γ treatment. In both cases this inducible gene was 'switched on' six hours post-IFN-γ therapy and remained `switched on' throughout the timepoints analysed for a period of 14 days of treatment with IFN-γ.

In conclusion, initial experiments have shown that daily therapy with human IFN-γ is the most effective. The two IFN-γ inducible genes investigated are both present in the treated tumours and, unlike many *in vitro* studies, do not appear to be transient but are maintained throughout a seven day daily treatment protocol. It is as yet unclear from

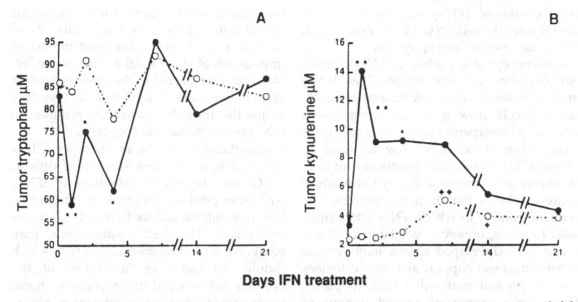

Figure 9.4 Measurement of tumour trytophan and kynurenine in the HU solid tumour xenograft following IFN-γ treatment. At appropritate timepoints (two hours, one day, two days, four days, seven days, 14 days, 21 days) tumours were excised and snapfrozen immediately. (A) = tumour tryptophan: open circles = diluent treated, closed circles = IFN-γ (1.5×10^5 U). (B) = tumour kynurenine: open circles = diluent treated, closed circles = IFN-γ (1.5×10^5 U). **different from diluent treated $p<0.001$. *different from diluent treated $p<0.005$.

our studies whether the induction of IDO is related to growth inhibition following IFN-γ treatment.

9.4 CLINICAL RELEVANCE OF THESE DATA

Malignant cells produce autocrine growth stimulating cytokines, they become independent of these autocrine cytokines, resistant to growth inhibitory cytokines or lose the ability to respond to these. Thus, the cytokine environment that surrounds a tumour is extremely abnormal. Moreover, recent research has highlighted the importance of survival cytokines that prevent apoptosis when growth conditions are unfavourable [26]. Thus, cancer can be considered as much a disease of unscheduled cell survival as uncontrolled cell proliferation. All forms of cytokine

therapy have the potential to perturb the abnormal cytokine milieu of an individual tumour. If we model the action of IFN-γ on an ovarian tumour, we would propose that within this microenvironment there are extracellular autocrine or paracrine growth stimulating cytokines; intracellular loops signalling cell growth; paracrine or autocrine cytokines that ensure survival of cells in unfavourable conditions and a lack of growth suppressive influences. When a sufficient concentration of IFN-γ is introduced into this environment, it acts (as has been shown in tissue culture) as a suppressive cytokine preventing proliferation, but apoptosis is inhibited by the presence of survival cytokines. The cells remain locked in G_1/G_0 until the suppressive influence is removed and then will start growing again.

However, if the tumour is very small and has not yet developed an adequate stroma to provide optimal nutritional support and survival cytokines, IFN-γ may do more than simply hold the cells in G_1/G_0. In this context, IFN-γ may well induce apoptosis.

This concept of the action of IFN-γ explains our experimental observations that IFN-γ therapy is directly cytotoxic for ovarian cancer xenograft cells growing as free floating tumour cell clumps intraperitoneally, but is only cytostatic when these cells grow as solid IP tumours. The tumour cell clumps do not have an appreciable stroma and may not produce many cytokines that inhibit apoptosis. The cytokine context in which IFN-γ acts against solid tumours, however, will be quite different. A well developed stroma may provide better nutritional support and more cytokines may be present that will inhibit apoptosis. Thus, the response of a solid tumour to IFN-γ will tend to be cytostasis rather than cytotoxicity.

In a multicentre trial of IP IFN-γ in chemoresistant ovarian cancer, there was a significant association between size of tumour and response with microscopic tumours being most likely to respond (Chapter 24). Microscopic tumours would be more likely to show apoptosis than cytostasis.

9.5 IMPLICATIONS FOR FUTURE THERAPEUTIC STRATEGIES

The ideas presented in this chapter suggest that the response of an ovarian tumour to IFN-γ is contextual and that larger tumours with well developed stromas are unlikely to respond to this cytokine except by reversible cytostasis. It is possible that chronic exposure to the cytostatic influence (which has not generally been modelled in tissue culture) may cause some cell death. In scheduling experiments in the ovarian cancer xenograft model, daily treatment with low doses resulted in a significantly longer survival than intermittent high dose therapy. This is an area that could be modelled further and may suggest the importance of slow release formulations that would allow chronic local exposure of the tumour area. However, the most important implication of this model is that an understanding, even partial, of the cytokine context of an individual tumour or tumour type may define therapies that switch the response to IFN-γ from cytostasis to apoptosis.

Identification of one or more cytokines involved in maintaining survival of cells in G_1/G_0 may suggest combinations of IFN-γ with other cytokines, or cytokine antagonists, that may shift the balance from cell survival to cell death. The best combinations may be IFN-γ and cytokine antagonists, which should not cause an 'unfolding' of the cytokine network and unacceptable systemic toxicity often generated by cytokine combinations. Our studies on cytokines in human tumour biopsies suggest TNF as a candidate cytokine for promotion of growth and survival of ovarian cancer cells *in vivo*. Therapy with IFN-γ combined with specific TNF antagonists is currently being evaluated in tissue culture and animal models of ovarian cancer.

REFERENCES

1. Old, L.J. (1985) Tumour necrosis factor (TNF). *Science*, **230**, 630.
2. Palladino, M.A., Refaat Shalaby, M., Dramer, S.M. *et al.* (1987) Characterization of the anti-tumour activities of human tumor necrosis factor alpha and the comparison with other cytokines: induction of tumor-specific immunity. *J. Immunol.*, **138**, 4023.
3. Creasey, A.A., Reynolds, M.T. and Laird, W. (1986) Cures and partial regression of murine and human tumors by recombinant human tumor necrosis factor. *Cancer Res.*, **46**, 5687–90.
4. Fiers, W. (1991) Tumor necrosis factor: characterisation at the molecular, cellular and *in vivo* level. *FEBS*, **285**, 199–212.
5. Sugarman, B.J., Aggarwal, B.B., Hass, P.E. *et al.* (1985) Recombinant human tumor necrosis factor-alpha: effects on proliferation of normal and transformed cells *in vitro*. *Science*, **230**, 943.

6. Dvorak, H.F. (1986) Tumours: wounds that do not heal. *N. Engl. J. Med.*, **315**, 1650–9.

7. Gerlach, H., Liebermann, H., Brett, J. *et al.* (1989) Growing/motile endothelium shows enhanced responsiveness to tumor necrosis factor/cachectin. *J. Exp. Med.*, **170**, 913–31.

8. Frater-Schroder, M., Risau, W. Hallaman, R. *et al.* (1987) Tumor necrosis factor type alpha, a potent inhibitor of endothelial cell growth *in vitro*, is angiogenic *in vivo*. *Proc. Natl. Acad. Sci. USA*, **84**, 5277–87.

9. Ito, A., Sato, T., Iga, T. and Mori, Y. (1990) Tumor necrosis factor bifunctionally regulates matrix metalloproteinases and tissue inhibitor of metalloproteinases (TIMP) production by human fibroblasts. *FEBS*, **269**, 93–5

10. Brenner, D.A., O'Hara, M., Angel, P. *et al.* (1989) Prolonged activation of jun and collagenase genes by tumor necrosis factor-alpha. *Nature*, **337**, 661.

11. Liotta, L.A. and Stetler Stevenson, W.G. (1991) Tumor invasion and metastasis: an imbalance of positive and negative regulation. *Cancer Res.*, **51**, 5054s–9s.

12. Malik, S.T.A., Griffin, D.B., Fiers, W. and Balkwill, F.R. (1989) Paradoxical effects of tumor necrosis factor in experimental ovarian cancer. *Int. J. Cancer*, **44**, 918–25.

13. Spriggs, D., Imamura, K., Rodriguez, C. *et al.* (1987) Induction of tumor necrosis factor expression and resistance in a human breast tumor cell line. *Proc. Natl. Acad. Sci. USA*, **84**, 6563–6.

14. Piguet, P.F., Ribaux, C. Karpuz, V. *et al.* (1992) Cellular origin of pulmonary tumor necrosis factor (TNF) during idiopathic pulmonary fibrosis. *Eur. Cytokine Netw*, **3**, 255 (abs).

15. Niitsu, Y., Watanabe, N., Neda, H. *et al.* (1988) Induction of synthesis of tumor necrosis factor in human and marine cells by exogenous recombinant human tumor necrosis factor. *Cancer Res.*, **48**, 5407–10.

16. Baiocchi, G., Kavanagh, J.J., Talpaz, M. *et al.* (1991) Expression of the macrophage colony stimulating factor and its receptor in gynecologic malignancies. *Cancer*, **67**, 990–6.

17. Abruzzo, L.V., Thornton, A.J., Liebert, M. *et al.* (1992) Cytokine-induced gene expression of interleukin 8 in human transitional cell carcinomas and renal cell carcinomas. *Am. J. Pathol.*, **140**, 365–73.

18. Aderka, D., Engelmann, H., Hirnik, V. *et al.* (1991) Increased serum levels of soluble receptors for tumor necrosis factor in cancer patients. *Cancer Res.*, **51**, 5602–7.

19. Allavena, P., Peccatori, F., Maggioni, D. *et al.* (1990) Intraperitoneal recombinant g-interferon in patients with recurrent ascitic ovarian carcinoma: modulation of cytotoxicity and cytokine production in tumor associated effectors and of major histocompatibility antigen expression on tumor cells. *Cancer Res.*, **50**, 7318–23.

20. D'Acquisto, R., Markman, M., Hakes, T. *et al.* (1988) A phase I trial of intraperitoneal recombinant g-interferon in advanced ovarian carcinoma. *J. Clin. Oncol.*, **6**, 689–95.

21. Pujade-Lauraine, E., Guastella, J.P., Colombo, N. *et al.* (1991) Intraperitoneal human r-IFN-gamma as treatment of residual carcinoma (OC) and laparotomy (SLL). *Proc. ASCO*, **10**, 195.

22. Ward, B.G, Wallace, K., Shepherd, J.H. and Balkwill, F.R. (1987) Intraperitoneal xenografts of human epithelial cancer in nude mice. *Cancer Res.*, **47**, 2662–7.

23. Malik, S.T.A., Knowles, R.G., East N. *et al.* (1991) Antitumor activity of γ-interferon in ascitic and solid tumor models of human ovarian cancer. *Cancer Res.*, **51**, 6643–9.

24. Ozaki, Y., Edelstein, M. and Duch, D. (1988) Induction of indoleamine 2,3 dioxygenase: a mechanism of the antitumour activity of interferon-γ. *Proc. Natl. Acad. Sci. USA*, **85**, 1242–6.

25. Takikawa, O., Kuroiwa, T., Yamazaki, F. and Kido, R. (1988) Mechanism of interferon-γ action. *J. Biol. Chem.*, **263**, 2041–8.

26. Evan, G.I. and Littlewood, T.D. (1993) The role of *c-myc* in cell growth. *Curr. Opin. Genet. Develop.*, **3**, 44–9.

Chapter 10

Growth factors and receptors in ovarian cancer

R. LEAKE, A. BARBER, O. OWENS, S. LANGDON and B. MILLER

10.1 INTRODUCTION

Repair of the normal ovarian epithelium, subsequent to the damage inflicted by ovulation, is thought to be carried out by epidermal growth factor (EGF) acting through its receptor (EGFR). In many tumour cells, it has been shown [1] that the role of EGF is taken by transforming growth factor-α (TGF-α). In breast cancer, there is firm evidence that over-expression of EGFR is associated with poor prognosis [2], implying a role for this receptor in promoting tumour progression. Thus, TGF-α may, through the EGF receptor, be a driving force in the growth of some ovarian cancers. If so, blocking either growth factor or receptor function may have therapeutic implications. This study set out to establish the levels and frequency at which TGF-α and EGFR can be detected in human ovarian epithelial cancers. Concurrently, in an effort to create model systems for testing potential drugs, ovarian cancer cell lines and xenografts were established and characterized in terms of sensitivity to EGF/TGF-α and the corresponding levels and frequency of detection of endogenous EGFR and TGF-α determined.

10.2 MATERIALS AND METHODS

Material was collected fresh from 52 women with normal ovaries (removed at hysterec-

tomy), 30 with benign ovarian tumours (removed at laparotomy) and 174 ovarian cancer samples were collected from 133 consecutive patients. Material was either assayed immediately or was snap frozen in liquid nitrogen. Storage studies [3] showed that there was no difference, within experimental error, between values obtained for TGF-α content or for EGFR content (determined by the ligand binding assay) between fresh and stored material.

10.2.1 EXTRACTION AND MEASUREMENT OF EGF AND TGF-α.

This was routinely carried out as follows. Frozen specimens were allowed to thaw on ice. Once thawed, excess water was carefully removed, then each specimen halved. Two samples were cut from each half and one placed in formal saline for pathological analysis; the other was used for immunohistochemical staining. The remaining tumour was minced, then homogenized in an ultra-turrax (2 × 15 second bursts with thorough cooling in between) in 5 ml/g wet weight of homogenizing buffer (20 mM HEPES, 2 mM EDTA, 0.5 mM PMSF, pH 7.4). A low speed pellet was retained for DNA analysis and a higher speed (12 000 g for one hour) supernatant added to two volumes of ice-cold alcohol (the pellet was retained for determination of EGF receptor – see below). After centrifugation of the supernatant/alcohol mix at 1000 g for 30 minutes, the supernatant was again recovered and added to four volumes of ice-cold ethyl acetate and stored at 4° overnight. A crude extract precipitated and was resuspended in 2 ml of 1 N acetic acid. This extract was stored at –70°C until assay. Batches of extracts were lyophilized, then resuspended each in 1 ml of radioimmunoassay (RIA) buffer (phosphate buffer at pH 7.4 containing 0.1% sodium azide, 0.15 M sodium chloride, 0.01 M EDTA and 0.5% BSA). Corresponding standards of human recombinant EGF and TGF-α were also prepared. Polyclonal antibodies (showing less than 0.01% crossreactivity) were supplied by ICI Pharmaceuticals, having been raised in sheep from synthetic peptides. The antibody dilutions (made fresh with RIA buffer) were 1:10 000–1: 20 000 for TGF-α and 1:100 000 for EGF (subject to some modification depending on the specific activity of the iodinated probe).

Iodination of rhEGF and TGF-α was carried out by an 'in-house' technique using iodogen and a Biogel P6 column. Full details are given in ref [3]. Labelled peptides were diluted with RIA buffer to give 30 000 cpm/ 250 μl. To every 1 ml of labelled peptide, 4 μl of sheep serum was added to reduce non-specific binding. Tumour extract (250 μl) was added in duplicate to eppendorfs, 250 μl primary antibody added followed by 250 μl of appropriate labelled peptide. Samples and standards were vortexed and incubated at 4°C for 48 hours. Secondary antibody (donkey/antisheep), at a dilution of 1:15, was added at a volume of 250 μl and each tube incubated for a further 24 hours at 4°C. All tubes were centrifuged (40 000 g for 20 minutes) and the pellet washed in RIA buffer, then counted in a gamma counter (60% efficiency). The peptide content was read from the appropriate standard curve.

10.2.2 MEASUREMENT OF EGFR

This was carried out on the pellet (membrane fraction) from the 12 000 g spin in the extraction described for EGF and TGF-α. Initially, this pellet was resuspended in RIA buffer, then stored at –70°C. All samples were screened by a single point assay to determine which samples should be subject to full Scatchard analysis. Prior to screening, eppendorfs were coated with RIA buffer to prevent EGF binding to the plastic. Membrane pellets were thawed on ice, then subjected to glass/teflon homogenization to re-establish a uniform suspension. Labelled mouse EGF (^{125}I from NEN), with a specific activity of 90– 180 μC/μg, was made to a final concentration of 1 nM. Total cpm were about 100 000/100 μl. Non-specific binding was determined by adding unlabelled mEGF at 100 nM final concentration. Membrane preparation (50 μl) was added, in duplicate, to precoated eppendorfs which then received 50 μl labelled EGF (1 nM) with or without 100 nM unlabelled mEGF. All samples were thoroughly vortexed. Placental membrane was run as internal positive control and the assay was subject to external quality assurance through the EORTC Receptor Group scheme. Incubation was for 2 hours at room temperature and the reaction stopped by adding ice-cold RIA buffer (750 μl). The eppendorfs were centrifuged at 40 000 g for 10 minutes at 4°C. The supernatant was aspirated off and the pellet counted, as before. The mean of each pair of results was taken and a difference of greater than 20% between total and non-specific counts was taken as justification to subject that membrane suspension to Scatchard analysis. Random samples which gave less than 20% competition on the screen were also subject to Scatchard analysis but none gave positive plots.

Scatchard analysis was carried out over 12 points of increasing concentration of labelled EGF (0.086–16.67 nM). Non-specific binding was ascertained by incubating three aliquots (50 μl) of membrane suspension at the top three concentrations of EGF plus 100-fold excess of unlabelled EGF. Incubation and termination were as for the single screen. Full practical details are given in ref [5]. Data were analysed using an 'in-house' program adapted from [4] and graphs constructed on an Apple Mackintosh. Individual components of binding were only recognized if five or more data points could be used to construct the line. The 'high affinity' component was defined as that with a K_d of higher affinity than 10^{-9} M and the lower affinity component as that with K_d equal to or lower than 10^{-9} M.

10.2.3 CELL LINE METHODOLOGY

Human ovarian adenocarcinoma cell lines PEO1, PEO4 and PEO14 were established from malignant effusions using ascitic filtrate to promote initial growth (for full details, see [6]). At a later stage, a platinum resistant variant of PEO1 was also established. Cells were routinely maintained at 37°C in a humidified atmosphere of 5% CO_2 in air in RPMI 1640 containing 10% heat-inactivated foetal calf serum (FCS) supplemented with streptomycin (100 μg ml^{-1}), penicillin (100 u ml^{-1}) and glutamine (2 mM). Cells were harvested by trypsinization and plated into 24-well plates at densities of about 4×10^4 cells per well (four wells per experimental condition) in RPMI 1640 without phenol red, plus 5% charcoal stripped FCS (CSFCS). After a further 24 hours, medium was removed, cells were washed with phosphate buffered saline and RPMI 1640 containing 5% CSFCS plus appropriate concentrations (range 0.001–10 nM) of human recombinant EGF or TGF-α added. This time point was designated day 0. Media including growth factors were replenished on days 2 and 5. Cells were harvested on days 0, 2, 5 and 7, then counted using a

Coulter Counter. For cell cycle distribution studies, cells were plated into 6-well plates and fed EGF or TGF-α, as previously described. Cells were harvested at 0, 12, 24, 36, 48 and 72 hours. Samples of approximately 10^6 cells were prepared from quadruplicate wells at each time point. Cells were treated with trypsin/detergent and the DNA stained with 100 μg ml^{-1} propidium iodide [7]. Analysis was performed using a FACScan flow cytometer (Becton Dickinson) equipped for doublet discrimination using Cellfit Software. All data were gated on forward and side scatter signals to exclude fragmented and clumped material and on a fluorescence width versus fluorescence area signal to exclude doublets.

EGFR content of cell lines was determined on harvested, washed cell pellets (obtained as already described). The cells were disrupted in ice-cold, Tris-buffered saline (TBS), pH7.4 using a sonicator and centrifuged at 105 000 g for 30 minutes at 4°C. The pellet was resuspended in TBS. An aliquot was removed for protein determination (Bradford method). EGF binding capacity was determined by incubating aliquots (100 μl) with 200 μl of a range (0–300 nM) of concentrations of unlabelled EGF and 100 μl of a fixed concentration (about 0.2 nM) of ^{125}I-EGF (equivalent to about 10 000 cpm) to give a final reaction volume of 400 μl for 90 minutes at 26°C. The reaction was terminated by ice-cold 0.5% (w/v) IgG followed by mixing and addition of 25% (w/v) polyethylene glycol. After further mixing, the bound and free ^{125}I-EGF were separated by centrifugation. The supernatant, containing the free component, was aspirated and the remaining pellet counted in a Gamma counter. After Scatchard analysis, plots were examined by the computer analysis method of Hetherington (see [2]). Measurement of EGFR by immunofluorescence utilized the EGFR1 murine monoclonal antibody raised against the A431 cell line and supplied by Dr Bill Gullick. Cells were

101

harvested and washed, as before. Aliquots of about 10^6 cells were incubated with EGFR1 antibody (diluted 1:5 in PBS/FCS) for 60 minutes. Cells were washed in PBS/FCS and incubated with sheep-antimouse fluorescein isothiocyanate (FITC) (1:20) for 60 minutes, then washed twice in cold PBS/FCS. All incubations were performed on ice. The cells were resuspended in PBS and analysed on a FACScan flow cytometer. To eliminate background fluorescence, cells were taken through the procedure with EGFR1 antibody omitted. A431 cells were used as positive controls and the small cell lung cancer cell line, H69 (known to be EGFR negative), was used as negative control (see [8]).

10.2.4   TYROSINE KINASE ACTIVITY

This was determined in cell lines as follows: cell pellets were harvested as previously described, then stored at $-20°C$ for 48 hours. Cell pellets were then lysed by resuspension in 50 mM Tris, 150 mM NaCl, 5 mM EDTA, 1% NP-40, 1 μg ml^{-1} aprotonin followed by homogenization using a Kontes glass/glass homogenizer. Homogenates were centrifuged first for 10 minutes at 1000 g, followed by 20 minutes at 12 000 g (all procedures at 4°C). For each pellet, this generated a crude nuclear fraction, a membrane fraction and a soluble (cytosol) fraction. Overall tyrosine kinase activity was determined using an ELISA kit developed by Rijksen (Utrecht), characterized in our laboratory and now retailed by European Diagnostica. This kit involves polyglu-tyr attached to multiwell plates. The tyrosines can be phosphorylated by aliquots of the test material, the number of tyrosines phosphorylated is then visualized by adding a mouse monoclonal antityrosine phosphate antibody, then adding an enzyme conjugated rabbit antimouse antibody. An internal standard is provided by prealiquoted amounts of phosphotyrosine. An additional positive control is provided by increasing amounts of

spleen extract. Samples were assayed in triplicate with intra-assay c. v. of <5%.

10.3   RESULTS

Measurable amounts of TGF-α were detected in normal ovary. Combining results, the median value found in proliferative ovaries was 0.38 ng mg^{-1} DNA, that in secretory ovaries was 0.75 and that in postmenopausal ovaries was 0.87. These results suggested that the changing levels of steroids during the ovarian cycle might influence overall levels of TGF-α in the ovary. In a small series of benign ovarian tumours, the range of TGF-α detected was large (range for mucinous cystadenomata was 0.3–195 ng mg^{-1} DNA) and no obvious trend was observed. In the ovarian epithelial cancers (174 samples from 133 patients), TGF-α was detectable in 88.5% of samples, whereas EGF was only detected in 27.6% of samples. TGF-α was also present at higher concentrations than EGF (TGF-α range was 0.04–33 ng mg^{-1} DNA, whereas EGF range was 0.03–2.5 ng mg^{-1} DNA – values were also expressed relative to protein content and to g wet weight but values expressed relative to DNA gave the closest to a normal distribution and were therefore selected as being most readily compared by standard statistical techniques. Overall incidence and median values for each major histological subgroup are shown in Table 10.1.

Because serous tumours were the most common, these were analysed separately. Of 109 samples, 92 contained detectable TGF-α (range 0.041–33 ng mg^{-1} DNA) at a median value of 1.18 ng mg^{-1} DNA. When subdivided according to the degree of differentiation, TGF-α content was found to be higher in well-differentiated tumours (median values were 0.75 for poorly differentiated, 1.36 for moderately differentiated and 3.14 for well-differentiated tumours). When subdivided according to oestrogen (ER) and

Table 10.1 TGF-α in ovarian epithelial cancer

	Serous	Endometrioid	Mucinous	Clear	Unclassified
% detectable	84	95	100	85	100
Median conc.	1.2	1.3	1.7	1.2	0.4

The table shows the frequency (%) at which TGF-α was detected in the different histological subgroups of human ovarian epithelial cancers. Median concentrations are quoted in ng mg^{-1} DNA

Table 10.2 Levels of TGF-α in relation to oestrogen and progesterone receptor status in serous ovarian cancers

Receptor status	TGF-α (ng mg $^{-1}$DNA)
ER+/PR+	5.8
ER+/PR–	0.45
ER–/PR+	2.1
ER–/PR–	0.74

Tumours were defined as positive for each receptor only if Scatchard analysis revealed >20 fmol mg^{-1} cytosol protein for the particular receptor and the dissociation constant indicated greater affinity than 7×10^{-10} M. Values quoted for TGF-α are median values for that category

progesterone receptor (PR) status (Table 10.2), the median level in ER+/PR+ tumours was much higher than that in other subgroups. As our previous definition of hormone sensitive disease [9] has required the presence of both ER and PR, these data are consistent with the idea that ovarian cancers secrete a basal level of TGF-α but that additional TGF-α may be secreted as a result of hormonal stimulation.

Presence of EGFR has been shown by Berchuck *et al.* [10] to be an indicator of poor prognosis. One explanation of this observation is that an autocrine or paracrine loop exists in (some) ovarian cancers in which TGF-α is secreted, then activates the EGFR. To test the reality of this, we measured EGFR in the membrane fraction of all biopsies processed for TGF-α determination. Frequency of detection of EGFR is shown in Table 10.3, in relation to histological subgroups. The cut-off for 'high' and 'low' affinity binding sites was taken arbitrarily at a K_d of 10^{-9} M. On this basis, tumours divided about equally into those containing only high affinity sites, those containing both sites and those containing only low affinity sites. TGF-α was present at similar concentrations in all three sets of tumours (data not shown). Until follow-up accumulates, it will not be

Table 10.3 Incidence and characteristics of the epidermal growth factor receptor in different histological subgroups of ovarian cancer

	Serous	Endometrioid	Mucinous	Clear	Undifferentiated
No. samples	114	20	11	14	19
No. EGFR +	46	8	4	6	9
% +ve	40.4	41	36.4	42.8	47.4
Lo affinity	17	4	2	2	6
Hi affinity	18	3	2	1	2
Lo + Hi affinity	11	1	0	3	1

Lo = low affinity binding; Hi = high affinity binding. The distinction between low and high affinity binding was made using a dissociation constant of 10^{-9} M as an arbitrary cut off.

Table 10.4 The relationship between EGF receptor content of ovarian cancers when determined by ligand binding assay and by immunohistochemistry

Tumour type (%)	No. of patients	No. of samples	Bio+/ IHC+	Bio–/ IHC–	Bio+/ IHC–	Bio–/ IHC+	Concordance
Serous	52	67	25	25	8	9	75
Endometrioid	10	10	2	2	4	2	40
Mucinous	6	6		5	1		83
Clear cell	7	8	3	3		2	75
Undifferentiated	10	14	7	5	2		86
Total	85	105	37	40	15	13	73

Bio = ligand binding assay; IHC = immunohistochemical assay

clear whether there is any biological significance to the presence of these receptors with apparently different binding affinities. The incidence of TGF-α is much higher than that of EGFR and one possible explanation for underestimation of EGFR is that there was no or insufficient exchange occurring during the assay and so 'filled' sites were not detected. Such sites should be detected by immunohistochemistry. As Table 10.4 shows, there are inconsistencies between EGFR determined by ligand binding and by immunohistochemistry. However, these differences cannot be explained solely by the blocking of the binding site, because some tumours were clearly positive by binding assay but negative on staining (epitope blocked by, for example, active internalization – see [11]).

The cell lines PEO1, PEO4 and PEO14 were tested as suitable models for study of the TGF-α/EGFR loop. All three cell lines were differentially growth stimulated by both EGF and TGF-α. The stimulation was reflected in a decreased proportion of cells in G1 phase and an increased proportion in S and G2 phases. Ligand binding assay revealed non-linear curves for all three cell lines. The dissociation constants for the three cell lines were similar (0.05–0.18 nmol l^{-1} for 'high' affinity and 2.0–4.8 nmol l^{-1} for 'low' affinity). High affinity receptors were present in greater concentration in PEO1 cells (high affinity sites at 22 fmol mg^{-1} protein and total binding 70 fmol mg^{-1} protein) than in the other two cell lines (PEO4 cells had 1.4 and 80 fmol mg^{-1} protein respectively, and PEO14 had 1.5 and 50 fmol mg^{-1} protein respectively.) PEO1 cells also showed the greatest median intensity of staining with the EGFR1 antibody, with about 90% of cells showing fluorescence in excess of background. In PEO4 and PEO14 cells, only about 66% of cells showed fluorescence above background.

Levels of tyrosine kinase activity were measured in both the cell lines and in xenografts set up in nude mice. Corresponding levels of TGF-α were measured. The recently acquired platinum resistant variant (PEO1 cddp) was included in these studies. The data in Figure 10.1 show that tyrosine kinase activity can be detected in the membrane fraction, the cytosol fraction and the nuclear fraction. The basal level of activity is always greatest in the platinum resistant variant. In all fractions, and in all cell lines tested, tyrosine kinase activity is stimulated by platinum. Figure 10.2 shows that the level of TGF-α detected is highest in the platinum resistant cell line. However, we cannot suppose that the tyrosine kinase activity is principally attributable to the TGF-α driven EGFR. Blocking experiments will be carried out to determine to what extent this loop

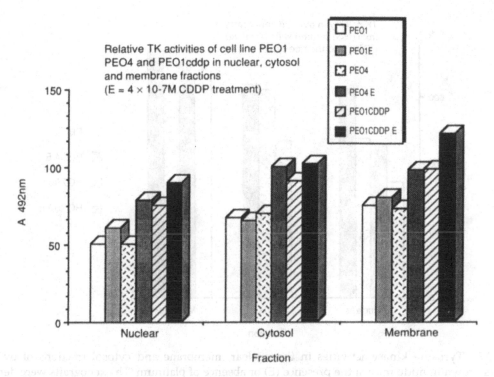

Figure 10.1 Relative tyrosine kinase activities of the different fractions obtained from the PEO1, PEO4 and PEO1 platinum resistant (PEO1CDDP) cell lines, grown in the presence (E) and absence of platinum drug.

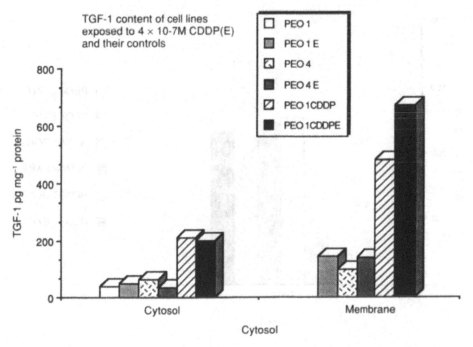

Figure 10.2 TGF-α content of the PEO1, PEO4 and PEO1 platinum resistant cell lines, grown in the presence (E) and absence of platinum.

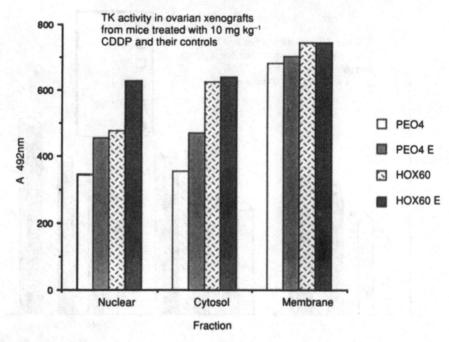

Figure 10.3 Tyrosine kinase activities in the nuclear, membrane and cytosol fractions of ovarian xenografts grown in nude mice in the presence (E) or absence of platinum. The xenografts were derived from the PEO4 cell line and directly from a human ovarian cancer (HOX60).

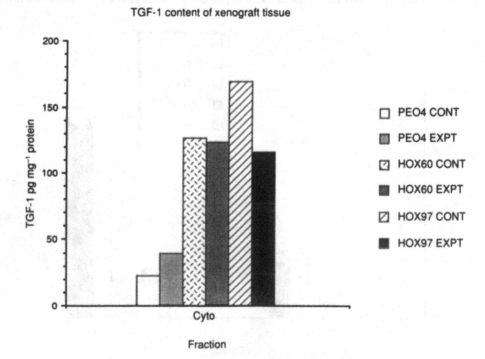

Figure 10.4 TGF-α content of the PEO4 cell line and of human ovarian cancers when grown as xenografts in nude mice in the presence (E) or absence of platinum.

contributes to the measured tyrosine kinase activity. To try to overcome the problems of cell culture conditions (a major problem when trying to study potential paracrine loops), the experiments were repeated in xenografts in nude mice and compared with the properties of directly established human ovarian xenografts. The results were very similar to the *in vitro* results in that tyrosine kinase activity was found at similar levels in cytosol, membrane and nuclear fractions of the xenografts (Figure 10.3) and again these were increased in the presence of platinum. The levels of TGF-α detected were much lower in the PEO4 xenograft than in the xenografts raised directly from human ovarian cancers (Figure 10.4). This reflects the relative levels of tyrosine kinase activity measured, but this does not prove the extent of the contribution of EGFR-linked tyrosine kinase activity.

10.4 DISCUSSION

Although TGF-α is found in about 90% of ovarian epithelial cancers, the incidence is similar in all histological subtypes and there is no clear correlation with prognosis. Since only about half (45%) of these tumours contain measurable EGFR, this is not surprising. The prognostic value of TGF-α content has not been separately determined in the EGFR-positive subgroup. Because EGF levels are higher in normal ovary but much lower than TGF-α in ovarian cancer, determination of EGF/TGF-α ratio in borderline or suspicious benign tumours might be worthwhile. However, the detection rate for EGF (found in only 28% of tumours) is low and so such an approach may be of limited use. A further complication arises from the fact that TGF-α may be upregulated in ER+/PR+ tumours. These are usually good prognosis tumours (see [9]) and so prognosis information may only be forthcoming if ER+/PR+ tumours are analysed separately from the rest.

Although EGFR has been associated with poor prognosis in ovarian cancer [10] this has not been accepted by all authors [12]. There is no convincing evidence for use of EGFR in patient management, such as exists for EGFR in breast cancer [2]. When EGFR is determined according to histological subgroup, there are no obvious differences between subgroups. Application of an arbitrary cut-off at a dissociation constant of 10^{-9} M shows that some tumours exhibit a single, high affinity binding site, while others have both and low affinity sites and a third group have only low affinity sites; however, these are relatively high affinity compared with most protein–protein interactions. More follow-up is required before the clinical significance, if any, of these different sites can be established in ovarian cancer. The demonstration that there are some differences in detection of EGFR when the ligand binding method is compared with immunohistochemistry reinforces the need to compare like methodologies only with like. The ideal solution would be the establishment of an index of receptor functionality, such as a rise in tyrosine kinase activity after stimulation with TGF-α.

To test out the reality of the TGF-α/EGFR autocrine/paracrine loop and to study the control of tyrosine kinase activity, we have established several human ovarian cancer cell lines and some human xenografts. These lines are all growth stimulated by TGF-α and all express both high and low affinity EGFR. The highest level of high affinity EGFR was found in the PEO1 cell line, which is the line for which a platinum resistant variant is available. Both TGF-α levels and tyrosine kinase levels are highest in this platinum resistant line (whether measured in cells grown *in vitro* or in xenografts). However, there is no direct evidence that the elevated levels of tyrosine kinase can be attributed to TGF-α stimulation of the EGFR. It was interesting to note that the levels of tyrosine kinase were further elevated in cell lines and in xenografts after exposure to platinum. One might speculate that anti-tyrosine kinase therapies might be useful in ovarian cancer, particularly in patients whose tumours have become platinum resistant. Blocking of the TGF-α/EGFR loop requires further testing *in vitro* and in the xenografts but the reality of inhibiting such a vital system in patients is questionable, unless a very specific targeting mechanism is employed.

ACKNOWLEDGEMENTS

The authors are most grateful for generous support from the Association for International Cancer Research and from ICI Pharmaceuticals (Zeneca). We should like to thank all our gynaecological and pathological colleagues for ongoing support, without which this work could not be attempted.

REFERENCES

1. Sporn, M.B. and Roberts, A.B. (1986) Peptide growth factors and inflammation, tissue repair and cancer. *J. Clin. Invest.*, **78**, 329–32.
2. Nicholson S., Sainsbury, J.R.C., Halcrow, P. *et al.* (1989) Expression of epidermal growth factor receptors associated with lack of response to endocrine therapy in recurrent breast cancer. *Lancet*, **i**, 182–4.
3. Owens, O.J., Stewart C. and Leake, R.E. (1991) Growth factors in ovarian cancer. *Br. J. Cancer*, **64**, 1177–81.
4. Leake, R.E., Cowan, S. and Eason, R. (1987) Computer program for Scatchard analysis of protein:ligand interaction. In *Steroid Hormones: A Practical Approach*, (eds B. Green and R.E. Leake), Oxford University Press, Oxford, pp. 93–7.
5. Owens, O.J., Stewart, C., Brown, I. and Leake, R.E. (1991) Epidermal growth factor receptors (EGFR) in human ovarian cancer. *Br. J. Cancer*, **64**, 907–10.
6. Langdon, S.P., Lawrie, S.S., Hay, F.G. *et al.* (1988) Characterization and properties of nine human ovarian adenocarcinoma cell lines. *Cancer Res.*, **48**, 6166–72.
7. Vindelov, L.L., Christenen, I.J. and Nissen, N.I. (1983) A detergent/trypsin method for the preparation of nuclei for flow cytometric analysis. *Cytometry*, **3**, 317–39.
8. Crew, A.J. Langdon, S.P., Miller E.P. and Miller, W.R. (1992) Mitogenic effects of epidermal growth factor and transforming growth factor-α on EGF-receptor positive human ovarian carcinoma cell lines. *Eur. J. Cancer*, **28**, 337–41.
9. Harding, M., McIntosh, J., Paul, J. *et al.* (1990) Oestrogen and progesterone receptors in ovarian tumours. *Cancer*, **65**, 486–92.
10. Berchuck, A., Rodriguez, G.C., Kael, A. *et al.* (1991) Epidermal growth factor receptor expression in normal ovarian epithelium and ovarian cancer. *Am. J. Obstet. Gynecol.*, **164**, 669–74.
11. Owens, O.J., Stewart, C., Leake, R.E. and McNicol, A.M. (1992) A comparison of biochemical and immunohistochemical assessment of EGFR expression in ovarian cancer. *Anticancer Res.*, **12**, 1455–8.
12. Bauknecht, T., Runge, M., Schwall, M. and Pfleiderer, A. (1988) Occurrence of epidermal growth factor receptors in human adnexal tumours and their prognostic value in advanced ovarian cancer. *Gynecol. Oncol.*, **29**, 147–57.

Chapter 11

Cell growth regulation in ovarian cancer: tyrosine kinases, tyrosine phosphatases and tumour necrosis factor-α

R.C. BAST JR, J. WIENER, S. KASSIM, S. WU, C.M. BOYER, K. DE SOMBRE, J.A. HURTEAU, G. RODRIGUEZ, G.B. MILLS and A. BERCHUCK

Since the last Helene Harris Symposium two years ago, epithelial ovarian cancer has been shown to be a clonal disease [1,2]. Consequently, multiple genetic changes within a single cell are thought to be required for malignant transformation. Such events are most likely to occur during the proliferation of surface epithelial cells to repair defects created by ovulation. Growth regulation of the normal surface epithelium is tightly controlled by several known growth factors [3].

Over the last several years, a number of groups including our own have compared growth regulation in normal and malignant epithelium [3]. Several changes have been associated with malignant transformation including:

1. Persistence of autocrine growth stimulation by transforming growth factor alpha (TGF-α) and epidermal growth factor (EGF) through the EGF receptor (EGFR) [4,5];
2. Interruption of an autocrine inhibitory loop mediated by transforming growth factor beta (TGF-β) [6];
3. Autocrine growth stimulation by macrophage colony stimulating factor through the c-*fms* receptor [7];
4. Paracrine stimulation by IL-1, IL-6 and TNF-α produced by macrophages [8];

5. Overexpression of HER-2/*neu* (c-*erb*B-2) in 30% of cases [9,10];
6. Mutation of p53 in up to half of patients with advanced disease [11].

Among the several molecular changes observed to date, a poor prognosis has been associated with the expression or overexpression of three transmembrane tyrosine kinase growth factor receptors. Shortened survival has correlated with the continued expression of EGFR, the overexpression of c-*erb*B-2 and the novel expression of c-*fms*. In the case of EGFR the effect is subtle [12] but in the case of overexpression of c-*erb*B-2 there is a 50% decrease in median survival [10] (Figures 11.1 and 11.2).

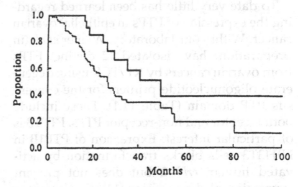

Figure 11.1 Prognosis of ovarian cancer patients with persistence (lower curve) or loss (upper curve) of EGFR expression.*

*Figure 11.1 is reproduced, with permission, from Berchuck, A. *et al.* (1991) *Am. J. Obstet. Gynecol.*, **164**, 669–74. See [12].

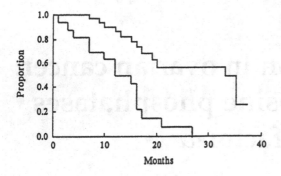

Figure 11.2 Prognosis of ovarian cancer patients with overexpression (lower curve) or normal (upper curve) expression of c-*erb*B-2 (HER-2/*neu*) [10].

11.1 PROTEIN TYROSINE PHOSPHATASES (PTPs) IN EPITHELIAL OVARIAN CANCER

Ligand induced activation of a receptor protein tyrosine kinase (PTK) leads to increased phosphorylation of intracellular proteins and of the cytoplasmic tail of the kinase. Removal of phosphate groups from phosphorylated tyrosine residues by PTPs can downregulate the growth stimulatory activity of these signalling pathways. Alternatively, removal of phosphate groups by PTPases may be required for repeated activation of PTK receptors.

To date very little has been learned regarding the expression of PTPs in epithelial ovarian cancer. Within our laboratory, Wiener *et al.* (in preparation) have isolated 12 distinct PTPs from ovarian cancers by RT/PCR using degenerate oligonucleotide primers for the consensus PTP domain (Table 11.1). These include both receptor and non-receptor PTPs. PTP1B is of particular interest. Expression of PTP1B in NIH3T3 cells blocks transformation by activated human *erb*B-2 but does not prevent expression of the receptor [13]. Our group is particularly interested in whether such inhibition occurs due to the activity of PTP1B directly upon the tyrosine kinase growth factor receptor or upon downstream substrates. Very

Table 11.1 PTPs isolated from ovarian cancers by PCR using degenerate oligonucleotide primers for the consensus PTP domain

Non-receptor:	T cell PTP
	PTP 2A
	PTP H1
	PTP 1C
	PTP 1B
Not yet classified:	PTP 1D
Receptor and receptor-like:	PTP-α
	PTP-Σ
	LAR
	PTP-γ
	PTP Mu pr
Other clones with partial homology to:	LCA (4 clones)
	PTP 1C (1 clone)

little, if any, PTP1B was detected in seven specimens of normal ovarian epithelium. In contrast, 43 (79.6%) of 54 ovarian tumors displayed increased PTP1B expression [14]. Marked overexpression of PTP1B was significantly associated with the expression of the p185$^{c-erbB-2}$, p170^{EGFR} and p165^{c-fms} PTKs. Northern analysis indicated that PTP1B mRNA could be detected in normal epithelium and could be expressed at different levels in ovarian carcinomas. Thus, the level of PTP1B protein observed does not appear to be regulated exclusively at the level of transcription. Currently, we are exploring the hypothesis that expression of PTP1B represents a compensatory mechanism that would balance the activity of receptor tyrosine kinases. One might, for example, predict that coexpression of PTP1B in cancers that overexpress c-*erb*B-2 could improve an otherwise poor prognosis.

11.2 THE ROLE OF TNF-α AND IL-1 IN OVARIAN TUMOR CELL GROWTH REGULATION

Working with Dr S. Ramakrishnan, our group had shown that macrophage colony stimulating factor (M-CSF) was produced both by malignant ovarian cancer cell lines [15] and by normal epithelial cells in culture [16]. In addition to possible autocrine growth stimulation through c-*fms*, M-CSF is a potent chemoattractant of macrophages. Consequently, cytokines produced by macrophages might also influence ovarian tumor growth. Wu *et al.* in our laboratory had shown that supernatants from human monocytes could stimulate the growth of epithelial ovarian cell lines [8]. Recombinantly derived interleukin 1, IL-6 and TNF-α each stimulated three of four cell lines that had been established in our laboratory [8]. Stimulation of growth with IL-1 or TNF-α also increased the endogenous expression of TNF-α mRNA and protein [17]. In the absence of exogenous IL-1 or TNF-α, little if any TNF-α mRNA expression could be detected in cultures of ovarian cancers or normal cells. By contrast, each of four highly purified specimens of tumor cells from ascites fluid exhibited detectable levels of TNF-α mRNA. When purified tumor cells taken from ascites were grown in culture for seven days, TNF-α expression was lost but could be reinduced by treatment with additional TNF-α or IL-1 [17]. Induction of TNF-α mRNA by IL-1 or TNF-α was both concentration and time dependent. The concentrations of IL-1 and TNF-α required to induce cell proliferation and endogenous TNF-α expression were comparable to those that have been observed in ascites fluids from a small fraction of patients. Increased steady state TNF-α mRNA levels appeared to result from new mRNA synthesis based on nuclear run-on assays.

Stimulation of tumor cell proliferation with TNF-α or IL-1 could be blocked with antibodies against TNF-α or with soluble TNF receptor [17]. To explore further the role of endogenous TNF-α expression, the TNF-α gene was placed in reversed orientation within the pcDVI expression vector [18]. Transfection of antisense resulted in markedly reduced expression of TNF-α in the presence

of IL-1. Proliferation of transfected cells could be stimulated with exogenous TNF-α, but not with exogenous interleukin-1α or β. Taken together, these data are consistent with a model similar to that described by Balkwill *et al.* [19,20], in which cytokines such as M-CSF produced by ovarian cancers attract macrophages which in turn generate TNF-α, IL-1 and other cytokines. Both TNF-α and IL-1 can stimulate endogenous production of TNF-α which acts as an autocrine stimulatory factor enhancing proliferation of tumour cells.

To determine whether stimulation by TNF-α might have a significant impact on tumor growth *in vivo*, studies were undertaken by Boyer *et al.* (in preparation) with OVCAR-3 human ovarian carcinoma xenografts in nude and scid mice. Animals were injected intraperitoneally with 3×10^7 OVCAR-3 tumor cells and were then treated biweekly for four weeks with IP injections of 0.25–2.5 μg of TNF-α. During the fifth week, animals were sacrificed. Injection with TNF-α markedly increased the formation of tumor nodules, consistent with Balkwill's earlier observations [20]. The weight of tumor nodules was increased 2.5–5-fold by TNF-α treatment. Consequently, repeated exposure to TNF-α *in vivo* could produce a substantial acceleration of tumor growth rate. Rodriguez *et al.* (in preparation) have found that treatment of OVCAR-3 with TNF-α *in vitro* increased their ability to invade matrigel membranes, possibly relating to the impact of TNF-α on the nude and scid mouse heterograft models.

Another important question is what fraction of freshly isolated human ovarian cancer cells can be stimulated rather than inhibited by TNF-α. Hurteau *et al.* in our laboratory have purified epithelial tumor cells from 15 cases of ovarian ascites (in preparation). Incubation with TNF-α stimulated the growth in 18%. If, however, tumor cells were grown in the presence of EGF, significant stimulation of proliferation was observed in 40%. Earlier studies by Salman *et al.* (personal communication) indicated that significant stimulation of clonogenic growth of ovarian cancer cells in soft agar was produced by TNF-α in 10% of cases.

Substantial heterogeneity in response to TNF-α has been observed by different investigators. In some cases tumor growth can be stimulated, whereas in other cases tumor growth can be inhibited. If stimulation occurs in a significant and identifiable fraction of patients with ovarian cancer, novel strategies for intervention could be evaluated. In addition to monoclonal antibodies and soluble receptors that bind to and neutralize the biological activity of TNF-α, there are multiple low molecular weight inhibitors of TNF expression or processing. One or more of these agents might inhibit the autocrine or paracrine stimulatory loops that stimulate ovarian tumor growth.

ACKNOWLEDGEMENTS

This work was funded in part by grants R01 39930 and R29 CA55640 from the National Cancer Institute, Department of Health and Human Services, Bethesda, MD. Jean A. Hurteau is a Research Fellow funded by the National Cancer Institute of Canada. The authors gratefully acknowledge the aid of the Helene Harris Memorial Trust in furthering our collaborative efforts.

REFERENCES

1. Mok, C.H., Tsao, S.W., Knapp, R.C. *et al.* (1992) Unifocal origin of advanced human epithelial ovarian cancers. *Cancer Res.*, **52**, 5119–22.
2. Jacobs, I.J., Kohler, M.F., Wiseman, R. *et al.* (1992) Clonal origin of epithelial ovarian carcinoma: analysis by loss of heterozygosity, p53 mutation and X-chromosome inactivation. *J. Natl. Cancer Inst.*, **84**, 1793–8.
3. Bast, R.C. Jr., Jacobs, I., Berchuck, A. (1992) Editorial: Malignant transformation of ovarian epithelium. *J. Natl. Cancer Inst.*, **84**, 556–8.
4. Rodriguez, G.C., Berchuck, A., Whitaker, R.S. *et al.* (1991) Epidermal growth factor receptor expression in normal ovarian epithelium and ovarian cancer. II. Relationship between receptor expression and response to epidermal growth factor. *Am. J. Obstet. Gynecol.*, **164**, 745–50.
5. Stromberg, K., Collins, T.J., Gordon, A.W. *et al.* (1992) Transforming growth factor-α acts as an autocrine growth factor in ovarian carcinoma cell lines. *Cancer Res.*, **52**, 341–7.
6. Berchuck, A., Rodriguez, G., Olt, G.S. *et al.* (1992) Regulation of growth of normal ovarian epithelial cells and ovarian cancer cell lines by transforming growth factor-β. *Am. J. Obstet. Gynecol.*, **166**, 676–84.
7. Kacinski, B.M., Carter, D., Mittal, K. *et al.* (1990) Ovarian adenocarcinomas express *fms*-complementary transcripts and *fms* antigen, often with coexpression of CSF-1. *Am. J. Pathol.*, **137**, 135–47.
8. Wu, S., Rodabaugh, K., Martínez-Maza, O. *et al.* (1992) Stimulation of ovarian tumor cell proliferation with monocyte products including interleukin-1, interleukin-6 and tumor necrosis factor-alpha. *Am. J. Obstet. Gynecol.*, **166**, 997–1007.
9. Slamon, D.J., Godolphin, W., Jones, L.A. *et al.* (1989) Studies of HER-2/*neu* proto-oncogene in human breast and ovarian cancer. *Science*, **244**, 707–12.
10. Berchuck, A., Kamel, A., Whitaker, R. *et al.* (1990) Overexpression of HER-2/*neu* is associated with poor survival in advanced epithelial ovarian cancer. *Cancer Res.*, **50**, 4087–91.
11. Marks, J.R., Davidoff, A.M., Kerns, B.J.M. *et al.* (1991) Overexpression and mutation of p53 in epithelial ovarian cancer. *Cancer Res.*, **51**, 2979–84.
12. Berchuck, A., Rodriguez, G.C., Kamel, A. *et al.* (1991) Epidermal growth factor receptor expression in normal ovarian epithelium and ovarian cancer. I. Correlation of receptor expression with prognostic factors in patients with ovarian cancer. *Am. J. Obstet. Gynecol.*, **164**, 669–74.
13. Brown-Shimer, S., Johnson, K.A., Hill, D.E. *et al.* (1992) Effect of protein tyrosine phosphatase 1B expression on transformation by the human *neu* oncogene. *Cancer Res.*, **52**, 478–82.

14. Wiener, J.R., Hurteau, J.A., Whitaker, R.S. *et al.* (1993) Overexpression of the protein tyrosine phosphatase PTP1B in human ovarian carcinomas. *Proc. Am. Assoc. Cancer Res.*, **34**, 527.

15. Ramakrishnan, S., Xu, F.J., Brandt, S.J. *et al.* (1989) Constitutive production of macrophage colony-stimulating factor by human ovarian and breast cancer cell lines. *J.Clin. Invest.*, **83**, 921–6.

16. Lidor, Y.J., Xu, F.J., Martínez-Maza, O. *et al.* (1993) Constitutive production of macrophage colony stimulating factor and interleukin-6 by human ovarian surface epithelial cells. *Exp. Cell Res.*, **207**, 332–9.

17. Wu, S., Boyer, C.M., Whitaker, R. *et al.* (1993) Tumor necrosis factor-alpha (TNF-α) as an autocrine and paracrine growth factor for ovarian cancer: monokine induction of tumor cell proliferation and TNF-α expression. *Cancer Res.*, **53**, 1939–44.

18. Wu, S., Meeker, W.A., Wiener, J.R. *et al.* (1994) Transfection of ovarian cancer cells with tumor necrosis factor-alpha (TNF-α) antisense mRNA abolishes the proliferative response to interleukin-1 (IL-1) but not TNF-α. *Gynecol. Oncol.*, in press.

19. Balkwill, F., Osborne, R., Burke, F. *et al.* (1987) Evidence for tumor necrosis factor/cachectin production in cancer. *Lancet*, **2**, 1229–32.

20. Malik, S.T.A., Naylor, M.S., Balkwill, F.R. (1992) Cytokines and ovarian cancer. In *Ovarian Cancer 2: Biology, Diagnosis and Management*, (eds F. Sharp, W.P. Mason and W. Creasman), Chapman & Hall, London, pp. 87–92.

Chapter 12

TNF, LT and IL-1 natural inhibitors (soluble receptors and receptor antagonists) in women with ovarian cancer

G. GRANGER, T. GATANAGA, R. BURGER, E. GROSEN, M. BERMAN and P. DiSAIA

Cell mediated immunity (CMI) is an important element of host antitumor resistance mechanisms. Tumor necrosis factor (TNF), lymphotoxin (LT) and interleukin-1 (IL-1) are key cytokines used by host effector lymphoid cells to orchestrate recognition, tissue destructive and inflammatory phases of these important reactions [1–4]. These molecules have multiple effects on cells *in vitro* and tissues *in vivo*. Some of these effects which are important for tumor regression are:

1. Cytolysis of certain transformed cells
2. Destruction of tumor blood vessels
3. Upregulation of surface proteins making tumor cells more immunogenic
4. Induce, recruit and activate host lymphoid cells to express antitumor activity
5. Induce inflammation
6. Leukocytosis [1–4].

It is clear that a major portion of the antitumor effects of these molecules involves activation of host antitumor mechanisms. However, low levels of TNF could induce localized effects in the tumor cell itself which could promote tumor growth.

Recent results indicate there are natural inhibitors that can control the biological activity of TNF, LT and IL-1 locally and systematically once they have been released by effector cells [1,2,5–7]. The mechanisms involved are not yet clearly understood, but cells can release the extracellular domain of both 55 and 75 kd TNF membrane receptors (TNFR). The soluble forms of TNFR are 30 and 40 kd respectively and have been termed TNF/LT binding proteins (TNF-BP) [5,6]. Many types of cells express both 55 and 75 kd TNF membrane receptors; however, one may predominate depending upon the cell type. Cells can also actively secrete an IL-1 receptor antagonist (IL-1RA) [1,2]. Both TNF-BP and IL-1RA can specifically bind to and block cytokine binding to specific cell membrane receptors. It is clear that the biologic activity of TNF, LT and IL-1 can be blocked by these inhibitors both *in vitro* and *in vivo* [1,2,7]. The interaction of cytokine and inhibitor is a stoichiometric reaction and inhibition occurs when there is a 3- to 5-fold molar excess of inhibitors over the level of cytokines. These soluble forms of membrane receptors are potent natural cytokine inhibitors. ELISA and immunohistochemical assays are now available to detect and establish levels of TNF, LT and IL-1 and their natural inhibitors. Thus, by measuring levels of the cytokines and their inhibitors, it is possible to establish the reactive status of a local tissue site and/or sample. For example, if the concentration of the TNF-BP or IL-R antagonist is in excess, the cytokine is not biologically active; however, if the cytokine is in excess, it would be active.

Our laboratory identified and characterized TNF-BP in the serum of patients with various types of cancer [7,9]. These BP are biologically active and block recombinant human TNF and LT activity *in vitro*. Similar results were subsequently reported by Aderka *et al.* [10]. We present results of our ongoing studies of natural inhibitors for TNF/LT and IL-1 in women with ovarian cancers that focus on the role of natural inhibitors as: a) a serum test that can be used to help detect women with ovarian cancer and monitor the response of this disease to therapy; and b) possible immunomodulatory agents in the interaction of the tumor with host effector mechanisms in the peritoneal cavity of these patients.

The results of serum testing are shown in Figure 12.1a and 12.1b [11].

ELISA measurement of 55 and 75 kd TNF-BP in serum can distinguish women with active disease from normal women and from women with inactive disease. These results are highly statistically significant. Table 12.1 is a comparison of the sensitivity, specificity and predictability of levels of TNF-BP when compared to CA-125 tested on the same samples. While the data are not shown, we found that serial serum TNF-BP levels can also be used to monitor residual disease and recurrence in women receiving therapy. Serum TNF-BP levels were equal to or more accurate than CA-125 levels assayed on the same samples. While not tumor specific, serum levels of TNF-BP, when used with other techniques, may provide a new method to both detect and monitor women with this disease. Finally, serum levels of TNF measured by ELISA in normal women and women with ovarian cancer are in the range of 20–30 pg/ml^{-1}. Comparison of TNF-BP and

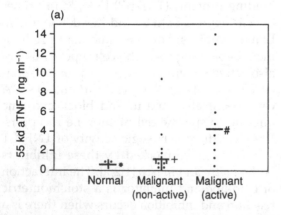 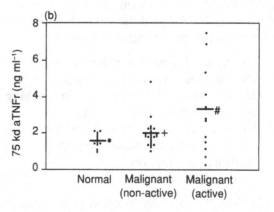

Figure 12.1 (a) Comparison of the mean serum levels of the 55 kd sTNFr between normal individuals *(0.065 ± 0.22 ng/ml), patients with non-active ovarian cancer + (1.17 ± 1.47 ng/ml, n.s.) and patients with active ovarian cancer, # (4.31 ± 4.61 ng/ml, $p<0.01$). Difference between non-active and active groups was significant at $p<0.01$. (b) Comparison of mean serum levels of the 75 kd sTNFr between normal individuals * (1.62 ± 0.37 ng/ml), patients with non-active ovarian cancer, +(2.02 ± 1.49 ng/ml, n.s.) and patients with active ovarian cancer, # (3.39 ± 1.49 ng/ml, $p<0.001$). Difference between non-active and active groups was significant at $p<0.001$.

Table 12.1 Comparison of the sensitivity, specificity and predictability of 55 and 75 kd TNF-BP and CA-125 values to distinguish between normal women and women with active disease.

	CA-125	55 kd sTNFr	75 kd sTNFr
Sensitivity	75%	83%	77%
Specificity	71%	71%	95%
+ Pred. value	43%	45%	83%
– Pred. value	91%	94%	95%

Table 12.2 Cytokine and cytokine inhibitors in malignant ascites.

Cytokine inhibitor	Mean concentration	Standard deviation	Range
TNF	Undetectable	N/A	N/A
LT	Undetectable	N/A	N/A
IL-1B	2.9 pg ml^{-1}	5.7	(0–17)
IFN-γ	69.4 pg ml^{-1}	121	(0–343)
55 kd sTNFr	2.6 ng ml^{-1}	0.5	(1.9–3.4)
75 kd sTNFr	4.3 ng ml^{-1}	0.5	(3.6–5.3)
IL-1ra	1.2 ng ml^{-1}	1.6	(0.04–7.4)
1L-6	3.3 ng ml^{-1}	4.6	(0.04–20.4)

TNF serum levels indicates the serum TNF is inactive, which was supported by the findings that these sera block TNF activity and fail to detect cytolytically active TNF in these samples.

Additional studies indicate that natural inhibitors for TNF, LT and IL-1 dominate the ascites from women with ovarian cancer [12]. Table 12.2 is a summary of results obtained from the ELISA analysis of ascites from 15 women. With the exception of IL-6, the levels of cytokines, i.e. TNF and IL-1 , are very low when compared to levels of 55 and 75 kd TNF-BP and IL-1 receptor antagonist. The molar excess of inhibitors supports the concept that the environment in the ascites is very inhibitory for these cytokines. Additional studies that prove this concept are: a) no cytolytically active TNF or LT was detectable in ascites samples; and b) the

ascites was inhibitory when added to recombinant human TNF and LT in *in vitro* assays.

Studies are ongoing to determine the cell and tissue source of these cytokine inhibitors in the ascites [12]. One to three day primary cultures of both ascites cells and solid tumor nodules from these women were established. Supernatants were collected and assayed for both cytokines and cytokine inhibitors. A partial summary is shown in Table 12.3. Cells in these cultures vary from patient to patient in their ability to spontaneously release TNF and IL-1; however, with the exception of patients 5 and 7, all samples release high levels of both TNF-BP and IL-RA. In additional studies, we found that human continuous ovarian carcinoma cell lines spontaneously produce high levels of TNF-BP *in vitro* [13]. Studies are underway to establish which cells in ascites and tumor nodules are

Table 12.3 Comparison of inhibitory activity with TNF receptor levels and TNF levels*

Patient/ culture source	Inhibitory activity**		TNF/LT receptor levels in pg ml^{-1}		TNF levels in pg ml^{-1}
	TNF	LT	55 kd	75 kd	
4. Ascites Cells	++++	++++	2000	4500	25
4. CFA†		+++	2100	4750	20
4. Solid tumor	+	++	2050	500	30
6. Solid tumor	++	++	2050	1250	40
7. Ascites cells	++	++	650	3100	1350
7. Solid tumor	+	++	<16	0	>1600
7. CFA	+	++	1600	3700	19
8. Solid tumor	+	+++	<16	<16	>1600
8. CFA	+	++++	3520	5500	22
9. Ascites cells	++	+++	700	1200	NA
9. CFA	+	+++	1700	1700	NA
10. CFA	+++	+++	1300	2100	NA
11. Solid tumor	lytic	lytic	<16	2150	NA
11. CFA	++	++	3700	5800	NA
55 kd			>10,000	0	
75 kd			0	>10,000	

* Samples of cell-free ascites and culture supernatants from both solid tumor and ascites cells were tested for the presence of the 55 and 75 kd TNF/LT receptors and TNF by ELISA. These results are in comparison to the inhibitory activity of the samples on the L929 *in vitro* cytolytic assay
** Refer to Table 12.2 for description of data from cytolytic assay
† Cell-free ascites

releasing these inhibitors and what stimulates inhibitor release over the levels of cytokines.

These studies indicate there are elevated levels of 55 and 75 kd TNF-BP in serum from women with ovarian cancer. Serum levels of 55 and 75 kd TNF-BP may be a new method, when used with other techniques, to both detect and monitor patients with ovarian cancer. The ascites in women with ovarian cancer also has high levels of TNF-BP and IL-1R antagonist and low levels of the corresponding cytokines. It appears these inhibitors are produced locally in the peritoneal cavity by both ascites cells and cells from solid tumor nodules.

Natural inhibitors for TNF/LT and IL-1 may have profound effects on the tumor–host interaction both locally and systemically. These inhibitors in ascites and serum may block the ability of TNF/LT and IL-1 released by effector cells in the ascites and solid tumor nodules to recruit and activate host antitumor mechanisms. In addition, these inhibitors could suppress cytokine production and activation of both lymphocytes and macrophages in the peritoneal cavity. These molecules create an environment in the peritoneal cavity that could be immunosuppressive and restrict TNF, LT and IL-1 effects to highly localized areas not accessible to these inhibitors. Thus, only low levels of TNF may be produced and only be effective in highly localized microenvironments not accessible to inhibitors. The end result could be an environment that is highly favorable for tumor progression and profoundly immunosuppressive. Additional studies are underway to further examine these issues.

REFERENCES

1. Dinarello, C. (1991) Interleukin-1 and inter-leukin-1 receptor antagonist. *Blood*, **77**, 1627–52.
2. Conti, P. (1991) Interleukin-1 and interleukin-1 receptor antagonist. *Ann. Med. Int.*, **142**, 521–5.
3. Beutler, B. and Cerami, A. (1989) The biology of cachectin/TNF a primary mediator of the host response. *Ann. Rev. Immunol.*, **7**, 625–55.
4. Old, L. (1990) Tumor necrosis factor. In *Tumor Necrosis Factor: Structure Mechanisms of Action, Role in Disease and Therapy*, (eds B. Bonavida and G. Granger), Karger, Basel, pp. 1–30.
5. Peetre, C., Thysell, H., Grubb, A. and Olsson, I. (1988) A TNF binding protein is present in human biological fluids. *Eur. J. Haematol.*, **41**, 414–19.
6. Engelmann, H., Aderka, D., Rubenstein, M. *et al.* (1989) A TNF binding protein purified to homogeneity protects cells from TNF toxicity. *J. Biol. Chem.*, **264**, 11974–80.
7. Gatanaga, T., Hwang, C., Kohr, B. *et al.* (1990) Purification and characterization of an inhibitor for TNF and LT from the serum ultrafiltrates from human cancer patients. *PNAS USA*, **87**, 8781–4.
8. Olsson, I., Gatanaga, T., Gullberg, U. *et al.* (1993) TNF binding proteins (soluble TNF receptor forms) with possible roles in inflammation and malignancy. *Eur. Cytokine Netw.*, **4**, 169–80.
9. Gatanaga, T., Lentz, R., Masunaka, I. *et al.* (1990) Identification of TNF-LT blocking factors in the serum ultrafiltrates of human cancer patients. *Lymphokine Res.*, **9**, 225–9.
10. Aderka, D., Englemann, H., Shemer-Avoni, Y. *et al.* (1992) Increased levels of soluble TNF receptors for TNF in cancer patients. *Cancer Res.*, **51**, 5602–7.
11. Grosen, E., Granger, G., Gatanaga, M. *et al.* (1993) Measurement of soluble receptors for TNF and LT in the sera of patients with gynecologic malignancy. *Gynecol. Oncol.*, in press.
12. Grosen, E., Yamamoto, R., Ioli, G. *et al.* (1992) Blocking factors for TNF and LT detected in ascites and released by short term cultures obtained from ascites and solid tumors in women with gynecologic malignancy. *Lymphokine Cytokine Res.*, **11**, 347–53.
13. Gatanaga, M., Gatanaga, T. and Granger, G. (1993) Production of TNF and LT binding proteins by human ovarian cancer cell lines *in vitro. Lymphokine Cytokine Res.*, **12**, 249–53.

Chapter 13

Activation of human ovarian cancer cells: role of lipid factors in ascitic fluid

Y. XU and G.B. MILLS

13.1 INTRODUCTION

Normal cells proliferate in response to injury or to replace cells with a limited survival time. This is true for cells in the hematopoietic system and epithelial cells of the skin and bowel. It has been estimated that 1 million cell divisions per second are required for the replacement of lost cells. The proliferation of normal cells is regulated by the action of a number of polypeptide and lipid factors called growth factors [1–8]. These growth factors bind to specific cell surface receptors and transmit activation signals across the cell membrane. These signals initiate a limited number of intracellular biochemical cascades which in turn communicate with the nucleus, eventually leading to cellular proliferation [5–8]. In addition to positive growth signals, a series of proteins is involved in limiting cellular proliferation [9–10]. Several of these, such as p53 and the product of the retinoblastoma gene (RB), are more commonly known as tumor suppressor genes [9,10]. Finally, some activated cells are sensitized to a physiological process known as programmed cell death or apoptosis [11–13]. Both the products of tumor suppressor genes and the products of the genes involved in programmed cell death must be overcome for a cell to divide.

Malignant cells can proliferate independent of the normal growth signals received from the extracellular environment [1–8]. However, in many cases, extracellular growth mediators can modify the proliferative response of malignant cells. Strikingly, the response of malignant cells to growth factors and growth inhibitors is frequently different from that of their normal counterparts. In the multistep process leading to cancer, it is likely that activation of growth factor signalling pathways, inactivation of tumor suppressor genes and bypassing of programmed cell death constitute at least three of these stages. Indeed, oncogenes, those genes which are associated with tumorigenesis, are either growth factors, growth factor receptors or components of the pathways activated by growth factors [1–8]. Oncogenes function as dominant mediators due to a 'gain of function' [1–8]. Proto-oncogenes, the normal cellular counterparts of oncogenes, can acquire an oncogenic function through mutation or aberrant production, resulting in elevated levels, aberrant time of production or production by inappropriate cells. In contrast, tumor suppressor genes must be inactivated by a 'loss of function' and therefore were frequently designated recessive oncogenes [9,10]. The p53 gene, which is a tumor suppressor and normally inhibits cellular growth by cell cycle arrest in G1, was first characterized as an oncogene. Once it became apparent that loss of p53 function played a role in tumor formation, p53 was reclassified as a tumor suppressor [9,10]. Similarly, BCL2, which functions to prevent programmed cell death, was initially characterized as an oncogene [11].

In ovarian cancer, it is possible that the process leading to malignancy is associated with cellular repair following ovulation [see references in 14–17]. Ovulation results in damage which is repaired, at least in part, by proliferation of surface ovarian epithelial cells. During this period, the ovarian epithelial cells not only proliferate but are exposed to a number of growth factors. In addition, the repair process may result in epithelial cells being trapped within the stroma of the ovary, exposing them to a different environment than they would normally experience on the ovarian surface. This may explain data which suggest that frequent ovulation is associated with an increased incidence of ovarian cancer and processes that prevent ovulation, such as the birth control pill or pregnancy, decrease the incidence of ovarian cancer [see references in 14–16]. Elegant studies in a rat model have demonstrated that increased number of cell divisions of cultured ovarian epithelial cells results in an increased ability to grow under conditions that are thought to be pathognomonic of transformation [16]. Thus, it appears that the 'wear and tear' associated with ovulation could lead to a decreased sensitivity to the processes regulating normal cell growth by activating proto-oncogenes, inactivating tumor suppressor genes or bypassing programmed cell death. This, in turn, may provide the first or an essential step in tumorigenesis of ovarian epithelium.

Because many tumor cells will grow at their site of origin (orthotopic) but not at other sites (ectopic), it is likely that paracrine factors play a major role in regulating tumor cell growth. Many different tumor derived growth factors including transforming growth factor alpha (TGF-α), transforming growth factor beta (TGF-β) and platelet derived growth factor (PDGF) have been identified in the supernatants of cultured tumor cells [1–8]. These factors frequently appear to be required for the *in vitro* and probably the *in vivo* growth of the tumor cells that produce them. Because interstitial fluid is present in small amounts and it is difficult to isolate, it has been difficult to characterize the growth factors to which tumor cells are normally exposed *in vivo*. Ascitic fluid from ovarian cancer patients provides a unique opportunity to characterize the environment of tumor cells *in vivo*. Ascitic fluid contains not only large numbers of viable tumor cells but also significant numbers of infiltrating hematopoietic cells and mesothelial cells [17–19]. Each of these cells is capable of producing factors that can alter the growth of the ovarian cancer cells [14,17–19]. We have demonstrated that the lymphoid cells in the peritoneal cavity are activated as evidenced by high levels of the soluble activation marker Tac in ascites and in serum of patients [17,20]. Ascitic fluid has been demonstrated to contain significant quantities of previously characterized growth factors including interleukins 1, 6, and 10, macrophage colony stimulating factor (mCSF), TGF-α, TGF-β and tumor necrosis factor alpha (TNF-α) [see references in 14, 17–19]. Each of these factors can increase the proliferation of at least some ovarian cancer cell lines and has the potential to induce proliferation of ovarian tumor cells *in vivo*. Thus, ascitic fluid may provide a 'window' to characterize the growth factors to which tumor cells are exposed *in vivo*.

13.2 OVARIAN CANCER ASCITES CONTAINS POTENT GROWTH FACTOR ACTIVITY

We have demonstrated that ascites from ovarian cancer patients contains potent growth factor activity [14,18,19]. Ascitic fluid from various ovarian cancer patients is able to support the proliferation of cell lines both from ovarian cancer and from other lineages at 10 to 1000-fold lower levels than fetal calf serum which is considered the 'gold standard' for growth factor containing media [18]. At high concentrations (5–10%), ascites from approximately 25% of patients is growth inhibitory for ovarian cancer cells. Nevertheless, on further dilution, ascites from these patients exhibits a potent growth supporting activity [18]. Human ovarian cancer ascites allows proliferation (colony formation or thymidine incorporation) of both freshly isolated ovarian cancer cells and ovarian cancer cell lines, but does not on its own induce proliferation of normal resting human peripheral blood lymphocytes [18,19]. However, ascites will allow the proliferation of activated peripheral blood lymphocytes or lymphoid cell lines. Therefore, at least in the case of lymphocytes, it appears that ascites permits expression of cell growth induced by other agents rather than directly inducing cell growth. Whether this reflects the effect of ascitic fluid on the growth of ovarian cancer cells remains to be determined. The growth promoting activity of ascites is not present at lower levels in ascites from patients with benign diseases including hepatic cirrhosis and idiopathic ascites [18]. Furthermore, normal peritoneal fluid or fluid from individuals with endometriosis has a lower level of activity in inducing proliferation of ovarian cancer cells.

To determine whether ascites may play a role in the *in vivo* growth of human tumor cells, we used the observation that many human ovarian adenocarcinoma lines, including the HEY cell line, will grow subcutaneously but not intraperitoneally in mice [21]. This appeared to be in contradistinction to the normal growth pattern of ovarian cancer cells that tend to remain restricted to the peritoneal cavity: spontaneous subcutaneous metastases

are uncommon. Furthermore, many tumors will grow in orthotopic sites but not ectopic sites. A short course of intraperitoneal injections of semipurified human ascitic fluid allowed the intraperitoneal growth of HEY ovarian cancer cells in immunodeficient nude mice [21]. In the absence of ascitic fluid from ovarian cancer patients or in the presence of ascitic fluid with inhibitory action on cell growth *in vitro*, intraperitoneal growth was not detected in nude mice injected with HEY cells. Ascites from mice that developed intraperitoneal tumors contained high levels of growth promoting activity for HEY cells *in vitro* [21]. In addition, HEY tumor cells isolated from the peritoneal cavity of the nude mice gained the ability to grow in the peritoneal cavity of additional mice in the absence of exogenous ascitic fluid [21]. Whether this represents selection of an existing subpopulation of cells or the acquisition of new properties has not been analysed.

13.3 SIGNAL TRANSDUCTION BY GROWTH FACTORS

As described above, transmembrane signals from both polypeptide and lipid growth factors converge on a limited number of intracellular activation cascades [1–8]. Although the initial signalling events may be different, the downstream activation cascades are often the same. The most immediate event following the activation of the receptors by their specific ligand appears to be activation of either intracellular kinases or activation of heterotrimeric GTP binding or G proteins [1–8]. Intriguingly, many of the growth factor receptors contain intrinsic kinase domains that directly link the receptor to an intracellular enzyme. However, in the case of receptors that link to G proteins and many of the receptors that activate intracellular kinases, the receptor and the intracellular mediator are encoded in two separate peptide chains [1–8].

123

Most of the receptors that link to intracellular G proteins have a conserved domain 7-membrane-spanning structure. Surprisingly, many of the growth factor receptors, regardless of whether they link to G proteins or to tyrosine kinases, stimulate the phosphoinositol pathway. The phosphoinositol pathway consists of hydrolysis of membrane phosphatidylinositols by a specific phospholipase C (PLC). With receptors that link to tyrosine kinases, PLCγ is activated by tyrosine phosphorylation and with receptors that link to G proteins, PLCβ is activated [1–8].

Both PLC forms induce the production of two intracellular second messengers, inositol trisphosphate and diacylglycerol. Inositol trisphosphate binds to and activates inositol triphosphate receptors in the endoplasmic reticulum resulting in release of calcium from intracellular stores that leads to a rapid increase in intracellular free calcium ($[Ca^{2+}]_i$). Diacylglycerol activates protein kinase C (PKC). Hydrolysis of membrane phosphatidylinositol bisphosphate by PLC appears to be the only source of inositol trisphosphate for changes in $[Ca^{2+}]_i$. In contrast, hydrolysis of several different membrane phospholipids can produce diacylglycerol. The bifurcating PLC pathway activates many of the intracellular events that lead to growth and proliferation [1–8]. In many cell types, receptor mediated signalling can be bypassed by pharmacological activation of increases in $[Ca^{2+}]_i$ and of PKC. Furthermore, many of the known tumor promoters are potent activators of PKC. Thus, these pathways appear to play a major role in cell activation and proliferation.

13.4 SIGNAL TRANSDUCTION BY ASCITIC FLUID

In all patients tested (>50), ascites from ovarian cancer stimulated a transient intracellular calcium release in freshly isolated ovarian cancer cells and cell lines [18]. This may be an acquired characteristic of the tumor cells as ascites does not appear to induce an increase in $[Ca^{2+}]_i$ in normal ovarian epithelial cells. Although ascites induces increases in $[Ca^{2+}]_i$ in mesangial cells, fibroblasts, *Xenopus* oocytes and some malignant lymphoid cell lines, ascites does not induce a change in $[Ca^{2+}]_i$ in peripheral blood lymphocytes or in lymphocytes isolated from the peritoneal cavity of ovarian cancer patients [18,19]. The calcium changing activity of ascites is not found or is present at much lower levels in ascites associated with benign diseases including hepatic cirrhosis and idiopathic ascites [18]. Furthermore, normal peritoneal fluid or fluid from individuals with endometriosis has a decreased ability to induce changes in $[Ca^{2+}]_i$ in ovarian cancer cells.

Ascitic fluid induces both release of calcium from intracellular stores and transmembrane uptake [18]. The calcium response to ascites is associated with phosphatidylinositol turnover and inositol trisphosphate production that is pathognomonic for activation of PLC [18]. In contrast, ascites does not induce detectable increases in tyrosine phosphorylation in ovarian cancer cells under conditions in which increases in tyrosine phosphorylation induced by epidermal growth factor or other ligands were readily detect- able. Furthermore, tyrosine kinase inhibitors that block increases in $[Ca^{2+}]_i$ mediated through tyrosine kinase coupled receptors [22,23] did not block calcium changes induced by ascites. Taken together, the data suggest that PLCβ rather than PLCγ is activated by ascites. They also suggest that ascites links to PLCβ through a receptor containing the 7-membrane-spanning motif through the intermediacy of a heterotrimeric G protein.

Ascites appears to signal $[Ca^{2+}]_i$ increases through binding and activating specific cell surface receptors. This hypothesis is supported by the observation that ascites increase $[Ca^{2+}]_i$ in a limited spectrum of cell lineages. In addition, growth factors can be eluted in many cases from their receptors by incubation at low pH. When fresh ovarian cancer cells were first incubated with ascites and then washed extensively in a buffer of neutral pH, the supernatant did not alter $[Ca^{2+}]_i$ in either fresh ovarian cancer cells or in HEY cells [18]. In contrast, when ovarian cancer cells were incubated with fresh ascitic fluid, washed extensively and then acid-treated, the acid eluate increased $[Ca^{2+}]_i$. Supernatants from similarly treated normal lymphoid cells did not alter intracellular calcium in ovarian cancer cells, suggesting that normal lymphoid cells not only do not respond but also do not express a high affinity receptor for the $[Ca^{2+}]_i$ mobilizing factor [18].

In light of its ability to increase $[Ca^{2+}]_i$ in ovarian cancer cells, its presence at high levels in ascitic fluid and the association of increases in $[Ca^{2+}]_i$ with action of growth factors, we have designated the factor which increases $[Ca^{2+}]_i$ in ascites fluid as ovarian cancer ascites factor (OCAF). To elucidate the relationship between OCAF and other growth promoting factors in ascites will require further purification and characterization of OCAF. Similarly, whether OCAF is the factor that induces proliferation of ovarian cancer cells in the nude mouse model [21] or in the *in vitro* models described above [18] will require further studies with purified material.

13.5 CHARACTERIZATION OF THE MEDIATOR THAT INCREASES $[Ca^{2+}]_i$

In order to further define the identity of OCAF, we have tested many known peptide growth factors and lipid mediators, as well as performing purification and enzymatic analysis. In most cases, we have used changes in $[Ca^{2+}]_i$ as assessed by cytofluorimetry with the intracellular calcium sensitive dye, indo-1

(Figure 13.1). This technique has the potential to be a sensitive assay to detect the presence of unique growth factors because:

1. Intracellular calcium release is associated with action of many growth factors;
2. Many cellular regulatory enzymes are sensitive to intracellular calcium concentrations;

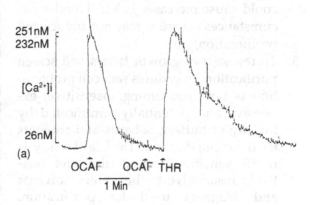

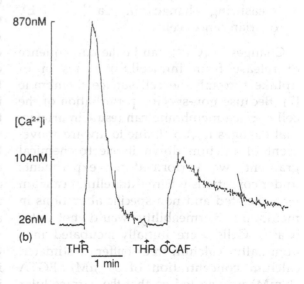

Figure 13.1 Effect of OCAF and thrombin on $[Ca^{2+}]_i$ in HEY cells. $[Ca^{2+}]_i$ response to sequential addition of the partially purified OCAF (10 μl) and thrombin (0.1 U) (a); or addition of thrombin followed by OCAF (b).

3. Calcium levels are tightly regulated and thus calcium has the potential to be a signalling molecule;

4. More than one growth factor activity may be required to induce a proliferative response so that a purified factor may induce a limited amount of cell proliferation because a required co-factor such as a competence or progression factor is missing. In contrast, a single growth factor could cause increases in $[Ca^{2+}]_i$ under circumstances where it may not induce cell proliferation;

5. To test known growth factors and screen purification procedures with cell proliferation is time consuming, insensitive, expensive and potentially complicated by toxicity of buffers, solvents and reagents used for purification. The $[Ca^{2+}]_i$ assay is rapid, sensitive, reproducible and relatively insensitive to the buffers, solvents and reagents used for purification. Therefore, we have screened known compounds and our purification procedure by measuring changes in $[Ca^{2+}]_i$ in HEY ovarian cancer cells.

Changes in $[Ca^{2+}]_i$ can be the consequence of release from intracellular stores or of uptake through the cell surface membrane [7]. Because non-specific perturbation of the cell surface membrane can result in artefactual changes in $[Ca^{2+}]_i$ due to inward movement of calcium down its electrochemical gradient, we performed the experiments under conditions where extracellular calcium was chelated and non-specific alterations in membrane permeability would not alter $[Ca^{2+}]_i$. Cells were initially incubated in a nominally calcium-free buffer (estimated calcium concentration of 50 μM). EGTA (1 mM) was added so that the extracellular free calcium was lower than 10 nM. Any observed increases in calcium are due to release from intracellular stores and are less sensitive to artefacts.

13.6 COMPARISON OF OCAF WITH POLYPEPTIDE GROWTH FACTORS AND HORMONES

The following peptide growth factors, vasoactive agents, hormones and neurotransmitters have been assessed in calcium release assays in HEY ovarian cancer cells: epidermal growth factor (EGF), TGF-α, TGF-β, insulin-like growth factor I and II (IGF-I and II), tumor necrosis factor alpha (TNF-α), PDGF, insulin, IL-1, 2 and 8, α and β interferons, leukemia inhibitory factor (LIF), acidic and basic fibroblast growth factor, fibrinogen, vasopressin, angiotensin, bombesin, bradykinin, estrogen, progesterone, testosterone, human chorionic gonadotropin, follicle stimulating hormone, luteinizing hormone and glucocorticoids. None of these factors induced a detectable increase in $[Ca^{2+}]_i$ under conditions wherein ascites fluid or semipurified OCAF induced marked changes. In addition, although OCAF desensitized its own activity (Figure 13.1), none of these factors altered the ability of OCAF to induce increases in $[Ca^{2+}]_i$. In support of the suggestion that OCAF was different from these polypeptide mediators, the effects of these factors on the proliferation of HEY cells were minor, being within two or three-fold of background. In contrast, ascites induced a five to tenfold increase in [^{3}H] thymidine incorporation. It remains to be determined whether the failure of these factors to induce marked increases in cellular proliferation indicates that ascites contains multiple additional growth factors or whether an appropriate combination of the factors listed above would be more efficacious.

Thrombin was the only peptide growth factor that stimulated a transient $[Ca^{2+}]_i$ increase in HEY cells. Thrombin is an intriguing mediator because it is a serine protease that functions by cleaving the terminus of its specific receptor [24]. The remainder of the receptor is then able to 'flip back' on itself and activate changes in $[Ca^{2+}]_i$. The functional portion of the receptor contains the 7-membrane-spanning motif and couples to a heterotrimeric G protein [24].

To address the question of whether OCAF is thrombin, homologous desensitization and inhibitor studies were performed. Figure 13.1 shows the $[Ca^{2+}]_i$ response to sequential addition of partially purified OCAF (10 μl) followed by thrombin (0.1 U) (A); or addition of thrombin followed by OCAF (B) to 10^6 indo-1-loaded HEY ovarian cancer cells suspended in 1.7 ml of buffer. A single administration of semipurified OCAF totally inhibits or desensitizes the response to additional OCAF. In contrast, the OCAF desensitized cells retain responsiveness to the effects of thrombin. The same was true when thrombin was added first. Pretreatment of thrombin and OCAF with 0.01 U of the specific thrombin inhibitor, antithrombin, blocked thrombin-induced calcium mobilization completely while OCAF induced increases in $[Ca^{2+}]_i$ were not affected, indicating that OCAF is not thrombin. Furthermore, a non-specific serine protease inhibitor PMSF totally blocked the action of thrombin without having any significant effects on the action of OCAF, suggesting that OCAF is not a serine protease.

13.7 OCAF APPEARS TO BE A LIPID

Although our original characterization suggested that OCAF could be a polypeptide [18], more extensive characterization suggests that it is a lipid and most likely a phospholipid with a glycerol backbone. Our initial confusion appears to have resulted from two factors. First, we have found that OCAF purifies as a protein through purification techniques including reverse phase chromatography, isoelectric focusing and other column chromatographic methods. Second, in solvent extraction tests, the OCAF activity in crude ascites partitioned into the aqueous phase (MeOH/H_2O phase), which is different from most other lipids. Both these observations are probably due to a tight association of OCAF with serum albumin and/or other proteins. It is even possible that OCAF has a specific protein carrier.

After a 20 000-fold increase in specific activity based on the $[Ca^{2+}]_i$ release activity and prot- ein concentration, we have found that OCAF is stable to the action of proteases including bromelain, carboxypeptidase Y, peptidase, pepsin, papain, pronase E, protease V8, proteinase K, stromelysin, thermolysin and trypsin. Furthermore, OCAF was stable under some quite drastic conditions, such as boiling, extremes of pH and detergent treatment that should destroy proteins. We have also found that this partially purified OCAF is soluble in 80% acetone and 100% MeOH, further suggesting that OCAF could be a lipid.

13.8 THE BIOLOGICAL SIGNIFICANCE OF LIPID MEDIATORS IN SIGNAL TRANSDUCTION AND CELL PROLIFERATION

Lipids had been thought to play primarily structural functions in biological systems. However, evidence implicating lipids in intracellular signalling functions (such as membrane phospholipids in intracellular $[Ca^{2+}]_i$ regulation, activation of PKC, regulation by arachidonic acid and its metabolites, prostaglandins and leukotrienes) has altered many of our original concepts [7,25,26]. In addition, more recent studies have demonstrated that phospholipids, such as platelet activating factor (PAF) and lysophosphatidic acid (LPA), have the potential to be extracellular growth factors acting on specific receptors inducing cell activation and cellular proliferation at very low concentrations [25,26].

PAF induces rapid increases in $[Ca^{2+}]_i$ through the apparent intermediacy of a heterotrimeric G protein and PLC [33,34].

Indeed, cloning of the PAF receptor demonstrated that it contains the 7-membrane-spanning motif and thus directly couples to an intracellular G protein [33,34]. The PAF receptor exhibits a high affinity and is also expressed on a limited number of cell types, perhaps explaining the response patterns of these cells.

LPA has been demonstrated to induce rapid increases in $[Ca^{2+}]_i$ through the intermediacy of G proteins and the phosphoinositol pathway [32,35,36]. Strikingly, LPA is much more efficient than EGF at inducing proliferation in fibroblasts, making it the most potent of known growth factors for fibroblasts. The relationship between LPA induced increases in $[Ca^{2+}]_i$ and proliferation is unclear; however, it is clear that LPA induced increases in $[Ca^{2+}]_i$ are not sufficient or obligatory for cell growth. Phosphatidic acid (PA) is a potent mitogen in fibroblasts and induces increases in $[Ca^{2+}]_i$ in some cell types [36]. However, whether some of the effects of PA are due to LPA contaminating commercial PA preparations is controversial.

Other lysophospholipids have been noted to have a variety of signalling activities. For example, lysophosphatidylcholine (LPC) and lysophosphatidylglycerol (LPG) have been shown to induce Ca^{2+} efflux from mitochondria [27]. LPC and lysophosphatidylinositol (LPI) stimulate insulin release from pancreatic islet cells [28]. Lysophosphatidylserine (LPS) has been shown to increase histamine release from mast cells through the intermediacy of PLC and the phosphoinositol pathway [29].

Sphingolipids, including gangoliosides, particularly sphingosine, sphingosine-1-phosphate and sphingosylphosphorylcholine (SPC), have also been shown to be involved in regulation of protein kinase C, growth factor receptor function and cell growth [30,31]. More recently, ceramide, a derivative of sphingomyelin, has been proposed to be the mediator of signalling through the IL1 and TNF-α receptors.

Several different classes of lipids have been demonstrated to be involved directly or indirectly in cell activation and proliferation. Several of these mediators are more effective than peptide growth factors at inducing cell growth. Some of the characterized lipids appear to signal through the intermediacy of PLCβ and $[Ca^{2+}]_i$, suggesting that this may be a common signalling pathway.

13.9 OCAF PURIFICATION

Unlike most other lipids, OCAF partitions into the aqueous/methanol phase in standard lipid purification protocols [37,38]. This could be due to a strong association between OCAF and human serum albumin and/or other proteins normally present in ascites. This may also be due to the association of OCAF with a specific carrier protein. It appears likely that this association is non-covalent; however, we cannot eliminate the possibility that OCAF is an unusual proteolipid. Due to its association with protein carriers, OCAF can be highly purified by a combination of columns designed for protein purification. Sequential passage over C8 reverse phase column, Prep-Cell (a preparative polyacrylamide electrophoresis column) in the presence of SDS, and reverse phase HPLC can lead to a greater than 20 000-fold increase in specific activity based on protein concentration with a minimal loss in total activity.

We have designed a simplified extraction strategy based on the unusual partitioning characteristics of LPA. First, OCAF is extracted with chloroform and methanol (MeOH) at neutral pH. More than 99% of proteins precipitate in this step. Following separation into two phases by addition of 0.88% KCl, OCAF partitions into the aqueous/MeOH phase. The aqueous phase is then extracted a second time by chloroform and MeOH at acidic pH. OCAF partitions into the acidic chloroform phase under these conditions. This material is further purified on a silica Sep-Pak column. At this point, OCAF is virtually free of protein and neutral lipids. This semipurified OCAF was used in the assays described below. These results suggest that i) OCAF is tightly associated with protein(s); ii) OCAF is probably negatively charged, most likely containing one or more phosphate groups; and iii) OCAF is extremely polar.

Preliminary results show that OCAF elicits the calcium release activity at nM to μM concentrations. LPA stimulates calcium release in the 0.2–100 μM range in HEY cells. OCAF is therefore more potent than LPA [32].

13.10 COMPARISON OF OCAF TO OTHER LIPID MEDIATORS

In order to determine whether OCAF is one of the known lipid mediators, we compared its activity to compounds that have been demonstrated to change $[Ca^{2+}]_i$ in other systems or were potential inducers of cellular proliferation or activation. These studies tested whether the lipid induced an increase in $[Ca^{2+}]_i$ in ovarian cancer cells or whether the mediator altered the ability of OCAF to induce increases in $[Ca^{2+}]_i$.

Each mediator was tested over a concentration range that included concentrations within or above the range reported to be effective in other systems. PAF, lyso-PAF, arachidonic acid, phosphatidic acid (PA), lysophospholipids such as LPC, LPE, LPI and LPG and sphingolipids such as sphingosine and ceramide failed to induce an increase in $[Ca^{2+}]_i$.

On the other hand, when added at concentrations between 0.2 and 50 μM, LPA (Figure 13.2), SPC (Figure 13.3) and LPS (not shown) elicit transient $[Ca^{2+}]_i$ elevations in HEY ovarian cancer cells that are very similar to that evoked by OCAF (Figure 13.1). The onset of the increase in $[Ca^{2+}]_i$ is rapid, with no

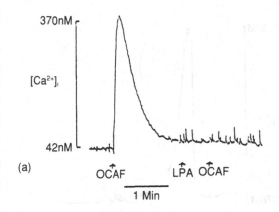

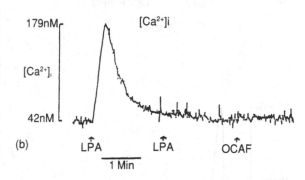

Figure 13.2 Cross inhibition of the $[Ca^{2+}]_i$ response induced by OCAF and LPA. (a) The fluorimetry trace shows the $[Ca^{2+}]_i$ response triggered by partially purified OCAF (10 μl), which inhibits the $[Ca^{2+}]_i$ response to subsequent addition of OCAF (20 μl) and LPA (10 μM); (b) LPA (10 μM) was added first as indicated, followed by additional LPA (20 μM) and OCAF (10 μl).

detectable delay (<10 seconds), reaching a peak within seconds after stimulation and returning to basal levels within two minutes. LPA with oleoyl, palmitoyl or stearoyl fatty acids at the sn-1 position was equally effective. In addition, LPA, SPC and LPS cross-inhibit increases in $[Ca^{2+}]_i$ induced by themselves, by OCAF and also by each other (Figures 13.2 and 13.3). Thus, signalling by each of these lipids undergoes homologous and heterologous desensitization. These data raise the possibility that OCAF is one of these lipid mediators. However, as these lipids mediate heterologous desensitization (that is,

129

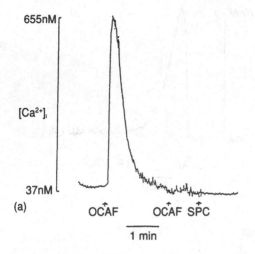

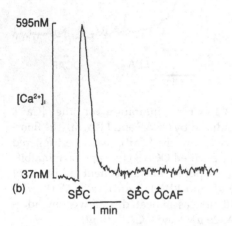

Figure 13.3 Cross inhibition of the $[Ca^{2+}]_i$ response induced by OCAF and SPC. (a) The trace shows the $[Ca^{2+}]_i$ response triggered by partially purified OCAF (10 μl), which inhibits the $[Ca^{2+}]_i$ response to subsequent addition of OCAF (20 μl) and SPC (10 μM); (b) SPC (10 μM) was added first as indicated, followed by additional LPA (20 μM) and OCAF (10 μl).

they desensitize each other), OCAF could just as readily be an independent mediator. It has not been determined whether the heterologous desensitization mediated by these lipids is due to binding to a single receptor, whether

they have separate receptors that converge on a specific intracellular mediator or whether signals transmitted through the receptors interact in such a way as to prevent signal transduction. However, examples of each of these three possibilities have been observed in other signalling pathways.

13.11   OCAF IS A UNIQUE PHOSPHOLIPID

Enzymatic digestions of OCAF and other lipids were performed in an attempt to determine whether OCAF could be LPA, SPC or LPS and to provide a better indication of the structure of OCAF (Table 13.1). LPC and thrombin were used as controls for enzyme activity and non-specific effects of the enzymatic reactions, respectively. The sites of action of phospholipases and the chemical structures of LPA, LPS and SPC, as well as PAF, are shown in Figure 13.4.

Table 13.1 $[Ca^{2+}]_i$ release after enzymatic digestions

Sample	Control	PLB	PLD
OCAF	++	−	−
LPA	++	−	++
LPC	−	−	++
LPS	++	−	++
SPC	++	++	−
Thrombin	++	++	++

OCAF: Partially purified OCAF
LPA: Lysophosphatidic acid (oleoyl, palmitoyl or stearoyl)
LPC: Lysophosphatidylcholine (oleoyl or palmitoyl)
LPS: Lysophosphatidylserine (mainly stearoyl)
SPC: Sphingosylphosphorylcholine

Phospholipase digestions were carried out in 10 mM HEPES, pH 7.4, with either 100 mM NaCl or 4 mM $CaCl_2$ at 37°C for 3 h. The reactions were stopped by freezing at −20°C. No further extraction was done and the mixtures were assayed for calcium release activity as described in [5]. The enzymes used were also incubated in the absence of substrate under the same conditions and no calcium release was observed

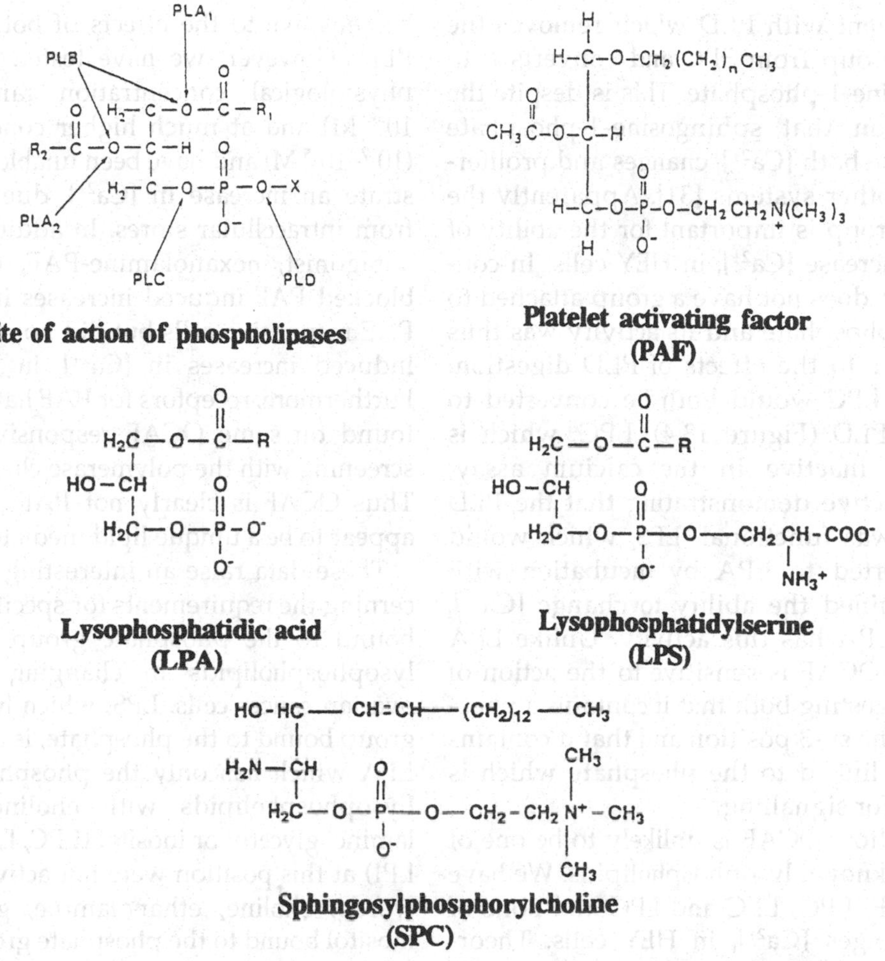

Site of action of phospholipases

Platelet activating factor (PAF)

Lysophosphatidic acid (LPA)

Lysophosphatidylserine (LPS)

Sphingosylphosphorylcholine (SPC)

Figure 13.4 The sites of action of phospholipases and chemical structures of LPA, LPS and SPC. R=fatty acid.

Phospholipase B (PLB) which has both phospholipase A1 and A2 activity, cleaves fatty acyl groups with an ester linkage at either sn-1 or sn-2 positions or both of lipids with a glycerol backbone (Figure 13.4). Both LPA and LPS possess a fatty acyl group with an ester linkage at the sn-1 position, but not the sn-2 position. The $[Ca^{2+}]_i$ changing activity of both LPA and LPS was sensitive to digestion with PLB (Table 13.1) indicating that a fatty acyl group present in the sn-1 position is necessary for their function. OCAF was similarly sensitive to the action of PLB suggesting that OCAF has a glycerol backbone with a

fatty acyl group linked by an ester bond at the sn-1 or sn-2 position or both which is essential for its ability to change $[Ca^{2+}]_i$ in ovarian cancer cells. In contrast, SPC was insensitive to PLB treatment. This was not surprising as, although SPC is a phospholipid, it does not have a glycerol backbone. In particular SPC does not contain a fatty acyl group with an ester bond recognized by PLB.

The non-specific PLD utilized herein can hydrolyse any group attached to phosphate at the sn-3 position in either glycerol phospholipids or sphingolipids. As indicated in Table 13.1, the activity of SPC was destroyed by treatment with PLD which removes the choline group from SPC and converts it to sphingosine-1-phosphate. This is despite the observation that sphingosine-1-phosphate can induce both $[Ca^{2+}]_i$ changes and proliferation in other systems [31]. Apparently the choline group is important for the ability of SPC to increase $[Ca^{2+}]_i$ in HEY cells. In contrast, LPA does not have a group attached to the sn-3 phosphate and its activity was thus insensitive to the effects of PLD digestion. LPS and LPC would both be converted to LPA by PLD (Figure 13.4). LPC, which is normally inactive in the calcium assay, became active demonstrating that the PLD enzyme was functional. LPS, which would be converted to LPA by incubation with PLD, retained the ability to change $[Ca^{2+}]_i$ because LPA has this activity. Unlike LPA and LPS, OCAF is sensitive to the action of PLD, suggesting both that it contains a phosphate at the sn-3 position and that it contains a moiety linked to the phosphate which is essential for signalling.

In addition, OCAF is unlikely to be one of the other known lysophospholipids. We have tested LPE, LPG, LPC and LPG and none of them changes $[Ca^{2+}]_i$ in HEY cells. Theoretically, digestion of any of these compounds or compounds with similar structure but different moiety attached to the phosphate with PLD will convert it to LPA, which is active in the $[Ca^{2+}]_i$ change assay in HEY cells. However, the activity of OCAF is destroyed by PLD, indicating that it is unlikely to be a lysophospholipid. Preliminary data showed that OCAF was partially sensitive to treatment with phospholipase A1 and phospholipase A2. This combined information indicates that OCAF is probably a phospholipid with a glycerol backbone. It may have a fatty acid linked to the sn-1 position through an ether bond and an acyl group at sn-2 position with an ester linkage.

From the structure presented in Figure 13.4, PAF, similar to OCAF, would be predicted to be sensitive to the effects of both PLB and PLD. However, we have tested PAF in its physiological concentration range (10^{-11}–10^{-8} M) and at much higher concentrations (10^{-7}–10^{-5} M) and have been unable to demonstrate an increase in $[Ca^{2+}]_i$ due to release from intracellular stores. In addition, a PAF antagonist, hexanolamine-PAF, completely blocked PAF induced increases in $[Ca^{2+}]_i$ in PAF responsive cells but did not alter OCAF induced increases in $[Ca^{2+}]_i$ in HEY cells. Furthermore, receptors for PAF have not been found on some OCAF responsive cells by screening with the polymerase chain reaction. Thus OCAF is clearly not PAF and would appear to be a unique lipid mediator.

These data raise an interesting point concerning the requirements for specific moieties bound to the phosphate group present in lysophospholipids in changing $[Ca^{2+}]_i$ in ovarian cancer cells. LPS, which has a serine group bound to the phosphate, is active, as is LPA which has only the phosphate group. Lysophospholipids with choline, ethanolamine, glycerol or inositol (LPC, LPE, LPG or LPI) at this position were not active. In other words, choline, ethanolamine, glycerol or inositol bound to the phosphate group are not permissive for activity of lysophospholipids, but serine or hydrogen is permissive. If LPS and LPA bind to the same receptor, then the serine group must not interfere with this interaction whereas choline, ethano- lamine, glycerol or inositol would appear to interrupt the interaction. Alternatively LPA and LPS may bind to different receptors. However, the choline group in SPC at the similar position was required for its activity. This suggests that SPC binds to a receptor due to a different structural requirement.

13.12 SUMMARY

In summary, the data indicate that OCAF is the factor responsible for the calcium releasing activity in ascites. We have tested many known lipid mediators for their ability to stimulate $[Ca^{2+}]_i$ release in HEY cells. Whilst most failed to elicit a response, LPA, LPS and SPC induced the characteristic transient $[Ca^{2+}]_i$ release observed with OCAF. Furthermore, there was heterologous desensitization of the response between these mediators and OCAF, suggesting that all four may act at a common point in eliciting changes in $[Ca^{2+}]_i$. Whether this represents a common receptor or a downstream mediator remains to be determined.

The enzymatic digestion experiments reported herein show that the $[Ca^{2+}]_i$ releasing activity of OCAF is sensitive to PLB and PLD. As shown in Table 13.1, the pattern of the enzyme sensitivity does not correlate with that of LPA, LPS or SPC. Thus it is unlikely that OCAF is one of these lipid mediators. The enzyme sensitivity of OCAF gives some clues as to its structure and studies are underway to elucidate this further.

If the activation of ovarian cancer cells by OCAF plays a major role in *in vivo* growth, it may be possible to design derivatives that prevent the interaction of OCAF with its receptor. In addition it may be possible to generate drugs which will interfere with the signalling pathway utilized by OCAF. Preliminary results suggest that high concentrations of some lipids can be growth inhibitory. Indeed, synthetic lipid mediators, particularly those which are non-metabolizable due to unusual lipid structures, are currently in phase I therapy trials as antineoplastic reagents at several centers [39].

ADDENDUM

We have subsequently found that the phospholipidase D (PLD) from Sigma Chemical Co. that we used for characterization of ovarian cancer ascites factor (OCAF) might be contaminated with PLA1 and PLA2 activities. We have since tested two other PLD preparations from Calbiochem and Boehringer and found that OCAF is insensitive to treatment with the PLDs. We have been able to confirm that these preparations do contain active PLD. This significantly changes the potential interpretation of our data as it is possible that OCAF is a form of lysophosphatidic acid (LPA). Indeed, mass spectrometric analysis of purified OCAF supports this contention. There is, however, a 100-fold discrepancy between the specific activity of commercially available LPA and purified OCAF, with OCAF being the more active. We are currently exploring the possibility that OCAF is an LPA containing an unusual fatty acyl side chain.

ACKNOWLEDGEMENTS

This work is supported by grants from the National Cancer Institute of Canada, Medical Research Council of Canada, Genesis Foundation and Johnson and Johnson PRI. Y.X. is the recipient of an NSERC Fellowship and G.B.M. of a Medical Research Council of Canada Scientist award. We thank the management and scientists of Allelix for support of some of this work, Alan Mellors for extensive advice and assistance and John Boynton, Chris May, Susan Campbell and Mary Hill for technical assistance.

REFERENCES

1. Rozengurt, E. (1992) Growth factors and cell proliferation. *Curr. Opin. Cell Biol.*, **4**, 161–5.
2. Bishop, M. (1991) Molecular themes in oncogenesis. *Cell*, **64**, 235–48.
3. Aaronson, S.A. (1991) Growth factors and cancer. *Science*, **254**, 1146–53.
4. Cross, M. and Dexter, T.M. (1991) Growth factors in development, transformation, and tumorigenesis. *Cell*, **64**, 271–80.
5. Boyle, W.J. (1992) Growth factors and tyrosine kinase receptors during development and cancer. *Curr. Opin. Oncol.*, **4**, 156–62.

6. Ullrich, A. and Schlessinger, J. (1990) Signal transduction by receptors with tyrosine kinase activity. *Cell*, **61**, 203–12.

7. Berridge, M.J. (1993) Inositol triphosphate and calcium signaling. *Nature*, **361**, 315–25.

8. Schmandt, R. and Mills, G.B. (1993) Genomic components of carcinogenesis. *Clin. Chem.*, **39**, 2375–85.

9. Marshall, C.J. (1991) Tumor suppressor genes. *Cell*, **64**, 313–26.

10. Weinberg, R.A. (1991) Tumor suppressor genes. *Science*, **254**, 1138–46.

11. Hockenberry, D.M., Nunez, G., Milliman, C. *et al.* (1990) Bcl-2 is an inner mitochondrial membrane protein that blocks programmed cell death. *Nature*, **348**, 334–6.

12. Grivell, L.A and Jacobs, H.T. (1992) Oncogenes, mitochondria and immortality. *Curr. Opin. Immunol.*, **1**, 94–6.

13. Williams, G.T. (1991) Programmed cell death: apoptosis and oncogenesis. *Cell*, **65**, 1097–8.

14. Mills, G.B., Hashimoto, S., Hurteau, J. *et al.* (1992) Regulation of growth of human ovarian cancer cells. In *Ovarian Cancer 2: Biology, Diagnosis and Management*, (eds. F. Sharp, Mason and W. Creaseman), Chapman & Hall, London, pp. 127–43.

15. Bast, R.C. Jr., Jacobs, I. and Berchuck, J.A. (1992) Malignant transformation of ovarian epithelium. *J. Natl. Cancer Inst.*, **84**, 556–8.

16. Godwin, A.K., Testa, J.R., Handel, L.M. *et al.* (1992) Spontaneous transformation of rat ovarian surface epithelial cells: association with cytogenetic changes and implications of repeated ovulation in the etiology of ovarian cancer. *J. Natl. Cancer Inst.*, **84**, 592–601.

17. Mills, G.B., Hashimoto, S., Hurteau, J.A. *et al.* (1992) Role of growth factors, their receptors, and signaling pathways in the diagnosis, prognosis, follow-up and therapy of ovarian cancer. *Diagn. Oncol.*, **2**, 39–54.

18. Mills, G.B., May, C., McGill, M. *et al.* (1988) A putative new growth factor in ascitic fluid from ovarian cancer patients: identification, characterization and mechanism of action. *Cancer Res.*, **48**, 1066–71.

19. Mills, G.B. and May C. (1989) Regulatory mechanisms in ascitic fluid. In *Ovarian Cancer: Biologic and Therapeutic Challenges*, (eds. F.

Sharp, W.P. Mason and R.E. Leake), Chapman & Hall, London, pp. 55–62.

20. Hurteau, J., Simon, H.U., Kurman, C. *et al.* (1993) Levels of the soluble interleukin 2 receptor alpha are elevated in epithelial ovarian cancer patients: evidence for activation of T lymphocytes and potential role in management of ovarian cancer. *Am. J. Obstet. Gynecol.*, in press.

21. Mills, G.B., May, C., Hill, M. *et al.* (1990) Ascitic fluid from human ovarian cancer patients contains growth factors necessary for intraperitoneal growth of human ovarian cancer cells. *J. Clin. Invest.*, **86**, 851–5.

22. Roifman, C.M., Chin, K., Gazit, A. *et al.* (1991) Tyrosine phosphorylation is an essential event in the stimulation of B lymphocytes by *Staphylococcus aureus* Cowan I. *J. Immunol.*, **146**, 2965–71.

23. Padeh, S., Levitzki, A., Mills, G.B. and Roifman, C.H. (1991) Activation of phospholipase C in human B cells is dependent on tyrosine phosphorylation. *J. Clin. Invest.*, **87**, 1114–18.

24. Vu, T.K., Hung, D.T., Wheaton, V.I. and Coughlin, S.R. (1991) Molecular cloning of a functional thrombin receptor reveals a novel proteolytic mechanism of receptor activation. *Cell*, **64**, 1057–64.

25. Needelman, P., Turk, J., Jakschik, B.A. *et al.* (1983) Arachidonic acid metabolism. *Ann. Rev. Biochem.*, **55**, 69–102.

26. Hanahan, D.J. (1986) Platelet activating factor: a biologically active phosphoglyceride. *Ann. Rev. Biochem.*, **55**, 438–509.

27. Lenzen, S., Gorlich, J.K. and Rustenbeck, I. (1989) Regulation of transmembrane ion transport by reaction products of phospholipase A2. I. Effects of lysophospholipids on mitochondrial Ca^{2+} transport. *Biochim. Biophys. Acta*, **982**, 140–6.

28. Metz, S.A. (1988) Mobilization of cellular Ca^{2+} by lysophospholipids in rat islets of Langerhans. *Biochim. Biophys. Acta*, **968**, 239–52.

29. Bellini, F., Viola, G., Menegus, A.M. *et al.* (1990) Signalling mechanism in the lysophosphatidylserine-induced activation of mouse mast cells. *Biochem. Biophys. Acta*, **1052**, 216–20.

30. Hannun, Y.A., and Bell, R.M. (1989) Functions of sphingolipids and sphingolipid breakdown products in cellular regulation. *Science*, **243**, 500–6.

31. Zhang, H., Desai, N.N., Olivera, A. *et al.* (1991) Sphingosine-1-phosphate, a novel lipid, involved in cellular proliferation. *J. Cell Biol.*, **114**, 155–67.

32. Van Corven, E.J., Groenink, A., Jalink, K. *et al.* (1989) Lysophosphatidate-induced cell proliferation: identification and dissection of signalling pathways mediated by G proteins. *Cell*, **59**, 45–54.

33. Honda, Z.I., Nakamura, M., Miki, I. *et al.* (1991) Cloning by functional expression of platelet-activating factor receptor from guinea-pig lung. *Nature*, **349**, 342–6.

34. Ye, R.D., Prossnitz, E.R., Zou, A. and Cochrane, C.G. (1991) Characterization of a human cDNA that encodes a functional receptor for platelet activating factor. *Biochem. Biophy. Res. Comm.*, **180**, 105–11.

35. Jalink, K., van Corven, E.J. and Moolenaar, W.H. (1990) Lysophosphatidic acid, but not phosphatidic acid, is a potent Ca^{2+}-mobilizing stimulus for fibroblasts. *J. Biol. Chem.*, **265**, 12232–9.

36. Van Corven, E.J., van Rijswijk, A., Jalink, K. *et al.* (1992) Mitogenic action of lysophosphatidic acid and phosphatidic acid on fibroblasts. *Biochem. J.*, **281**, 163–9.

37. Bligh, E.G. and Dyer, W.J. (1959) A rapid method of total lipid extraction and purification. *Can. Biochem. Physiol.*, **37**, 911–17.

38. Kates, M. (1978) *Techniques of Lipidology*, 2nd edn. Elsevier, Amsterdam.

39. Bittman, R., Byun, H.S., Mercier, B. and Salari, H. (1993) 2'-(Trimethylammonio)ethyl-4-(hexadecyloxy)-3(S)-methoxybutane-phosphate: a novel potent antineoplastic agent. *J. Med. Chem.*, **36**, 297–9.

Part Three
Early Ovarian Cancer and Borderline Tumours

Chapter 14

Update on early ovarian cancer and cancer developing in benign ovarian tumors

R.E. SCULLY, D.A. BELL and G.M. ABU-JAWDEH

Because advances in therapy have failed to make a significant impact on the survival of patients with ovarian cancer, recent attention has been devoted to early detection of this disease in the hope of improving survival. Very little is known, however, about the clinicopathological features of early ovarian cancer and whether early diagnosis and treatment will result in a major improvement in prognosis.

Several definitions of early ovarian cancer have been proposed: cancer confined to the ovary; cancer less than 5 cm in diameter, and stages I and IIA disease completely resected. In order to investigate the microscopic features and the behavior of the earliest form of ovarian cancer detectable by pathological examination, we restricted a recent investigation [1] to ovarian carcinomas that had not been recognized preoperatively, intraoperatively or even pathologically on gross examination of the ovary but were discovered only on microscopical examination. Twelve cases of this type were retrieved from the consultation practice of one of us (RES) and two from the files of the Massachusetts General Hospital. The patients ranged in age from 27 to 65 (mean 50) years. Three women had a family history of ovarian cancer, six did not and the family history was unknown or unreliable in the remaining cases. All the tumors were incidental findings in patients operated on because of a gynecological indication that did not include a suspicion of ovarian cancer.

The tumors ranged in size from microscopic to 7 mm in diameter. All of them were unilateral and four appeared to be multifocal. Surface involvement was found in five of the 13 cases in which its presence or absence could be determined (Figure 14.1). Ten carcinomas were serous, one endometrioid, one clear cell and two undifferentiated. The preoperative serum CA-125 level was normal in the four women in the above series in whom it was measured preoperatively close to the time of the oophorectomy. Follow-up data of two or more years' duration were available for 10 of the 14 patients. Five of the seven whose diagnoses had been made at the time of oophorectomy were alive without recurrence 2–12 years postoperatively. One was alive with recurrent tumor and one had died of tumor. Two of the three women whose ovarian tumors had been diagnosed for the first time on retrospective microscopic examination of previously removed ovaries after the development of peritoneal carcinomatosis six, seven and 10 years subsequently died and the third was alive with recurrent tumor. There were no differences in the clinical or

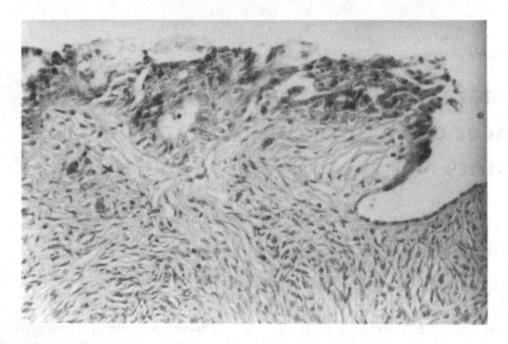

Figure 14.1 Early *de novo* carcinoma confined to surface of ovary. Normal surface epithelium is present at the far right.(H & E, × 125).

pathological features of the cases whether or not the patients had a family history of ovarian cancer.

Several conclusions can be drawn from the results of this study. Firstly the location of the early tumors supports the speculation that epithelial cancers of the ovary can arise *de novo* from surface epithelium or its inclusions. Secondly, early *de novo* cancers as defined in this study can be fatal. Also some early ovarian cancers may be stage III almost from their inception instead of passing through an orderly sequence from stage I to stage III, as generally assumed. Tiny potentially fatal cancers of the type reported almost certainly could not have been discovered by currently available techniques for early detection of ovarian cancer – transvaginal ultrasound examination and measurement of CA-125 levels in the serum. In the three cases in which the tumor was discovered after the development of peritoneal carcinomatosis the long intervals between the first and second tumors suggests that the peritoneal tumors may have been second primary tumors rather than recurrent ovarian cancers. The alternative explanation is that microscopic deposits of carcinoma on the peritoneum may survive for years in a dormant state before becoming clinically evident. Clonality studies may be necessary to answer this question.

It may be argued that this series of 14 cases is small and possibly not representative of ovarian cancer of the type encountered clinically. However, if one excepts the three cases in which the ovarian tumors were discovered retrospectively there is no reason to believe that the cases were sent for consultation except for their microscopic size.

Since the great majority of ovarian and other pelvic lesions that have been detected by transvaginal ultrasound examination in the course of screening women for ovarian cancer have been benign, some gynecologists, instead of exploring patients with lesions considered to be almost certainly benign on the basis of their ultrasonic appearance, have been following them with repeated ultrasound examinations. This approach has highlighted the question of a second source of epithelial cancers, namely, benign epithelial lesions. There is circumstantial evidence that the latter may become malignant. The prevalence of benign epithelial tumors in first degree and second degree relatives of patients with ovarian cancer is five times as great as it is in patients without this background [2]. Ovarian carcinomas occur at an average age 10–15 years earlier than benign tumors of the same cell type [3] and pathologists are well aware of the occasional presence of cytologically benign, borderline and malignant epithelium within the same ovarian tumor specimen. No one until recently, however, has made a quantitative study of the association of benign, borderline and malignant elements in specimens of ovarian carcinoma.

In an investigation from the University of Kentucky [4], 28 of 31 (90%) mucinous carcinomas were found to contain benign-appearing epithelium and in eight of these cases (26% of the total), a transition was observed between the two types of epithelium. Benign epithelium was found in 22 of 39 (56%) serous carcinomas, with a transition observable in 11 of these tumors (28% of the total). In a study in our laboratory of 189 epithelial cancers of the ovary from 156 patients [5], benign epithelium was identified in 74% of mucinous carcinomas, 46% of endometrioid carcinomas and 39% of clear cell carcinomas. In contrast benign epithelium was encountered in only 15% and 31% of serous carcinomas and mixed serous–transitional cell carcinomas, respect-

ively. In the cases of serous carcinoma and mixed serous–transitional cell carcinoma the benign epithelium invariably occupied 25% or less of the tumor and it was difficult to be certain in most cases whether the benign epithelium was residual surface epithelium, the epithelium of a surface inclusion or the residuum of a serous cystadenoma. In contrast, there was a significant component of benign epithelium (over 25%) in the mucinous carcinomas in 48% of the cases and the benign epithelium was predominant in 22%. Analogous figures for endometrioid and clear cell adenocarcinomas were 33% and 6% and 32% and 5%, respectively. Transitions between the benign and malignant epithelium appeared to be present in 8% of the serous carcinomas, 18% of the mixed serous–transitional cell carcinomas, 52% of the clear cell carcinomas, 57% of the endometrioid carcinomas and 80% of the mucinous carcinomas. These findings, in conjunction with those of our previous study of *de novo* carcinomas, suggest that the great majority of serous carcinomas arise *de novo* from the surface epithelium and its inclusions, that a sizeable proportion of mucinous carcinomas arise from mucinous cystadenomas and that smaller proportions of endometrioid and clear cell carcinomas arise from pre-existing benign lesions such as endometriosis as well as benign tumors of the same cell types.

The great rarity of mucinous metaplasia of the surface epithelium and mucinous epithelial inclusions as well as an absence of mucinous carcinomas in our small series of *de novo* carcinomas of the ovary provide further evidence that at least some mucinous tumors of the ovary may be of germ cell rather than surface epithelial origin. The very high reported association of endometriosis with endometrioid carcinoma and clear cell carcinoma (28% and 49%, respectively) in contrast to its very low frequency in association with serous and mucinous carcinomas of the ovary

(3% and 4%, respectively) [6] furnishes strong evidence that endometriosis of the ovary is a precancerous lesion and the numerous reports in the literature of cancer developing in endometriosis after unopposed estrogen replacement therapy [7] suggest that the latter is not optimal treatment for a patient with known residual endometriosis in the pelvis. The carcinomas that were associated with benign epithelium (with the exception of a small group of endometrioid carcinomas associated with adenofibromas, which occur mainly in elderly women and are probably overrepresented in a consultation file) were diagnosed on an average of 7–16 years earlier than the carcinomas unassociated with a benign component. This suggests that the epithelium of a cystadenoma or other benign epithelial lesion may be at higher risk for the development of cancer than surface epithelium or the epithelium of its inclusions. Similarly, the presence of a significantly higher frequency of tubal metaplasia of surface epithelial inclusions in the ovaries contralateral to carcinomas of the ovary supports the contention that müllerian differentiation may be a precursor of carcinomas [8, D.A. Bell and R.E. Scully, personal observation].

Some authors [9,10] have questioned whether the finding of benign epithelium in association with carcinomas of the ovary indicates an origin of the carcinoma from the benign epithelium or, in contrast, maturation of the malignant epithelium into benign-appearing epithelium. The latter explanation is based on the observation that metastatic adenocarcinomas, particularly from the gastrointestinal tract and pancreas to the ovary

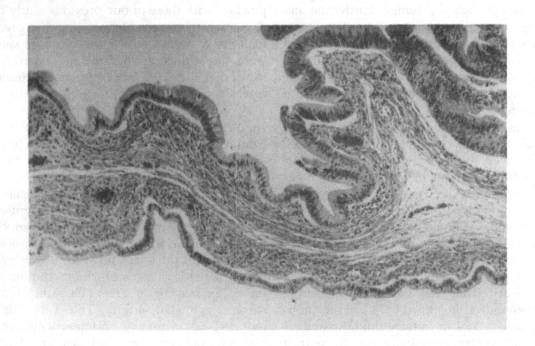

Figure 14.2 Ovary. Metastatic adenocarcinoma from large intestine. The upper cyst is lined by benign appearing epithelium that has undergone a gradual transition on the right side to highly atypical epithelium. The lower cyst is lined by slightly atypical appearing epithelium (H & E, × 75).

[11], may contain cysts lined by benign-appearing epithelium, under those circumstances obviously reflecting maturation of malignant epithelium. In the metastatic tumors, the benign-appearing epithelium typically lines cysts in a diffuse distribution, sometimes with a gradual transition to atypical or malignant epithelium (Figures 14.2 and 14.3). Since a similar maturation of the malignant epithelium is rarely seen in the extra-ovarian primary tumor in these cases, it is possible that either pressure of the cyst contents or the presence of some unknown substance within the cyst fluid or in the surrounding stroma induces diffuse maturation of the malignant epithelium. In contrast, in at least some cases of primary ovarian carcinoma associated with benign epithelium, the carcinoma occupies only a minor component of an otherwise benign-appearing tumor and arises more or less abruptly within a cyst lined by otherwise benign epithelium, the usual finding in cases in which carcinoma in other organs is generally conceded to arise on a background of benign epithelium. It is doubtful that pathologists, by examining routine sections of ovarian carcinomas, will be able to distinguish reproducibly maturation of malignant epithelium into benign-appearing epithelium from an origin of carcinoma from benign epithelium in all cases and additional research will be necessary to determine the true frequency of transformation of benign ovarian epithelial lesions into carcinomas. Ultrasonographic follow-up of benign-appearing ovarian cystic tumors may help to solve the problem but because of the average 10–15 years' age difference of patients with benign and malignant ovarian epithelial tumors, demonstration of a benign

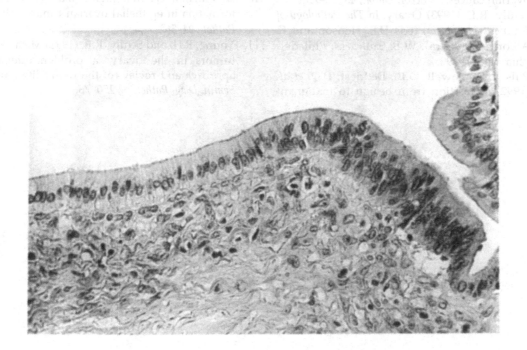

Figure 14.3 Ovary. Metastatic adenocarcinoma from large intestine. The cyst lining has undergone a transition from benign appearing epithelium (left) to stratified, atypical epithelium (right) (H & E, × 25).

to malignant sequence may require prolonged follow-up examination. The use of newly evolving techniques, including immunohistochemical demonstration of oncogenes and antioncogenes and molecular genetic investigation, should be applied to malignant, atypical-appearing and benign-appearing epithelium in both primary and metastatic carcinomas of the ovary to elucidate the relationship of these types of epithelium and to determine with greater accuracy the frequency of development of ovarian carcinomas from benign epithelium, both neoplastic and non-neoplastic.

REFERENCES

1. Bell, D.A. and Scully, R.E. (1994) Early *de novo* ovarian carcinoma: a study of 14 cases. *Cancer*, **73**, 1859–64.

2. Bourne, T.H., Whitehead, M.J., Campbell, S. *et al.* (1991) Ultrasound screening for familial ovarian cancer. *Gynecol. Oncol.*, **43**, 92–7.

3. Scully, R.E. (1993) Ovary. In *The Pathology of Incipient Neoplasia*, (eds D.E. Henson and F. Albores-Saavedra), W.B. Saunders, Philadelphia, pp. 279–93.

4. Puls, L.E., Powell, D.E., DePriest, P.D. *et al.* (1992) Transition from benign to malignant epithelium in mucinous and serous ovarian cystadenocarcinoma. *Gynecol. Oncol.*, **47**, 53–7.

5. Abu-Jawdeh, G.M., and Scully, R.E. Association of surface epithelial–stromal carcinomas of ovary with benign epithelial tumors and non-neoplastic lesions. In preparation.

6. Russell, P. (1979) The pathological assessment of ovarian neoplasms. 1: Introduction to the common 'epithelial' tumors and analysis of benign 'epithelial' tumors. *Pathology*, **11**, 5–26.

7. Reimnitz, C., Brand, E., Nieberg, R.K. and Hacker, N.F. (1988) Malignancy arising in endometriosis associated with unopposed estrogen replacement. *Obstet. Gynecol.*, **71**, 444–7.

8. Mittall, K.R., Zeleniuch-Jacquette, A., Cooper, J.L. and Demopolis, R.I. (1993) Contralateral ovary in unilateral ovarian carcinoma. A search for preneoplastic lesions. *Int. J. Gynecol. Pathol.*, **12**, 59–63.

9. Fox, H. (1993) Pathology of early malignant change in the ovary. *Int. J. Gynecol. Pathol.*, **12**, 153–5.

10. Austin, R.M. (1993) Benign to malignant transformation in epithelial ovarian tumors. *Hum. Pathol.*, **24**, 562.

11. Young, R.H. and Scully, R.E. (1991) Metastatic tumors in the ovary: a problem-oriented approach and review of the recent literature. *Semin. Diag. Pathol.*, **8**, 250–76.

Chapter 15

Spontaneous transformation of the ovarian surface epithelium and the biology of ovarian cancer

H. SALAZAR, A.K. GODWIN, L.A. GETTS, J.R. TESTA, M. DALY,
N. ROSENBLUM, M. HOGAN, R.F. OZOLS and T.C. HAMILTON

The ovary is perhaps one of the more complex organs of the human body with two major normal physiological functions: (1) the production of steroid hormones and (2) the timely release of ova. These functions are accomplished by numerous different cell types from which tumors may arise (Figure 15.1). The majority of the ovarian neoplasms (80–90%) are believed to arise from the cells which cover the ovarian surface [1–3]. These so-called common epithelial tumors of the ovary display a range of histological features which allow them to be classified according to their histological similarities with the epithelial components characteristic of different müllerian structures. Thus, serous tumor epithelia are similar to fallopian tube epithelia; the epithelia of endometrioid tumors recapitulate the epithelia of the endometrium and its neoplasms, while those of mucinous tumors usually show features identical to either endocervical or intestinal epithelia [1–3]. Important embryological relationships exist between the ovarian surface epithelium and the epithelial lining of the fallopian tubes, endometrium and endocervix that can explain the histogenetic basis for the various histological subtypes of these common epithelial tumors of the ovary. The surface epithelial cells are a modified peritoneal

mesothelium which originates from the same celomic epithelium which during embryonic development invaginates lateral to the gonads to form the paramesonephric or müllerian duct system of the embryo. From this, ultimately, the fallopian tubes, the uterus (endometrium and endocervix) and at least part of the vagina differentiate [4]. Hence, a strong histogenetic basis for the histological subtypes of epithelial ovarian tumors is evident.

Given that the majority of ovarian cancers arise from the surface epithelium, it is important to define what features or functions of this cell type may make it susceptible to malignant transformation. In those species studied, there are various levels of evidence to suggest that the surface epithelium, through production of proteolytic enzymes, participates in synergism with follicular factors in the breakdown of the follicle wall necessary for ovulation [5,6]. The wound created at the ovarian surface by ovulation is then repaired by growth of the surface epithelial cells. It is this latter normal process about which there has been much speculation in regard to its potential role in malignant transformation [7–9]. For example, nulliparity, which is a risk factor for ovarian cancer, would result in incessantly repetitive ovulation and therefore, the

145

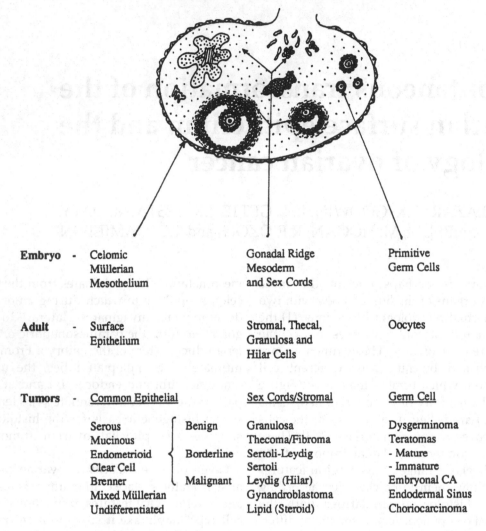

Embryo -	Celomic Müllerian Mesothelium	Gonadal Ridge Mesoderm and Sex Cords	Primitive Germ Cells
Adult -	Surface Epithelium	Stromal, Thecal, Granulosa and Hilar Cells	Oocytes
Tumors -	<u>Common Epithelial</u>	<u>Sex Cords/Stromal</u>	<u>Germ Cell</u>

Common Epithelial		Sex Cords/Stromal	Germ Cell
Serous	Benign	Granulosa	Dysgerminoma
Mucinous		Thecoma/Fibroma	Teratomas
Endometrioid	Borderline	Sertoli-Leydig	- Mature
Clear Cell		Sertoli	- Immature
Brenner	Malignant	Leydig (Hilar)	Embryonal CA
Mixed Müllerian		Gynandroblastoma	Endodermal Sinus
Undifferentiated		Lipid (Steroid)	Choriocarcinoma

Figure 15.1 Histogenesis of ovarian neoplasms.

need for frequent cycles of cell division by surface epithelial cells. Obviously, whenever DNA replication occurs there is an increased risk of mutations, some of which could yield malignant transformation. It is, then, significant that ovarian surface epithelial cells replicate as generative stem cells, that is, division of a surface epithelial cell yields daughter cells with equal potential for additional growth. This pattern of growth creates the potential for accumulation of subpopulations of cells with the same mutation. Based on

information suggestive of a major role for tumor suppressor genes in many, if not most, human cancers, it is of note that if such a mutation were within a tumor suppressor gene, the probability of a second similar mutation in a cell with only one remaining normal allele for the putative tumor suppressor gene would be increased by the presence of multiple cells with only one normal allele of that gene (Figure 15.2). This would be analogous to the classical model of tumor suppressor gene inactivation described in the

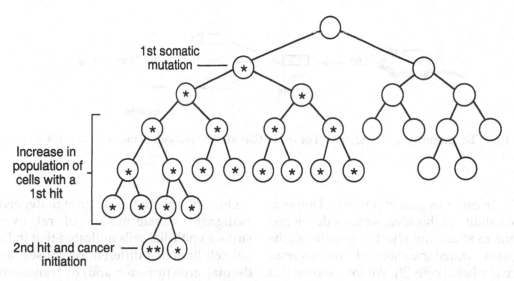

Figure 15.2 Accumulation of genetic damage in ovarian surface epithelial cells. Note that subsequent requirements for growth of a surface epithelial cell with a single somatic or germ line mutation in a tumor suppressor gene will yield subpopulations of cells with that same lesion. Hence, a second mutation in the remaining normal allele of the gene may be all that is required to initiate the malignant cascade.

development of retinoblastoma [10,11]. It may also be of significance that during the course of reproductive life, the ovarian surface epithelium may become entrapped within the ovarian cortex and form surface epithelial inclusion cysts, resembling glandular structures. This process places the ovarian surface epithelial cells within these cysts in closer proximity to the growth factor and steroid hormone producing components of the ovary, hence increasing the probability of mutations in these cells because of increased mitotic activity within inclusion cyst epithelia. An indication that components within the cortex do indeed influence surface epithelial cells within inclusion cysts is evident from a change in morphology of these normally unremarkable cells to cells with features similar to fallopian tubal, endometrial or endocervical epithelia. There is also much direct evidence in support of a role for many growth factors and hormones in normal and neoplastic ovarian surface epithelial cell growth and function (Table 15.1).

Although the concept that repetitious ovulation contributes to ovarian cancer etiology has been embellished since its first publication [7,8], there has been little if any direct experimental proof supportive of this hypothesis, except for limited experimental work in fowl using fluorescent light to stimulate prolonged superovulation which results in tumors similar to those that occur spontaneously in humans

Table 15.1 Growth factors and hormones involved in regulation of growth and function of the normal or neoplastic ovarian surface epithelium

Receptors		Growth effects	
Estrogen	[12–15]	Estrogen	[14,16–18]
Progestagen	[19,20]	Androgen	[19,20,21]
Androgen	[14,20]	IL-1	[22]
FMS	[23]	CSF-1	[23]
ERB-b2	[24]	EGF	[9,25–27]
EGF/TGFα	[25–27]	TGFβ	[9,28]
LH	[29,30]	LH	[21,31]
FSH	[30]	FSH	[21,31]

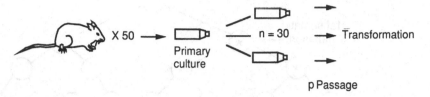

Figure 15.3 Diagrammatic representation of the initiation of 30 individual rat ovarian surface epithelial cell lines.

[32, 33]. In order to gain experimental support for the validity of this idea, we have developed a means to study the effect of growth on the malignant transformation of rat ovarian surface epithelial cells [9]. We have shown that ovarian surface epithelial cells may be readily removed from rat ovaries by selective trypsin treatment [9]. These cells readily adapt to tissue culture and rapidly grow to cover the surface of the culture flask as if to repair a wound at the ovarian surface. Once confluent, the cells discontinue growth and will remain as a quiescent but viable cobblestone-like monolayer for many months. Alternatively, mimicking frequent ovulations, cells may be required to undergo repeated cycles of proliferation by subculture of cells at frequent intervals. We have compared the phenotypes of these cells which have undergone a substantial requirement for growth to those which have remained as a confluent monolayer culture for an extended period of time. We observed that cells subjected to growth stress frequently develop the full malignant phenotype, including the capacity for substrate independent growth and tumorigenicity in athymic mice. Hence, we have added direct experimental evidence to the concept that the repetitive requirement for growth, as occurs with uninterrupted ovulation, may contribute to malignant transformation. This concept is now supported further by clinical reports of borderline common epithelial ovarian tumors in individuals subjected to superovulation as a part of therapy for infertility [34].

Our original studies on growth dependent malignant transformation of rat ovarian surface epithelial cells indicated that individual cell lines had different responses to epidermal growth factor and/or transforming growth factor β and also produced different tumor histological types [9]. The tumorigenic phenotypes were associated with cytogenetic and molecular/genetic changes consistent with tumor suppressor gene loss and oncogene activation [9]. Based on these initial findings, we designed experiments to determine the frequency of malignant transformation on a larger number of individual rat ovarian surface epithelial cell cultures and to determine the patterns of growth factor responsiveness and tumor histology. To this end, we established 30 individual cell lines from rat ovarian surface epithelial cells (Figure 15.3), subjected them to the repeated requirement for growth by frequent subculturing and then examined the cells for markers of malignant transformation, that is, substrate independent growth and tumorigenicity, and epidermal growth factor effects on substrate independent growth. These data are summarized in Table 15.2. Those cell lines which were most efficient at tumor formation have been selected for more detailed study in efforts to define the molecular genetic bases for their phenotypes. It is of note that the tumors produced by these cell lines in athymic mice showed a wide range of histological patterns, from well-differentiated papillary serous tumors

Table 15.2 Manifestation of features indicative of transformation in rat ovarian surface epithelial cells

Cell line #	Passage	Tumorigenicity**	Substrate independent growth		
			Passage	No exogenous EGF	+EGF
1	37S	–	35S	29	46
2	41S	1/2+	39S	89	69
3	41S	1/2+	39S	<20	<20
4	40S	++	39S	117	30
*5	40S	–	39S	<20	42
6	39S	1/2+	39S	<20	51
7	39S	++	39S	<20	141
*8	40S	+++	39S	186	867
*9	39S	+++	39S	124	1318
*10	40S	+++	39S	66	149
11	39S	–	38S	<20	<20
*12	40S	+++1/2	39S	<20	381
13	37S	1/2+	35S	<20	36
*14	37S	+++1/2	35S	144	1229
*15	49S	–	42S	<20	<20
*16	40S	–	39S	<20	<20
*17	39S	–	38S	<20	258
18	48S	++	38S	341	418
*19	52S	+++1/2	42S	44	96
20	48S	+	42S	<20	<20
*21	39S	–	39S	<20	<20
*22	40S	–	39S	377	488
*23	39S	++	39S	1402	1110
24	39S	1/2+	39S	<20	<20
25	39S	–	39S	<20	60
*26	40S	+++	39S	44	39
27	40S	–	39S	<20	31
28	40S	–	39S	<20	218
29	40S	–	39S	<20	27
30	40S	+	39S	<20	95

* Cell lines selected for further study
** 5×10^6 cells were suspended in 0.1 ml matrigel for subcutaneous injection into female athymic nude mice

and well-differentiated glandular tumors to very poorly differentiated tumors which appeared predominantly as sheets of undifferentiated malignant cells with occasional signet ring like cells. These cells were shown to be mucicarmine positive. It was of particular note that one cell line was only capable of tumor formation upon intraperitoneal transplantation. These cells had a tendency to home to regions of the small intestine where they produced solid tumor which impeded bowel motility with associated morbidity, as is often a characteristic of clinical ovarian cancer. This tumor was predominantly solid and undifferentiated but had foci showing mucinous glands differentiated along intestinal rather than endocervical, endometrioid or serous patterns (Figure 15.4).

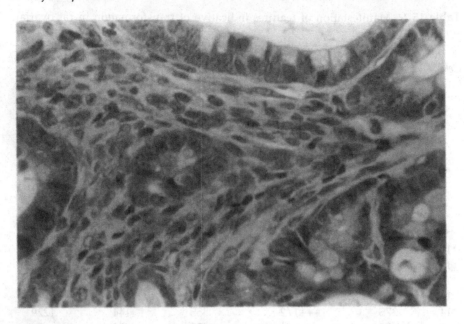

Figure 15.4 Invasive neoplastic glands with enteric differentiation (note numerous 'goblet' cells) and strands of undifferentiated tumor with pleomorphic nuclei (clone 7 IP, ×400).

Table 15.3 Relationship between cytogenetic abnormalities and tumor differentiation

Histology	Number alterations	Number markers	Number tumors with polyploid clones	Number tumors with dmin/hsr
Undifferentiated	4–8 (avg. 6.2)	0–3 (avg. 1.8)	2	3
Differentiated	1–3 (avg. 2.0)	0	0	0

We have now initiated cell lines from these tumors which vary in degree of differentiation in order to determine the cytogenetic and molecular genetic changes which contribute to tumor initiation, progression and histological subtypes. Cytogenetic evaluation has been completed and shows a remarkable correlation with tumor differentiation (Testa, Getts, Salazar *et al.*, in preparation). Well and moderately differentiated tumors have few cytogenetic abnormalities, while undifferentiated tumors have multiple and complex changes reminiscent of those characteristic of human ovarian carcinomas (Table 15.3). Cytogenetic observations of particular note include the findings of homogeneously staining chromosomal regions and double minute chromosomes in undifferentiated tumors

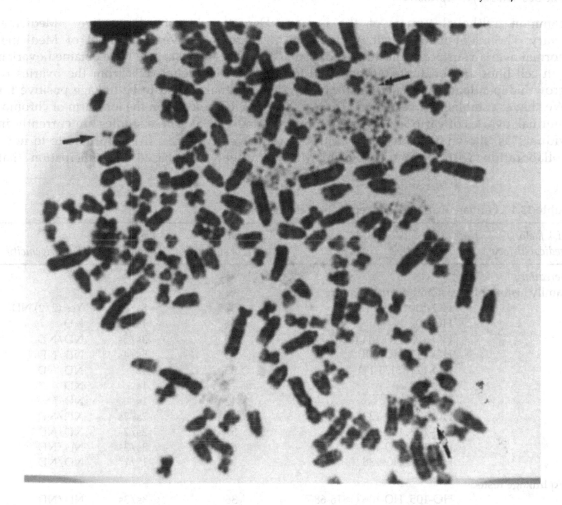

Figure 15.5 Metaphase spread of a cell line derived from a tumor produced in an athymic mouse by subcutaneous injection of a transformed rat ovarian surface epithelial cell line. Note karyotypic complexity and numerous double minute chromosomes (representative examples shown by arrows).

(Figure 15.5). These changes are hallmarks of gene amplification and suggest the possibility of oncogene amplification as a contributor to tumor progression. Our current strategy to identify the material amplified in these samples is to utilize chromosomal microdissection. We believe that this model of experimental ovarian cancer has the potential to provide leads as to genes involved in disease initiation, progression and histological differentiation. Using this model system, we can compare the cytogenetic and molecular genetics between individual tumors as well as follow the development of the malignant phenotype as the normal rat ovarian surface epithelial cells progress through the multiple steps leading to malignant transformation.

In addition to our investigation of the above described experimental model of ovarian cancer development, we also have a major interest in the direct study of the normal human ovarian surface epithelium and the common epithelial tumors of the human ovary. The major focus of our work on the normal ovarian surface epithelium is to establish cell lines and evaluate the potential for growth dependent malignant transformation. We have established cell lines from the 'normal' ovaries of various categories of individuals as shown in Table 15.4. Through collaboration with Henry T. Lynch, MD,

Department of Preventive Medicine, Creighton University School of Medicine, Omaha, Nebraska, we have obtained ovarian surface epithelial cells from the ovaries of individuals found to be linkage positive for the BRCA1 locus on the long arm of chromosome 17 [35]. These studies are currently in their early stages. It is appropriate to note, however, that based on anticipation that

Table 15.4 Human ovarian surface epithelial cell lines

Risk factor/ medical history	Patient ID #	Age of patient at time of surgery	Passage#* in vitro	Tumorigenicity
Hereditary				
Family history of breast and ovarian cancer:				
	HO-100**, HO-101	32	8s/3s	Yes (2/2) ND
	HO-102	33	1s	ND
	HO-103, HO-104 (3261-77)	40	3s/5s	ND/ND
	HO-117, HO-118	30	5s/4s	ND/ND
	HO-121 (3173-11)	33	4s	ND/ND
	HO-128		1s	ND
	HO-129	42	1s	ND
	HO-131, HO-132	42	2s/2s	ND/ND
	HO-133, HO-134	57	2s/2s	ND/ND
	HO-135, HO-136	60	3s/3s	ND/ND
	HO-137, HO-138		1°/1°	ND/ND
17q linkage tested:				
	HO-105, HO-106 (1816-686)	36	3s/3s	ND/ND
	HO-107, HO-108 (1816-680)	42	3s/2s	ND/ND
	HO-113, HO-114 (1816-575)	29	3s/3s	ND/ND
	HO-119 (1234-190)***	50	3s	ND
*Non-hereditary***				
Cancer; free of ovarian disease:				
Endometrial	HO-201	70	1s	ND
Endometrial	HO-202†		78s	Yes (6/6)
Cervical	HO-203†		74s	Yes (6/6)
Endometrial	HO-204, HO-205	63	2s/2s	ND/ND
Lyomyoma	HO-206, HO-207†	65	2s/3s	ND/ND
Endometrial	HO-208	46	2s	ND
Endometrial	HO-210, HO-211	52	2s/2s	ND/ND
Endometrial	HO-212, HO-213	79	1s/1s	ND/ND
Ovarian cancer:				
Unilateral	HO-301	68	1s	ND

Table 15.4 *Continued*

Risk factor/ medical history	Patient ID #	Age of patient at time of surgery	Passage#* in vitro	Tumorigenicity
Normal; non-cancer related oophorectomy:				
	HO-400, HO-401	50	3s/3s	ND/ND
	HO-402, HO-403		2s/3s	ND/ND
	HO-404, HO-405	48	3s/3s	ND/ND
	HO-407	58	5s	ND
	HO-408	63	2s	ND
	HO-410	49	2s	ND
	HO-411, HO-412	46	1s/3s	ND/ND
	HO-413, HO-414	46	2s/2s	ND/ND

*   Present number of times cells were subcultured *in vitro* as a split ratio of 1:5. One subculture results in 3 to 4 doublings

**   Detailed family pedigrees were taken by a trained research nurse from women undergoing surgery. A record was made whether a first degree relative (mother, sister or daughter) or second degree relatives had developed ovarian or breast cancer. Those with no clear inheritance pattern, i.e. there was no evidence of the dominant inheritance of either ovarian or breast cancer, were classified as non-hereditary. Those with a strong family history of breast/ovarian cancer and/or obligate 17q12-q21 gene carriers were classified as hereditary

***   Patient was linkage 17q with unilateral ovarian cancer. Cells were isolated from the unaffected ovary following surgery

†   Show capacity for substrate independent growth (i.e. growth in soft agarose)

ND   Not determined

human ovarian surface epithelial cells will be more refractory to transformation than similar rat cells, we are utilizing two complementary approaches to aid in this process: SV40 immortalization to increase the growth potential of the cells [36] and insertional mutagenesis [37,38]. This latter approach has particular relevance to ovarian surface epithelial cell lines derived from obligate carriers of the putative ovarian/breast cancer predisposing gene at the BRCA1 locus as, theoretically, the only requirement for initiation of the cascade of events leading to malignancy will be the inactivation of the remaining normal allele of this gene.

In addition to the study of the normal human ovarian surface epithelium, we are producing molecular karyotypes of individual human ovarian tumors by examining multiple loci on each chromosomal arm for loss of heterozygosity using combinations of restriction polymorphism analysis and microsatellite analysis. For example, we have examined normal and tumor DNA samples from 40 patients with ovarian cancer for loss of heterozygosity (LOH) at 15 loci on chromosome 17 (four on 17p and 11 on 17q). LOH on 17p was 54% (21/39) for informative 17p13.1 and 17p13.3 markers. Using four polymorphic markers flanking the familial breast/ovarian cancer susceptibility locus (BRCA-1) on 17q12-q21, LOH was 58% (23/40), with one tumor showing telomeric retention. Evaluation of a set of markers positioned telomeric to BRCA1 resulted in the highest degree of LOH, 73% (29/40), indicating that a candidate locus involved in ovarian cancer may reside distal to BRCA1. Deletion mapping of seven cases showing limited LOH on 17q revealed a common region of deletion on the long arm, distal to GH and proximal to D17S40 which spans approximately 8 cM (Figure 15.6). These results suggest that a potential tumor suppressor

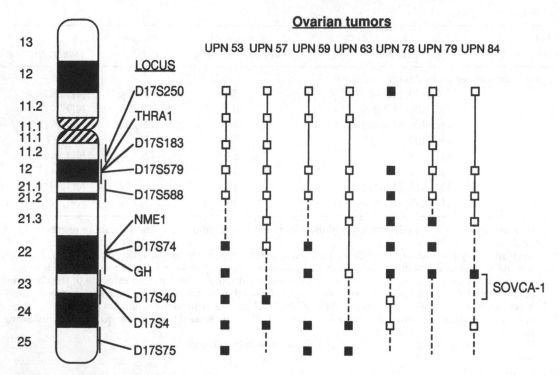

Figure 15.6 Allelic deletion patterns of ovarian tumors for the long arm of chromosome 17. DNA samples from normal blood and ovarian tumor tissue were typed with RFLP DNA markers, dinucleotide and tetranucleotide repeats on chromosome 17q. For each tumor, all informative loci are shown. ■, constitutional heterozygosity with LOH; □ constitutional heterozygosity with no LOH; blank spaces, homozygous. With the assumption that alleles in all regions between loci showing allelic loss are lost, solid lines indicate retained regions of chromosomes 17q and open areas show regions of allelic loss. Dashed lines represent regions that are uncertain in tumors with loss of heterozygosity for some loci.

gene involved in ovarian carcinogenesis is located on the distal portion of chromosome 17q and is distinct from the BRCA1 gene. We refer to this candidate locus at 17q22-q23 as SOVCA1 (for sporadic ovarian cancer 1).

During the course of our studies, Jacobs *et al.* [39] reported the identification of a common region of deletion in sporadic epithelial ovarian tumors which maps distal to BRCA1. This region spans 16 cM and was defined by the NME1 and the GH loci. Our results position this candidate ovarian cancer locus at a more distal location with respect to Jacobs' work. The discrepancy between the region identified by Jacobs and by us may be the result of the relatively small number of

informative samples and useful polymorphic markers available to define a common region of deletion within this distal portion of 17q. For example, if tumor UPN 63 were excluded from our study, the common region of loss would extend proximally to D17S74 and would thereby overlap the region identified by Jacobs (Figure 15.6). Out of 40 tumors studied, only seven showed LOH while retaining heterozygosity at other loci. Of these, only one tumor (UPN 84) possessed an interstitial deletion, while five of the remaining six cases showed telomeric deletions, most likely the result of mitotic recombination. It is apparent that unless a very large number of tumors is thoroughly studied, it will be difficult to accurately define the boundaries of this putative ovarian cancer locus. Therefore, further studies are needed to provide a more precise map of the chromosome 17q22-q23 locus before identification of the candidate ovarian cancer gene by positional cloning can be initiated.

Our studies on experimental models of ovarian cancer and on human tumors suggest several preliminary conclusions. It is obvious that clinical ovarian cancer is a complex disease but it may be more appropriate to consider it a complex of diseases, with many possible molecular genetic routes to disease initiation, progression and tumor phenotype. The development of these relevant experimental models is allowing longstanding hypotheses, including the role of repetitive ovulation in ovarian cancer etiology, to be tested. The integration of what we are learning about the ovarian surface epithelium with emerging views on cancer etiology and progression, that is, the frequent involvement of tumor suppressor genes, suggests that we may soon have a clearer understanding of ovarian cancer pathogenesis and clinical course.

REFERENCES

1. Scully, R.E. (1977) Ovarian tumors – a review. *Am. J. Path.*, **87**, 686–720.
2. Bell, D.A. (1991) Ovarian surface epithelial–stromal tumors. *Hum. Path.*, **22**, 750–62.
3. Langley, F.A. and Fox, H. (1987) Ovarian tumours: classification, histogenesis and aetiology. In *Obstetrics and Gynaecologic Pathology*, (ed. H. Fox), Churchill Livingstone, London.
4. Cormack, D.H. (1987) *Ham's Histology*, 9th edn, J.B. Lippincott, Philadelphia.
5. Bjersing, L. and Cajander, S. (1975) Ovulation and the role of the ovarian surface epithelium. *Experientia*, **31**, 605–8.
6. Hamilton, T.C. (1992) Ovarian cancer. Part I: Biology. *Curr. Probl. Cancer*, **16**, 1–57.
7. Fathalla, M.F. (1971) Incessant ovulation – a factor in ovarian neoplasia? *Lancet*, **2**, 163.
8. Fathalla, M.F. (1972) Factors in the causation and incidence of ovarian cancer. *Obstet. Gynecol. Survey*, **27**, 751–68.
9. Godwin, A.K., Testa, J.R., Handel, L.M. *et al.* (1992) Spontaneous transformation of rat ovarian surface epithelial cells: association with cytogenetic changes and implications of repeated ovulation in the etiology of ovarian cancer. *J. Natl. Cancer Inst.*, **84**, 592–601.
10. Knudson, A.G. (1978) Retinoblastoma: a prototypic hereditary neoplasm. *Semin. Oncol.*, **5**, 57.
11. Godwin, A.K., Hamilton, T.C. and Knudson, A.G. (1992) Oncogenes and anti-oncogenes in gynecologic malignancies. In *Gynecologic Oncology: Principles and Practice*, (eds W.J. Hoskins, C.A. Perez and R.C. Young) J.B. Lippincott, Philadelphia, pp. 87–116.
12. Stein, K.F. and Allen, E. (1942) Attempts to stimulate proliferation of the germinal epithelium of the ovary. *Anat. Rec.*, **82**, 1–9.
13. Hamilton, T.C., Davies, P. and Griffiths, K. (1981) Androgen and estrogen binding of cytosols of human ovarian tumors. *J. Endocrinol.*, **90**, 421–31.
14. Adams, A.T. and Auersperg, N. (1983) Autoradiographic investigation of estrogen binding in cultured rat ovarian surface epithelial cells. *J. Histochem. Cytochem.*, **31**, 1321–5.
15. Isola, J., Kallioniemi, O.P., Korte, J.M. *et al.* (1990) Steroid receptors and Ki-67 reactivity in ovarian cancer and in normal ovary: correlation with DNA flow cytometry, biochemical receptor assay and patient survival. *J. Path.*, **162**, 295–301.
16. Nash, J.D., Ozols, R.F., Smith, J.F. *et al.* (1989) Estrogen and anti-estrogen effects on the growth of human epithelial ovarian cancer *in vitro*. *Obstet. Gynecol.*, **73**, 1009.
17. Sawada, M., Terada, N., Wada, A. *et al.* (1990) Estrogen and androgen-responsive growth of human ovarian adenocarcinoma heterotransplanted into nude mice. *Int. J. Cancer*, **45**, 359–63.
18. Geisinger, K.R., Berens, M.E., Duckett, Y. *et al.* (1990) The effects of estrogen, progesterone, and tamoxifen alone and in combination with cytotoxic agents against human ovarian carcinoma *in vitro*. *Cancer*, **65**, 1055–61.
19. Hamilton, T.C., Behrens, B.C., Louie, K.G. *et al.* (1984) Induction of progesterone receptor with

17β-estradiol in human ovarian cancer. *J. Clin. Endocrinol. Metab.*, **59**, 561–3.

20. Slotman, B. and Rao, B. (1988) Ovarian carcinoma (a review). *Anticancer Res.*, **8**, 417–34.

21. Simon, W.E., Albrecht, M., Hansel, M. *et al.* (1983) Cell lines derived from human ovarian carcinomas: growth stimulation by gonadotropic and steroid hormones. *J. Natl. Cancer Inst.*, **70**, 839–45.

22. Yee, D., Morales, F., Hamilton, T.C. *et al.* (1991) Expression of IGF-I, its binding proteins, and its receptor in ovarian cancer. *Cancer Res.*, **51**, 5107–12.

23. Kacinski, B.M. and Chambers, S.K. (1991) Molecular biology of ovarian cancer. *Curr. Opin. Oncol.*, **3**, 889–900.

24. Slamon, D., Godolphin, W., Jones, L. *et al.* (1989) Study of the Her-2/*neu* protooncogene in human breast and ovarian cancer. *Science*, **244**, 707–12.

25. Berchuck, A., Rodriguez, C.G., Kamel, A. *et al.* (1991) Epidermal growth factor receptor expression in normal ovarian epithelium and ovarian cancer. *Am. J. Obstet. Gynecol.*, **164**, 669–74.

26. Rodriguez, G.C., Berchuck, A., Whitaker, R.S. *et al.* (1991) Epidermal growth factor receptor expression in normal ovarian epithelium and ovarian cancer. II. Relationship between receptor expression and response to epidermal growth factor. *Am J. Obstet. Gynecol.*, **164**, 745–50.

27. Bauknecht, T., Runge, M., Schwall, M. *et al.* (1988) Occurrence of epidermal growth factor receptors in human adnexal tumors and their prognostic value in advanced ovarian carcinomas. *Gynecol. Oncol.*, **29**, 147–57.

28. Marth, C., Lang, T., Koza, A. *et al.* (1990) Transforming growth factor-beta and ovarian carcinoma cells: regulation of proliferation and surface antigen expression. *Cancer Letters*, **51**, 221–5.

29. Rajaniemi, H., Kauppila, A., Ronnberg, L. *et al.* (1981) LH(hCG) receptor in benign and malignant tumors of human ovary. *Acta Obstet. Gynecol. Scand.*, (Suppl.) **101**, 83.

30. Stouffer, R.L., Grodin, M.S., Davis, J.R. *et al.* (1984) Investigation of binding sites for follicle-stimulating hormone and chorionic gonadotropin in human ovarian cancers. *J. Clin. Endocrinol. Metab.*, **59**, 441–6.

31. Nicosia, S.V., Johnson, J.H. and Streibel, E.J. (1985) Growth characteristics of rabbit ovarian mesothelial (surface epithelial) cells. *Int. J. Gynecol. Pathol.*, **4**, 58–74.

32. Wilson, J.E. (1958) Adenocarcinomata in hens kept in a constant environment. *Poultry Sci.*, **37**, 1253.

33. Fredrickson, T.N. (1987) Ovarian tumors of the hen. *Envir. Health Persp.*, **73**, 35–51.

34. Nijman, H.W., Burger, C.W., Baak, J.P.A. *et al.* (1992) Borderline malignancy of the ovary and controlled hyperstimulation: a report of 2 cases. *Eur. J. Cancer*, **28A**, 1971–3.

35. Narod, S.A., Lynch, H.T., Conway, T. *et al.* (1991) Familial breast–ovarian cancer locus on chromosome 17q12-q23. *Lancet*, **338**, 82–3.

36. Wu, S.Q., Storer, B.E., Bookland, E.A. *et al.* (1991) Non-random chromosome losses in stepwise neoplastic transformation *in vitro* of human uroepithelial cells. *Cancer Res.*, **51**, 3323–6.

37. Bodine, D.M., McDonagh, K.T., Brandt, S.J. *et al.* (1990) Development of a high-titer retrovirus producer cell line capable of gene transfer into rhesus monkey hematopoietic stem cells. *Proc. Natl. Acad. Sci. USA*, **87**, 3738–42.

38. Kolberg, R. (1992) Gene-transfer virus contaminant linked to monkeys' cancer. *J. NIH Res.*, **4**, 43–4.

39. Jacobs, I.J, Smith, S.A., Wiseman R.W. *et al.* (1993) A deletion unit on chromosome 17q in epithelial ovarian tumors distal to the familial breast/ovarian cancer locus. *Cancer Res.*, **53**, 1218–21.

Chapter 16

Human ovarian surface epithelium: growth patterns and differentiation

N. AUERSPERG, S.L. MAINES-BANDIERA and P.A. KRUK

16.1 INTRODUCTION

The ovarian surface epithelium (OSE) is the modified pelvic mesothelium that covers the ovary. It comprises only a minute fraction of the total ovarian mass but it is thought to be the source of most human ovarian carcinomas, including those varieties that contribute most to cancer mortality [1]. The precise causes of ovarian cancer are not known. However, it is likely that important clues will be obtained by a thorough understanding of the development, structure and functions of the surface epithelium from which these neoplasms arise.

Early in development, the future OSE forms part of the epithelial lining of the intraembryonic coelom. It is thus an epithelium of mesodermal origin. The gonadal blastema arises, in part, by the proliferation and differentiation of the coelomic epithelium in the presumptive gonadal area. This gonadal area lies near the region where invagination of the coelomic epithelium gives rise to the müllerian (paramesonephric) duct which, in turn, differentiates into the epithelia of the oviduct, uterus and upper vagina. Hence, these epithelia and the OSE are embryologically closely related. The OSE cells also take part in the formation of the somatic components of the ovarian cortex. They undergo intense mitotic activity during the fourth and fifth month of fetal development, possibly in response to steroid hormones [2,3]. The downgrowths of OSE which penetrate into the fetal ovary give rise to the presumptive granulosa cells [4], perhaps with contributions by the mesonephric tubules [5]. Thus, the celomic epithelium which gives rise to the OSE has the capacity to differentiate along many different pathways. The re-expression of this capacity probably contributes to the striking variety of phenotypes found among OSE derived ovarian carcinomas and to their frequent differentiation along the lines of müllerian duct derivatives.

The implication of OSE as the source of the common human ovarian cancers is based mainly on the frequent histopathological demonstration of premalignant and early malignant changes in the OSE, sometimes in direct continuation with fully malignant tumors [6]. Early malignant changes occur characteristically in OSE lined clefts and inclusion cysts rather than on the ovarian surface. This location has given rise to speculations that early carcinogenetic events might be influenced by the stromal microenvironment which surrounds the cysts but is separated from OSE on the ovarian surface by the tunica albuginea [7] or by secretory products (OSE or stroma derived) that accumulate in the confined cystic spaces but diffuse into the pelvic cavity from the ovarian surface.

In recent years, methods have been established to grow human OSE in tissue culture [8–10]. This experimental system has made it possible to characterize the properties of this epithelium and to begin to investigate the specific physiological and pathological conditions underlying early carcinogenic changes. This chapter summarizes some of the information that has been obtained by this approach.

16.2 GROWTH PATTERNS

In vivo, OSE forms a simple squamous-to-cuboidal epithelium with a basement membrane which, in turn, overlies a dense, collagenous tunica albuginea. This layer separates the epithelium from the underlying ovarian stroma. The epithelial phenotype which OSE exhibits *in vivo* tends to modulate to an atypical, fibroblast-like form *in vitro* — either gradually, under standard culture conditions [8], or more rapidly in response to epidermal growth factor [9] (Figure 16.1). Such phenotypic plasticity is also observed in cultures of other simple epithelia of mesodermal origin, e.g. endothelium, and may reflect a relatively labile state of determination as compared to other, more highly specialized epithelia. It also indicates that the phenotypic expression of normal OSE is highly responsive to changes in the environment of the cells.

A major factor in the regulation of all epithelial phenotypes is reciprocal interactions between the epithelium and its underlying extracellular matrix (ECM). Importantly, the capacity of epithelia to take part in these interactions is characteristically altered or impaired in malignancy. Our investigations of normal OSE in culture showed that its phenotype is profoundly influenced by interac-

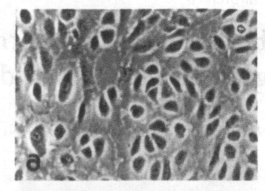

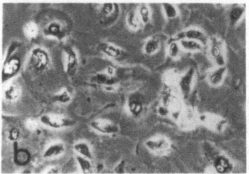

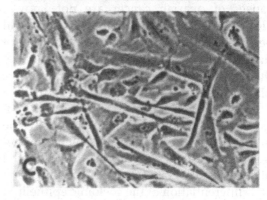

Figure 16.1 Morphological variation among cultures of human ovarian surface epithelium in low passage. (a) Compact, cobblestone monolayer; (b) flat epithelial monolayer; (c) atypical growth with cellular overlap and fibroblast like features. The cultures are grown in medium 199:MCDB 105 with 15% fetal bovine serum. In (c), epidermal growth factor (20 ng ml^{-1}) and hydrocortisone (0.4 μg ml^{-1}) were added five days previously [9]. (Phase contrast microscopy, ×150).

tions with ECM and that, in turn, OSE can modify its adjacent matrix through synthesis, lysis and physical restructuring.

We compared the morphology and growth patterns of OSE cells cultured on plastic, rat tail tendon derived collagen gel, fibrin clots and Matrigel (a basement membrane like matrix [11]) [12,13]. Within two days of culture on the various substrata, OSE cells showed consistent changes in morphology. On plastic and fibrin clots, the cells formed flat cobblestone, epithelial monolayers. However, on fibrin clots the cells were less cohesive than on plastic. It is tempting to speculate that this *in vitro* response to fibrin mimics the *in vivo* response of OSE at the ovulatory wound edges, which involves the migration of dispersed OSE cells onto the ovulatory fibrin clot. On collagen gels, OSE cells attached and spread but assumed a spindle shaped morphology suggestive of epithelio–mesenchymal conversion (Figure 16.2). This phenotypic plasticity may be related to the close developmental relationship of ovarian stroma and surface epithelium, both of which are derived from the gonadal ridge. It may be a new example of epithelial–mesenchymal conversion similar to the epithelial–mesenchymal conversions that can be induced by suspending embryonic anterior lens epithelial cells [14], adult thyroid follicular cells [15] or Madin-Darby canine kidney cells [16] within collagen gels. On Matrigel, the OSE cells formed aggregates that were joined to each other via branching structures. Granular areas near OSE cells suggested degradation of the matrix. This impression was supported by scanning electron microscopy and paraffin sections which showed that OSE aggregates became embedded and completely covered by Matrigel. Eventually, the aggregates invaded the matrix and finally attached and spread on the underlying plastic (Figure 16.3) [12,13]. The behaviour of OSE aggregates in Matrigel is reminiscent of differentiation and/or

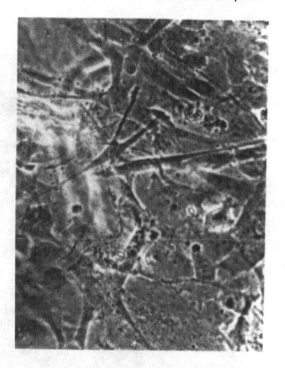

Figure 16.2 Ovarian surface epithelium grown on collagen gel for one week. The cells were originally epithelial but subsequently underwent mesenchymal conversion and some of them invaded the gel. (Phase contrast microscopy, ×180.)

morphogenesis *in vivo*, as seen in sex cord formation and müllerian duct formation. It is important to note that this form of invasiveness appears to be part of the normal OSE phenotype and must be distinguished from those aspects of invasiveness that are acquired with malignancy. Therefore, OSE cells can be added to the increasing list of normal cell types capable of invading Matrigel [17].

When OSE cells were seeded onto collagen gels that contain a rat OSE derived, collagenous ECM [18], they spread over this complex matrix and contracted it into irregular round structures which were a fraction of their

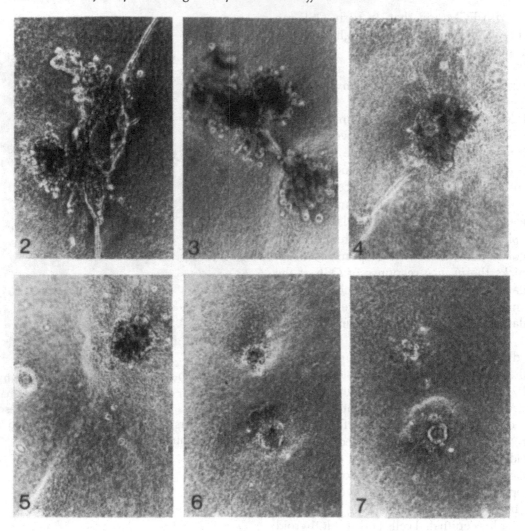

Figure 16.3 Ovarian surface epithelium grown on Matrigel [11]. The numbers on the panels indicate the number of days since passage. Over seven days, the cells, which were seeded onto the surface of the gel, formed aggregates and invaded the matrix. (Phase contrast microscopy, ×150.)

original size. The majority of cells lined the surface of these 'organoids' as well as clefts that had formed as a result of the contraction (Figure 16.4). The degree to which OSE cells contracted organoids was directly related to the number of OSE cells seeded. Thus, OSE cells have the capacity to physically remodel ECM [19]. While the exact mechanism of gel contraction is unknown, the morphological events associated with organoid contraction by the OSE cells appear to be the same as those described for fibroblast mediated collagen gel contraction [20] suggesting, perhaps, that contraction occurs by the same process in

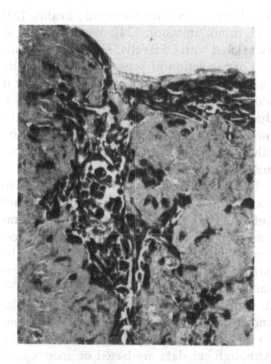

Figure 16.4 Ovarian surface epithelial cells, grown on a composite matrix of rat OSE derived ECM and collagen gel, contract the matrix and invade clefts. (H&E, ×140.)

that different substrata induce changes in the morphology and growth patterns of OSE cells that have counterparts *in vivo* during various morphogenetic processes.

The different OSE morphologies on the various substrata did not translate into the expression of different integrins at the cell surfaces [13]. The integrin profile of OSE cells cultured for 48 hours on plastic, collagen gel, fibrin clot and Matrigel was the same among early and late passage OSE cells, between cobblestone and atypical (fibroblast-like) OSE cells, and between OSE cells and their SV40 immortalized counterparts [12]. VLA-6 and B4, comprising a laminin receptor, were absent in all cases. With the exception of collagen gels, receptors for vitronectin (VNR), collagen, fibronectin and laminin (VLA-2, -3, -5) were present in all cases. Integrin expression was almost always greatest on plastic and least or absent on collagen gels. Time course immunoprecipitation studies of integrin expression clearly showed downregulation of integrin expression of OSE cells maintained on collagen gels.

Growth curves on the different substrata showed that plastic supported intense OSE cell proliferation, while collagen gels and fibrin clots supported little or no growth. On Matrigel, the cell numbers eventually decreased to below the initial seeding values [13].

Since the morphological data suggested that OSE cells invade Matrigel, the cultures were examined for the production of proteolytic enzymes which may degrade ECM [13]. Analyses of conditioned culture medium from all substrata demonstrated that normal OSE secrete a chymotrypsin-like peptidase with phenylalanine specificity and an elastase-like peptidase with alanine specificity. The levels of chymotrypsin-like activity and elastase-like activities were inversely related to cell growth. Thus, OSE cells appear to constitutively produce these proteases, although the amount of protease production

both systems. Further, the VLA-2 and possibly the VLA-5 integrins appear to play a role in fibroblast mediated collagen gel contraction [21,22]. Interestingly, OSE cells express VLA-2 and VLA-5 (see below), so that these integrins may function cooperatively to mediate organoid contraction via interactions between OSE cells and ECM. Since the ability of OSE cells to contract ECM parallels the fibroblast model of wound repair, it is also tempting to speculate that perhaps cyst formation and the ovarian shrinkage observed with age are facilitated in part by the matrix remodelling capabilities of OSE cells.

These results reflect the dynamic nature of OSE as well as its plasticity and heterogeneity both *in vivo* and *in vitro*. They demonstrate is influenced by the culture substratum. Major bands of gelatinolytic activity were consistently found in the conditioned medium of OSE maintained on the various substrata. A 30 kd gelatinase was expressed exclusively by OSE cells while a 42 kd gelatinase produced by OSE cells may be similar to a 42 kd gelatinase present in serum. Essentially all gelatinolytic activity was abolished following incubation of the zymograms with EDTA, indicating that these gelatinases are metalloproteases. OSE cells did not secrete plasminogen activator at levels detectable in casein agarose diffusion plate assays. The lack of plasminogen activator detection may be due to the presence of plasminogen activator inhibitor which was demonstrated by immunofluorescence staining. These results may have implications for normal ovarian functioning such as the initiation and repair of ovulation and for normal development such as sex cord formation. Like the ability to invade Matrigel, protease production appears to be part of the normal OSE phenotype and not one acquired with malignant progression. However, the 72 kd and/or the 94 kd type IV collagenase, recognized to be important for wound healing [23] and tumor invasion [24], were not found associated with OSE cells. The exact mechanism of regulation of protease production by OSE cells remains unknown. However, it would be interesting to see if protease production by OSE cells is under the same hormonal influences as proteases produced by other ovarian cell types such as the granulosa and thecal cells [25,26].

Human OSE also has the capacity to secrete ECM. It was found to produce not only the epithelial basement membrane components, such as laminin, but also macromolecules that are classically considered to be part of the stromal or fibroblastic phenotype such as collagen types I and III (Figure 16.5). A similar capacity for combined epithelial and stromal ECM synthesis has been demonstrated previously for OSE of the rat [27]. Although our data are based on matrix synthesis in culture, there is no reason to believe that OSE cells might not have the ability to express a similar phenotype *in vivo*. While in the human papillary outgrowths of normal OSE are scarce [3,28], OSE is greatly amplified and forms papillae with stromal cores in

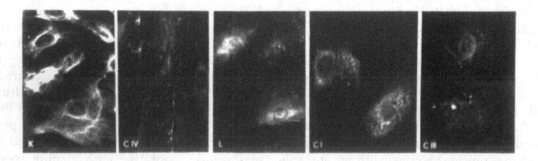

Figure 16.5 Parallel cultures of ovarian surface epithelial cells were stained by immunofluorescence for keratin (K) to confirm their epithelial phenotype and for components of the extracellular matrix. The cells produce the epithelial matrix components collagen type IV (CIV) and laminin (L), as well as the stromal components, collagen types I (CI) and III (CIII). (Immunofluorescence microscopy, ×150).

a high proportion of serous ovarian tumors. Thus, *in vivo*, increased numbers of OSE cells are accommodated on the limiting ovarian surface through the formation of papillae. It is tempting to speculate that the deposition of an ECM by OSE cells might, at least in part, provide the stromal cores for papillae that occur physiologically and pathologically. Such a capacity of ovarian cells to form a collagenous matrix autonomously would render the cells less dependent on stroma contributed by normal connective tissue cells and might therefore be an important factor for ovarian neoplastic progression. In the normal ovary, the capacity of OSE to secrete stromal matrix suggests that this epithelium may contribute directly to the postovulatory repair of the underlying stroma, including the tunica albuginea.

16.3 DIFFERENTIATION

In the mature woman, the OSE is a monolayered squamous-to-cuboidal, keratin positive epithelium. The cells are attached to a basement membrane and are joined by gap junctions, focal tight junctions and simple desmosomes. There are no known tissue specific differentiation markers that characterize OSE. In culture, therefore, a series of less specific markers is required to distinguish OSE cells from possible cell contaminants, to monitor the degree to which they retain their *in vivo* phenotype and to investigate markers of neoplastic progression. The identification by markers is important because morphologically, the epithelial form of OSE cells is indistinguishable from vascular endothelial and extraovarian mesothelial cells, while atypical OSE cells resemble fibroblasts (Figures 16.1 and 16.2). The following markers were evaluated by immunofluorescence microscopy, histochemistry and Western blotting.

In our hands, one the most reliable characteristics of OSE is the presence of keratin, which distinguishes these cells from other ovarian cells. OSE expresses keratins type 7, 8, 18 and 19 [29] and thus differs from granulosa cells which only contain very low amounts of keratins 8 and 18 [30,31]. OSE tends to become keratin negative with time in culture and, frequently, not all cells are positive even in early passage. Another useful marker developed to identify epithelial cells is 2G3 [32]. This antibody recognizes a subpopulation of OSE cells which overlaps but is not identical to the keratin positive cells. The accuracy of OSE identification is therefore improved with combined staining for keratin and 2G3. Keratin positive extraovarian mesothelial cells may contaminate biopsy specimens in the form of adhesions. In contrast to these mesothelial cells, OSE cells express 17-hydroxysteroid dehydrogenase and, occasionally, mucin [8,29]. Another contaminant that is difficult to distinguish from OSE morphologically is vascular endothelial cells. In OSE cultures, these cells can originate in cut surfaces of ovarian biopsy specimens and in capillaries that form on the ovarian surface in conjunction with adhesions. Most endothelial cells lack keratin. In addition, factor VIII proved to be useful for their identification since it is consistently positive in endothelial cells and negative in OSE. The markers that help distinguish OSE cells from fibroblasts are keratin and laminin, which persist in a proportion of OSE cells even after these assume atypical fibroblast-like shapes. E-cadherin, an adhesion molecule for most epithelia [33], was absent in normal OSE cultures but was present in cultures of the ovarian carcinoma lines OVCAR-3 and CAOV3 [34,35] (Figure 16.6). Interestingly, E-cadherin was also not detected in the OSE of cryostat sections of normal ovaries but was expressed in cysts that were lined with atypical and, sometimes,

CA125 positive epithelium (Figure 16.7). It should be noted that E-cadherin is a normal component of oviductal and endometrial epithelium. These observations suggest that E-cadherin expression may represent an early marker of neoplastic transformation in the OSE [36].

An important component of differentiation is the capacity of cells to produce autocrine and paracrine regulatory factors. Carcinoma cells frequently secrete such factors, in particular peptide growth factors, which maintain and stimulate the proliferation of the malignant cells by autocrine mechanisms [37,38]. The capacity to produce such growth stimulatory agents may be a normal cell property retained during malignant transformation, or it may be acquired in the course of carcinogenesis. There is increasing evidence that normal OSE cells also produce a variety of agents with growth regulatory capabilities. OSE cells secrete TGFβ which acts as an autocrine growth inhibitor for OSE and some ovarian cancers [39] and amphiregulin which appears to control OSE and ovarian cancer cell proliferation in a complex, dose dependent manner [40,41]. Amphiregulin has homology with epidermal growth factor which is a potent mitogen for OSE cells [9,42]. Recently, we identified a number of cytokines by bioassays, combined with antibody mediated inactivation, in media conditioned by

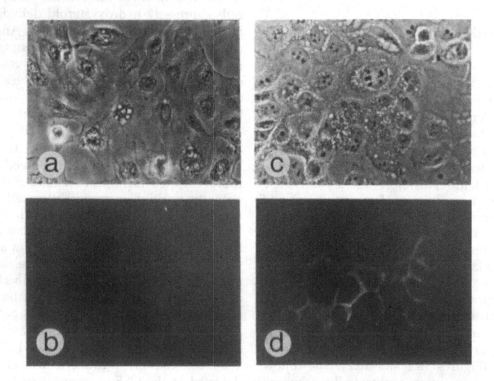

Figure 16.6 E-cadherin expression in culture by ovarian surface epithelial cells (a,b) and by ovarian carcinoma cells (c,d). (Phase microscopy (a,c) and immunofluorescence microscopy (b,d), ×200).

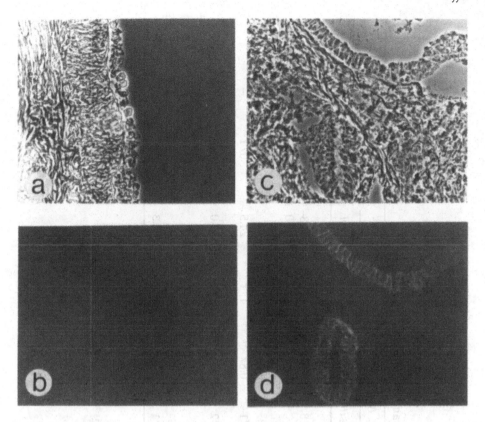

Figure 16.7 E-cadherin expression in ovarian cryostat sections showing surface epithelium (a,b) and two inclusion cysts (c,d). (Phase microscopy (a,c) and immunofluorescence microscopy (b,d), ×200).

normal OSE cells [43]. The cytokines that were identified include IL-1 and IL-6, as well as M-CSF, G-CSF and GM-CSF (Table 16.1). These results are important for several reasons: first, it has been shown that some ovarian cancer cells secrete IL-1, IL-6, GM-CSF and M-CSF and growth stimulation of ovarian carcinoma cells by IL-1, IL-6 and GM-CSF has been reported [reviewed in 37,43]. Importantly, levels of M-CSF in blood and ascitic fluid appear to correlate with a poor prognosis in ovarian cancer [44,45], as does overexpression of the M-CSF receptor [46]. The detection of these cytokines as products

of normal OSE suggests possible autocrine loops that may be important in ovarian carcinogenesis and indicates that their secretion by ovarian cancer cells represents the retention of normal cell properties rather than the acquisition of new characteristics with malignant progression. Finally, much information has accumulated which shows that IL-1 and IL-6, in particular, affect steroidogenesis by normal follicular cells and probably influence the proteolytic and protein synthetic activities associated with ovulation, atresia and luteolysis [43]. Thus, OSE derived cytokines may play a role in the regulation of normal

Table 16.1 Cytokine secretion by normal ovarian surface epithelium and its abnormal derivatives

Type of OSE cells	IL-1		IL-6		M-CSF		G-CSF		GM-CSF	
	No. positive	U/ml*	No. positive	U/ml	No. positive	U/ml	No. positive	U/ml	No. positive	U/ml
Normal, low passage**	4/4	2.5–38.7	5/5	1920–11,720	6/8	13.0–178.0	6/6	3.8–3000.0	4/6	0.065–1.5
Atypical, low passage +	1/1	1.3	1/1	870	1/1	0.87	1/1	24.5	0/1	–
IOSE line‡	1/2	7.9	2/2	484–618	0/2	–	1/2	193.0	0/2	–
Ovarian carcinoma lines §	0/2	–	1/1	100	1/1	21.0	1/2	0.3	ND	

*   For confidence limits, see ref [43]
** Cultures in passages 2–4, from normal ovaries
⁺   Asymptomatic clinically, but OSE cells were ciliated and CA125 positive
‡   Two lines of low passage OSE cells immortalized with SV40 early genes [12]
§   CaOV₃ and OVCAR3 [34,35]

ovarian differentiation and function through paracrine regulatory mechanisms.

16.4 CONCLUSION

The improved methodology now available to culture human OSE cells has made possible in depth studies of its biology. Results to date indicate that this epithelium is far more complex and physiologically versatile than would be predicted from its inconspicuous appearance. It is possible that its structural simplicity, compared to most other epithelia, is an expression of limited determination and is related to its competence for phenotypic plasticity. Their mesodermal origin and close developmental relationship to stromal cells appear to confer on OSE cells the capacity to express this plasticity by modulating between epithelial and fibroblastic phenotypes, as shown by their tendency to modulate towards a stromal phenotype under standard culture conditions and by their capacity to undergo epithelio–mesenchymal conversion upon interactions with specific substrata. The same phenotypic plasticity may, however, permit OSE to assume the abnormal phenotype of müllerian duct derived epithelia, a change that appears to correlate with the onset of neoplastic progression. Phenotypic plasticity renders cells adaptable to varying conditions and changing environments. Perhaps a loss of such plasticity by the more complex, atypical epithelium which lines pre-neoplastic inclusion cysts is related to its eventual transformation to malignancy.

The role of normal OSE in the remodelling of the ovarian cortex appears to be broader than is generally assumed. It involves synthetic, physical and proteolytic functions which may influence ovulation and the repair of ovulatory defects, as well as the ovarian shrinkage and cyst formation which occur with age. Furthermore, while proteolytic activities and invasiveness are characteristics of the malignant phenotype, they also appear to be part of the normal OSE phenotype. Perhaps aberrations in these normal functions contribute to the propensity of OSE cells to undergo malignant transformation. The discovery that OSE cells secrete biologically active cytokines suggests that OSE products are an integral part of the network of hormones and short range acting factors which regulate normal ovarian physiology. In addition, it is reasonable to suspect that these products may play a role in the progression of ovarian carcinogenesis.

ACKNOWLEDGEMENTS

The work described in this chapter was supported by grants to N.A. from the Medical Research Council of Canada, the National Cancer Institute of Canada and the BC Health Research Foundation. N.A. is the recipient of a research associateship from the National Cancer Institute of Canada and P.A.K. received a studentship from the BC Foundation for Non-Animal Research.

REFERENCES

1. Yancik, R. (1993) Ovarian cancer: age contrasts in incidence, histology, disease stage at diagnosis, and mortality. *Cancer*, **71**, 517–23.
2. Gondos, B. (1975) Surface epithelium of the developing ovary. *Am. J. Pathol.*, **81**, 303–20.
3. Nicosia, S.V. (1983) Morphological changes in the human ovary throughout life. In *The Ovary*, (ed. G.B. Serra), Raven Press, New York, pp. 57–81.
4. Motta, P.M. and Makabe, S. (1982) Development of the ovarian surface and associated germ cells in the human fetus. *Cell Tiss. Res.*, **226**, 493–510.
5. Byskov, A.G. (1986) Differentiation of mammalian embryonic gonad. *Physiol. Rev.*, **66**, 71–117.
6. Godwin, A.K., Testa, J.R. and Hamilton, T.C. (1993) The biology of ovarian cancer development. *Cancer*, **71**, 530–6.

7. Heinonen, P.K., Koivuls, T., Rajameinir, H. and Pystynen, P. (1986) Peripheral and ovarian venous concentrations of steroid and gonadotropin hormones in postmenopausal women with epithelial ovarian tumors. *Gynec. Oncol.*, **25**, 1–10.

8. Auersperg, N., Siemens, C.H. and Myrdal, S.E. (1984) Human ovarian surface epithelium in primary culture. *In Vitro*, **20**, 743–55.

9. Siemens, C.H. and Auersperg, N. (1988) Serial propagation of human ovarian surface epithelium in tissue culture. *J. Cell. Physiol.*, **134**, 347–56.

10. Kruk, P.A., Maines-Bandiera, S.L. and Auersperg, N. (1990) A simplified method to culture human ovarian surface epithelium. *Lab. Invest.*, **63**, 132–6.

11. Kleinman, H.K., McGarvey, M.L., Liotta, L.A. *et al.* (1982) Isolation and characterization of type IV procollagen, laminin, and heparin sulfate proteoglycan from the EHS sarcoma. *Biochem.*, **21**, 6188–93.

12. Maines-Bandiera, S.L., Kruk, P.A. and Auersperg, N. (1992) Simian virus 40-transformed human ovarian surface epithelial cells escape normal growth controls but retain morphogenetic responses to extracellular matrix. *Am. J. Obstet. Gynecol.*, **167**, 729–35.

13. Kruk, P.A., Uitto, J., Firth, J.D., Dedhar, S. and Auersperg, N. (1994) Dynamic interactions between human ovarian surface epithelial cells and adjacent extracellular matrix. Submitted.

14. Greenburg, G. and Hay, E.D. (1986) Cytodifferentiation and tissue phenotype change during transformation of embryonic lens epithelium to mesenchyme-like cells *in vitro*. *Develop. Biol.*, **115**, 363–79.

15. Greenburg, G. and Hay, E.D. (1988) Cytoskeleton and thyroglobulin expression change during transformation of thyroid epithelium to mesenchyme-like *cells*. *Development*, **102**, 605–22.

16. Zuk, A., Matlin, K. and Hay, E.D. (1989) Type 1 collagen gel induces Madin-Darby canine kidney cells to become fusiform in shape and lose apical–basal polarity. *J. Cell. Biol.*, **108**, 903–20.

17. Noel, A.C., Calle, A., Emonard, H.P. *et al.* (1991) Invasion of reconstituted basement membrane matrix is not correlated to the malignant metastatic cell phenotype. *Cancer Res.*, **51**, 405–14.

18. Kruk, P.A. and Auersperg, N. (1994) A line of rat ovarian surface epithelium (ROSE) provides a continuous source of complex extracellular matrix. *In Vitro Cell. Develop. Biol.*, in press.

19. Kruk. P.A. and Auersperg, N. (1992) Human ovarian surface epithelial cells are capable of physically restructuring extracellular matrix. *Am. J. Obstet, Gynecol.*, **167**, 1437–43.

20. Bell, E., Ivarsson, B. and Merrill, C. (1979) Production of a tissue-like structure by contraction of collagen lattices by human fibroblasts of different proliferative potential *in vitro*. *Proc. Natl. Acad. Sci. USA*, **76**, 1274–8.

21. Clark, R.A.F. (1990) Fibronectin matrix deposition and fibronectin receptor expression in healing and normal skin. *J. Invest. Dermatol.*, **94**, 1285-134-S.

22. Schiro, J.A., Chan, B.M.C., Roswsit, W.T. *et al.* (1991) Integrin VLA-2 mediates reorganization and contraction of collagen matrices by human cells. *Cell*, **67**, 403–10.

23. Granada, J.L., Lande, M.A. and Karvonen, R.L. (1990) A human cartilage metalloproteinase with elastolytic activity. *Connect. Tissue Res.*, **24**, 249–63.

24. Liotta, L.A., Rao, C.N. and Barsky, S.H. (1983) Tumor invasion and the extracellular matrix. *Lab. Invest.*, **49**, 636–49.

25. Curry, T.E., Dean, D.D., Sanders, S.L. *et al.* (1989) The role of ovarian proteases and their inhibitors in ovulation. *Steroids*, **54**, 501–21.

26. Ny, T., Bjersing, L., Hsueh, A.J.W. and Loskutoff, D.J. (1985) Cultured granulosa cells produce two plasminogen activators and an antiactivator, each regulated differently by gonadotropins. *Endocrinol.*, **116**, 1666–8.

27. Auersperg, N., MacLaren, I.A. and Kruk, P.A. (1991) Ovarian surface epithelium: autonomous production of connective tissue-type extracellular matrix. *Biol. Reprod.*, **44**, 717–24.

28. Nicosia, S.V. (1987) The aging ovary. *Med. Clin. N. Am.*, **71**, 1–9.

29. Auersperg, N., Kruk, P.A. and Maines-Bandiera, S.L. (1994) Characterization of cultured human ovarian surface epithelial cells: phenotypic plasticity and premalignant changes. *Lab. Invest.*, in press.

30. Czernobilsky, B. (1985) Co-expression of cytokeratin and vimentin filaments in mesothelial, granulosa, and rete ovarii cells of the human ovary. *Eur. J. Cell Biol.*, **37**, 175–90.

31. Czernobilsky, B., Moll, R., Franke, W.W. *et al.* (1984) Intermediate filaments of normal and neoplastic tissues of the female genital tract with emphasis on problems of differential tumor diagnosis. *Pathol. Res. Pract.*, **179**, 31–7.

32. Frankel, A.E., Ring, D.B., Tringale, F. and Hsieh-Ma, S.T. (1985) Tissue distribution of breast cancer-associated antigens defined by monoclonal antibodies. *J. Biol. Response Mod.*, **4**, 273–86.

33. Eidelman, S., Damsky, C.H., Wheelock, M.J. and Damjanov, I. (1989) Expression of the cell–cell adhesion glycoprotein cell-CAM 120/80 in normal human tissues and tumors. *Am. J. Pathol.*, **135**, 101–10.

34. Hamilton, T.C., Young, R.C., McKoy, W.M. *et al.* (1983) Characterization of a human ovarian carcinoma cell line (NIH:OVCAR-3) with androgen and estrogen receptors. *Cancer Res.*, **43**, 5379–89.

35. Fogh, J. and Tremple, G. (1975) New human tumor cell lines. In *Human Tumor Cells in Vitro*, (ed. J. Fogh), Plenum Publishers, New York, pp. 115–60.

36. Maines-Bandiera, S.L. and Auersperg, N. (1993) Progression of E-cadherin expression in normal human ovarian surface epithelial cells and ovarian carcinomas. *Proc. Am. Assoc. Cancer Res.*, **34**, 32.

37. Berchuck, A., Kohler, M.F., Boente M.P. *et al* (1993) Growth regulation and transformation of ovarian epithelium. *Cancer*, **71**, 545–51.

38. Mills, G.B., Hashimoto, S., Hurteau, J. *et al.* (1992) Regulation of growth of human ovarian cancer cells. In *Ovarian Cancer 2: Biology, Diagnosis and Management*, (eds F. Sharp, W.P. Mason and W. Creasman), Chapman & Hall, London, pp. 127–45.

39. Berchuck, A., Rodriguez, G., Olt, G. *et al.* (1992) Regulation of growth of normal ovarian epithelial cells and ovarian cancer cell lines by transforming growth factor-β. *Am. J. Obstet. Gynecol.*, **166**, 676–84.

40. Johnson, G.R., Saeki, T., Auersperg, N. *et al.* (1991) Response to and expression of amphiregulin by ovarian carcinoma and normal ovarian surface epithelial cells: nuclear localization of endogenous amphiregulin. *Biochem. Biophys. Res. Commun.*, **180**, 4481–8.

41. Johnson, G.R., Kannan, B., Shoyab, M. and Stromberg, K. (1993) Amphiregulin induces tyrosine phosphorylation of the epidermal growth factor receptor and p185^erbB2. *J. Biol. Chem.*, **268**, 2924–31.

42. Rodriguez, G.C., Berchuck, A., Whitaker, R.S. *et al.* (1991) Epidermal growth factor receptor expression in normal ovarian epithelium and ovarian cancer. *Am. J. Obstet. Gynecol.*, **164**, 745–50.

43. Ziltener, H.J. Maines-Bandiera, S., Schrader, J.W. and Auersperg, N. (1993) Secretion of IL-1, IL-6 and colony stimulating factors by human ovarian surface epithelium. *Biol. Reprod.*, **49**, 635–41.

44. Kacinski, B.M., Stanley, E.R., Carter, D. *et al.* (1989) Circulating levels of CSF-1 (M-CSF) a lymphohematopoietic cytokine may be a useful marker of disease status in patients with malignant ovarian neoplasms. *Int. J. Radiation Oncol. Biol. Phys.*, **17**, 159–64.

45. Price, F.V., Chambers, S.K., Chambers, J.T. *et al.* (1993) Colony-stimulating factor-1 in primary ascites of ovarian cancer is a significant predictor of survival. *Am. J. Obstet. Gynecol.*, **168**, 520–7.

46. Kacinski, B.M., Carter, D., Mittal, K. *et al.* (1990) Ovarian adenocarcinomas express *fms*-complementary transcripts and *fms* antigen, often with coexpression of CSF-1. *Am. J. Pathol.*, **137**, 135–47.

Chapter 17

Management of low malignant potential ovarian tumors

W.R. ROBINSON

17.1 INTRODUCTION

The recognition of low malignant potential (LMP) or borderline ovarian tumors as a distinct pathological entity by the International Federation of Gynecology and Obstetrics was an attempt to add a needed degree of precision to the diagnosis of ovarian tumors [1]. Despite this widely accepted improvement in histological diagnostic criteria, the behavior and prognosis of LMP tumors remain unpredictable and the appropriate treatment continues to be debated. The uncertainty in therapeutic decision making is complicated by several factors. The diagnosis of an LMP tumor is rarely made preoperatively, so the initial treatment plan is often made in the operating room by physicians unaccustomed to treating ovarian malignancies. Consultation with clinicians more experienced with these tumors is frequently not feasible. In addition, histological diagnosis by rapid frozen section of LMP tumors is often difficult and unreliable. Finally, the postoperative treatment of LMP tumors in the United States has been characterized by a wide variety of regimens, making comparisons of long term outcomes difficult.

This chapter will outline the current thinking regarding the management of LMP tumors. A consensus of opinion has developed regarding some topics; however for others, attempts to draw conclusions or make statements have been limited by a lack of documented information. Since these tumors have only been specifically recognized for 32 years and the long term outcome associated with them may require a decade or longer to evaluate fully, it is likely to be several more years before most questions regarding treatment and its effect on prognosis are answered.

17.2 PREOPERATIVE EVALUATION

Approximately 15% of all ovarian epithelial malignancies are LMP tumors [2]. It is often difficult or impossible to predict the histological diagnosis preoperatively in a patient who presents with an adnexal mass. Benign, LMP and malignant ovarian tumors overlap considerably in their clinical characteristics. This overlap requires the clinician to utilize multiple diagnostic modalities in the preoperative evaluation, but not to rely on any one too heavily. Patient age, physical examination, pelvic/abdominal ultrasound and tumor markers (most notably CA-125) are all important in the work-up of a patient with an adnexal mass prior to surgery. The question of whether a patient with a pelvic mass should be referred to someone specifically trained in treating ovarian malignancies cannot be answered by utilizing a rigid set of diagnostic criteria. A careful analysis of all available information and assessment of the physician's own technical capabilities are required to make that decision. Liberal use of preoperative consultation with physicians more experienced in treating these tumors will facilitate appropriate management decisions. Ultimately, physicians treating these patients must rely on seasonal clinical judgement with the aid of available diagnostic tools and consultative services to outline the appropriate treatment plan and carry it out. Whether the patient should be treated by an oncologist can only be decided on an individual basis.

17.2.1 PATIENT AGE

Multiple studies have demonstrated that LMP tumors occur more commonly in younger patients than frank malignancies. Marino and Jaffe showed that women aged 30–40 years are more frequently diagnosed with LMP tumors than older women, who are more often diagnosed with frank malignancies [3]. The mean age in three cumulated studies was 43 years [4,5,6]. Table 17.1 presents a comparison of patient ages with either benign, LMP or malignant tumors [7]. LMP tumors tend to be diagnosed at an age intermediate to benign and malignant tumors as the data from this population based study show.

Table 17.1 Age at diagnosis (from [7])

Age in yrs	<20	20–39	40–49	≥50
Benign	7%	41%	36%	16%
LMP*	<1%	44%	44%	11%
Malignant	<1%	11%	49%	39%

* Low malignant potential

17.2.2 PHYSICAL EXAMINATION

The characteristics of patients with LMP tumors on physical examination have been less well documented than some other features, primarily due to the difficulty in making the diagnosis preoperatively and the resulting lack of precise recording of physical characteristics for study purposes. Some generalizations do seem to be valid, however.

The physical findings associated with LMP tumors are usually intermediate between benign and malignant tumors. Benign adnexal masses tend to be smaller, more mobile, cystic and unilateral, while malignant tumors are more likely to be bilateral, solid, fixed and larger. LMP tumors rarely fit either pattern precisely. Bilateral ovarian involvement by LMP tumor has been found in approximately 25% of cases in a summary of data from several recent reports [8–11]. Benign ovarian tumors have been reported to be bilateral in only 15% of cases [12].

17.2.3 IMAGING STUDIES

Imaging studies of adnexal masses are sometimes helpful, although less frequently than one would hope. Ultrasound may help differentiate cystic from solid masses in cases where physical examination is difficult or inconclusive. Ultrasound may also reveal internal septa or small solid areas in an

Table 17.2 Ultrasound description of ovarian masses (from [14])

	Benign	LMP*	Malignant	Total
Unilocular cysts	295	0	1 (0.3%)	296
Multilocular cysts	191	18	20 (8%)	229
Solid tumors	48	1	31 (39%)	80

* Low malignant potential

ovarian mass. These findings have not proven to be reliable predictors of malignancy, however. Buy *et al.* found that ultrasound suggested malignancy in only 36% (five of 14) LMP tumors preoperatively [13]. The data in Table 17.2 correlate ultrasound findings with histological diagnosis. Solid areas within a tumor were shown to be the most frequent predictor of frank malignancy by abdominal ultrasound. However, the predictive value of ultrasound for LMP tumors in this study was poor [14].

Another recently developed technique has been utilized to evaluate adnexal masses, namely color Doppler sonography using a transvaginal probe, which has been used to delineate benign and malignant masses of the ovary [15,16]. A recent report from Fleischer *et al.* [17] used pulsatility indices of the ovarian vessels to predict whether a tumor was benign or malignant. This report described a 100% negative predictive value for malignancy, but only a 73% positive predictive value, suggesting that approximately one in four masses predicted to be malignant by this technique were in fact benign. The use of color flow Doppler ultrasonography for prediction of LMP tumors is being evaluated and remains uncertain, although this appears to be a promising imaging modality.

Other imaging studies such as intravenous pyelogram, barium enema and barium swallow are best used in cases where specific symptoms related to the gastrointestinal or urinary systems are noted. Since LMP tumors rarely involve these systems directly, the usefulness of these studies is limited. Computerized tomography (CT) scans and magnetic resonance imaging (MRI) can identify unsuspected metastatic disease such as liver metastasis or lymphatic involvement. However, these findings are also unusual in LMP tumors. Therefore, these studies are not routinely recommended in the evaluation of an adnexal mass.

17.2.4 TUMOR MARKERS

Serum CA-125 has been shown to correlate well with disease status, response to treatment and survival in patients with frankly malignant ovarian tumors. The role of CA-125 as a screening tool is limited, however. Finkler *et al.* [18] showed a positive predictive value of 94% and a negative predictive value of 80% for malignancy in postmenopausal patients with adnexal masses. However, for premenopausal patients, which will include the majority of LMP tumor patients, the positive and negative predictive values were only 36% and 82% respectively.

It is not surprising then that the role of CA-125 determination in LMP tumors is less well established. A report by Mogensen *et al.* [19] showed five of five LMP tumors and 38 of 41 malignant tumors to have preoperative CA-125 levels >35 u/nl. Rice *et al.* [20] demonstrated elevated CA-125 levels in 75% of LMP tumors with advanced stage (6/8) and 87.5% of serous cell types (7/8), whereas no patients with stage I disease (0/5) or mucinous tumors (0/5) had elevated levels. Tholander *et al.* [21] obtained several tumor markers in 26 patients with LMP tumors preoperatively. This report showed a sensitivity of 58% for CA-125 and tissue polypeptide antigen. Carcinoembryonic antigen (CEA) had an overall sensitivity of only 27%.

To summarize, patient age, physical findings, imaging studies and tumor markers provide useful information. All of these factors may serve to increase the level of suspicion and may alter the surgical approach to the patient. However, none of these, either alone or in combination, can be used as a reliable predictor of LMP tumor. It is necessary for the surgeon to approach the patient with a suspicious adnexal mass prepared for the diagnosis of LMP tumor or low grade malignancy by having an alternative surgical strategy dependent on intraoperative findings.

17.3 OPERATIVE MANAGEMENT

The surgical approach employed to treat an adnexal mass suspicious for LMP tumor should consist of several steps, some of which the surgeon may need to alter during the procedure. The trend in gynecological surgery toward the use of the Pfannenstiel skin incision has expanded over the last decade to include nearly all laparotomies for benign conditions. While the Pfannenstiel incision is certainly adequate for removal of most primary ovarian lesions, complete surgical staging is nearly impossible utilizing this incision. It is therefore important for the surgeon to consider the use of a low midline incision when operating on a patient with a suspicious adnexal mass.

There are no definite criteria for the use of a midline incision. The diagnosis of LMP tumor is too unpredictable to set precise guidelines for the type of incision. In general, the higher the index of suspicion, the more strongly the physician should consider midline incision. After the incision is made, any ascitic fluid found should be collected and sent for cytological analysis. If none is present, pelvic washings should be obtained using 100–200 ml of heparinized normal saline. These washings may be set aside until the primary ovarian mass is excised and a diagnosis is obtained via rapid frozen section analysis. If the lesion is unquestionably benign, the washings may be discarded. Otherwise this fluid should be sent for cytological analysis. A finding of tumor cells in the washings or ascitic fluid changes the stage of disease and possibly the prognosis and treatment.

The most important component of the assessment and treatment of a suspected or proven LMP tumor may be a thorough and accurate pelvic and abdominal exploration by the surgeon. This information is crucial in planning the subsequent operative procedure as well as evaluating the need for postoperative therapy. The presence of extraovarian metastatic disease, peritoneal adhesions or other abdominal or pelvic pathology should be clearly stated in the operative report, particularly if the surgeon is considering referral of the patient for postoperative therapy. The exploration should include palpation of the uterus, adnexa, pelvic peritoneum, sigmoid colon, the pelvic and aortic nodal chains, paracolic gutters, the small intestines and their mesentery, the transverse colon and omentum and the liver and diaphragms. This type of thorough exploration demands the midline incision. Most surgical or gynecological oncologists would find it difficult to believe an adequate exploration of upper abdominal structures such as the liver and diaphragms had been performed using a Pfannenstiel incision.

The primary ovarian lesion should usually be treated by unilateral salpingo-oophorectomy (USO). Tasker and Langley [22] followed 19 patients treated with USO with no decrease in survival over a nine year period. Robinson *et al.* [11] showed that in 19 cases of LMP tumor where a clinically uninvolved ovary was sampled or removed, none of these ovaries contained tumor. Conservative therapy consisting of unilateral adnexectomy therefore appears to be effective treatment. Although the trend in recent years has been toward using cystectomy for benign ovarian lesions, there is little information regarding this approach in LMP tumors. Lim-Tan *et al.* [9] evaluated 35 LMP tumor patients treated with cystectomy alone and found no decrease in survival after an average follow-up of 7.5 years. However, if the resection margin of the cyst was involved with disease or more than one cyst had to be removed, the tumor almost always persisted or recurred. Although these authors appeared to feel comfortable with a frozen section diagnosis of negative margins, it seems unlikely that diagnoses of these lesions made in a community hospital setting (where many if not most are initially treated) will be as confident. Until more extensive information regarding long term follow-up of LMP tumors treated with cystectomy alone is available, it seems prudent to limit its use to patients strongly desirous of childbearing whose contralateral ovary is surgically absent. Since this situation should routinely be known preoperatively, the surgeon may discuss the treatment options with the patient in advance and plan accordingly.

In the patient who is not desirous of childbearing, hysterectomy with bilateral salpingo-oophorectomy is entirely appropriate. Obvious metastatic disease may not be an indication for hysterectomy, however. If the uterus and contralateral ovary are not clinically involved, there is no strong evidence that their removal will be of benefit in a patient with LMP tumor [23]. Even if chemotherapy is required, fertility may be retained and numerous normal pregnancies have resulted following ovarian and other malignancies treated with multiple drug combinations [24,25].

Another important consideration in the management of LMP tumor intraoperatively is the reliability of frozen section diagnosis. Reports by Baak *et al.* [26] and Stalsberg *et al.* [27] showed disagreement among pathologists on the grading of LMP tumors and low grade malignancies in 30–40% of cases, based on permanent sections. TwaalFhoven *et al.* [28] reported a positive predictive value of 100% in frankly malignant ovarian tumors, and 92% in benign lesions, but only 62% for borderline tumors. Large mucinous tumors were shown to be particularly difficult to evaluate. In addition, multiple reports have shown that 17–30% of tumors diagnosed as LMP by frozen section are upgraded to frankly malignant on permanent analysis [11,28]. The surgeon should therefore be aware that a significant margin of error exists in evaluating LMP tumors by frozen section.

17.4 SURGICAL STAGING

The diagnostic and therapeutic value of surgical staging procedures has long been recognized for frankly malignant ovarian tumors. These procedures have routinely included omentectomy, paracolic gutter and diaphragm biopsies, pelvic and aortic lymph node sampling and peritoneal washings. The utility of these procedures in cases of LMP tumor is less certain. Most LMP tumors present as stage I lesions clinically, although since full surgical staging has frequently been omitted, the possibility exists that some tumors are incorrectly staged. Multiple recent reports have addressed this issue. In cases of LMP tumor where surgical staging has been performed, 12.5%–29% have been upstaged based on unsuspected histopathological findings [8,11,20,29–31] (Table 17.3). In addition, the patients were only partially staged in several of these series. Diaphragm biopsies and lymph node sampling were the procedures most frequently not done.

Table 17.3 LMP ovarian tumors upstaged by histopathological findings

Source	Total	Upstaged	%
Nation *et al.* [30]	55	7	12.7
Yazigi *et al.* [10]	29	7	24
Massad *et al.* [8]	31	9	29
Leake *et al.* [31]	27	6	22
Snider *et al.* [29]	26	5	19
Robinson *et al.* [11]	40	5	12.5
Total	208	39	18.7

17.5 LAPAROSCOPIC TREATMENT OF LMP TUMORS

The role of laparoscopy in gynecology has expanded rapidly as equipment, techniques and the confidence of surgeons have improved. Adnexal masses are frequently evaluated and treated using the laparoscope, often at considerable savings of time and morbidity to the patient. Reports of laparoscopically treated LMP tumors have appeared in the literature [32,33]. Given the lack of certainty in diagnosis of LMP tumors preoperatively, it seems likely that more of these lesions will be managed using laparoscopy. Based on current information, it does not appear prudent to recommend laparoscopy as a primary approach to LMP tumors. The possibility of tumor rupture or spillage is significant. In fact many laparoscopists routinely puncture cystic tumors prior to removal. The effect of spillage of LMP tumors intraoperatively is uncertain, although the spread of malignant cells is theoretically possible [34,35]. In addition, most laparoscopists are not technically capable of performing surgical staging procedures. Given the high yield of surgical staging mentioned previously it seems reasonable to recommed that suspicious masses be carefully considered preoperatively for laparotomy and that LMP tumors diagnosed at laparoscopy be treated with immediate laparotomy for which the patient should be prepared preoperatively.

In summary, the procedures listed in Table 17.4 represent a reasonable surgical approach to a patient with a suspicious adnexal mass. A midline incision greatly facilitates access in the event that surgical staging is necessary. Pelvic washings will alter the stage if positive. Exploration of the abdominal cavity remains the most important step as all further procedures are affected or determined by what is found. The decision to preserve the uterus and contralateral ovary should largely be based on reproductive considerations. The usefulness of additional surgical staging procedures is clear from a diagnostic standpoint. Almost one patient in five (18.7%) was found to have unsuspected disease in the series listed in Table 17.3. The decision to perform surgical staging in presumed stage I LMP ovarian

Table 17.4 Suggested surgical approach to suspicious adnexal masses

1. Consider midline incision
2. Obtain pelvic washings
3. Thorough abdominal and pelvic exploration
4. Unilateral salpingo-oophorectomy or abdominal hysterectomy and bilateral salpingo-oophorectomy (cystectomy in rare cases)
5. Frozen section analysis of the primary lesion
6. Surgical staging for LMP or malignant tumors

tumor appears warranted for several reasons. The presence of so-called invasive or destructive metastatic implants appears to be associated with a poorer prognosis stage-for-stage and is regarded by some clinicians as an indication for adjuvant postoperative chemotherapy [36,37]. Such lesions may be overlooked if surgical staging is not done. In addition, the unreliability of frozen section diagnosis of LMP tumor, with a 17–30% chance of frank malignancy on permanent analysis, makes accurate staging very desirable. Finally, stage alone seems to be the most significant determinant of long term survival [38–40].

Accurate knowledge of the stage of disease would result in both the physician and patient being better prepared to make decisions regarding subsequent treatment.

17.6 POSTOPERATIVE MANAGEMENT

The role of adjuvant postoperative therapy for LMP tumors has been evaluated by several authors. Creasman *et al.* [4] of the Gynecologic Oncology Group (GOG) reported on 55 patients. In this study, surgical intervention alone appeared to be equivalent to surgery plus chemotherapy or radiation as measured by 3–5 year survival rates, particularly in stage I disease. Many other reports have come to the same conclusion [5,30,41]. The role of adjuvant therapy in advanced stage lesions is less clear. Fort *et al.* [42] reported on 19 patients with residual disease postoperatively who were treated with chemotherapy, radiation or a combination of the two. Twelve of 19 were free of disease at second look laparotomy. In contrast, Yazigi *et al.* [43] reported on eight stage III patients with residual disease treated with cisplatin based combination chemotherapy. Seven of eight had tumor at second look surgery. A GOG study reported negative second look procedures in six of 15 cases treated with cisplatin combination therapy [44].

In view of the documented toxicity of chemotherapy in LMP tumor patients, which has included several deaths, and the conflicting evidence regarding efficacy, it seems appropriate to limit the use of postoperative chemotherapy to selected patients [5,45]. Until a randomized controlled trial of adjuvant chemotherapy for LMP tumors is completed, it is recommended that postoperative cisplatin based combination chemotherapy be used only in those patients with unresectable lesions or those with resected destructive or invasive metastatic implants, which may represent a more aggressive form of the disease [46,47].

17.7 SECOND LOOK SURGERY

The outcome of second look surgery in patients with LMP tumors is predictable based on the stage of disease. A series of nine reports showed an overall rate of 38% positive second look procedures (range 12.5%–100%). Stage I or II lesions, however, had positive second looks in only 14.9% of cases. In stage III and IV lesions positive second looks were noted in 54% of cases (Table 17.5) [5,8,30,41–45,48].

The findings obtained during second look laparotomy have significant influence on prognosis in patients with frankly malignant ovarian cancer. Determination of prognosis becomes less important in LMP tumor patients since the five year survival approaches or exceeds 90% even in stage III disease with a positive second look [43,44]. A more useful approach may be to consider second look surgery after a longer time interval than has traditionally occurred following treatment for ovarian cancer, since patients with metastatic LMP disease may have only a 50–60% 10 year survival [22,46]. The presence

Table 17.5 Outcome of second look laparotomy by stage of disease in LMP ovarian tumors

Source	Stage I & II		Stage III & IV		Overall
	All cases	Positive	All cases	Positive	
Fort *et al.* [42]	13	1	11	2	12.5%
Hopkins *et al.* [48]	12	0	8	3	15%
Chambers *et al.* [5]	6	1	4	1	20%
Massad *et al.* [8]	4	0	4	2	25%
Chien *et al.* [41]	3	1	7	3	40%
Krepart *et al.*	6	1	4	4	50%
Sutton *et al.* [44]	–	–	14	8	57%
Yazigi *et al.* [43]	–	–	9	7	77%
O'Quinn *et al.* [45]	3	3	7	7	100%
Totals	47	7 (14.9%)	68	37 (54%)	38%

of disease at re-exploration 5–7 years after initial therapy may therefore be a more accurate prognostic indicator.

It is also possible that second look procedures may be more important therapeutically than for prognosis in LMP tumor patients. In the absence of clear evidence supporting the use of chemotherapy for recurrent LMP tumor, surgical resection remains the only proven method of eradicating visible disease. Second look operations in presumably disease-free individuals may allow for detection of small lesions prior to widespread metastasis or extension to vital organs not easily resected. Unlike frankly malignant ovarian tumors, for which secondary debulking has minimal benefit and effective chemotherapeutic regimens exist, recurrent LMP tumors appear to be best treated primarily by aggressive and possibly multiple surgical resections [49,50].

17.8 COMMENTS

The inability to confidently diagnose LMP tumors preoperatively dictates that many or most will continue to be treated initially in a community hospital setting by physicians without specific training in oncology. This situation allows for great variation in initial surgical treatment. Patients are frequently not referred to tertiary centres or are referred postoperatively. This problem, plus the possibly decade-long time period required for accurate determination of outcome for these tumors, makes prospective study of these lesions difficult.

The fact that these tumors are often treated by primary care gynecologists also points out the need for standardization of the treatment recommendations and education of those physicians managing LMP tumor patients. The GOG is presently evaluating the efficacy of surgical staging of LMP tumors with a prospective study of clinical outcome. Due to the long follow-up necessary information from this study will not be finalized for several years. Other specific problems being addressed by various investigators are the role of CA-125 and color flow Doppler imaging in screening and diagnosis and the effect of adjuvant chemotherapy on outcome.

A uniform approach to work-up and initial surgical treatment would greatly facilitate decisions regarding postoperative care. Also, the small subset of LMP tumor patients who have poor outcomes may be identified earlier in the course of the disease by the information obtained from complete surgical staging. Evaluation of adjuvant chemotherapy or other treatment modalities in this group would appear to have the greatest potential impact on overall survival.

REFERENCES

1. Santesson, L. and Kottmeier, H.L. (1978) General classification of ovarian tumors. In *Ovarian Cancer, Vol. II*, (eds F. Gentil and A.C. Sunquierra), Springer-Verlag, New York, pp. 1–8.
2. Colgan, T.J. and Norris, H.J. (1983) Ovarian epithelial tumors of low malignant potential: a review. *Int. J. Gynecol. Pathol.*, **1**, 367–82.
3. Merino, M. and Jaffe, G. (1993) Age contrast in ovarian pathology. *Cancer*, **71**, 537–44.
4. Creasman, W.T., Park, R., Norris, H. *et al.* (1982) Stage I borderline ovarian tumors. *Obstet. Gynecol.*, **59**, 93–6.
5. Chambers, S.T., Merino, M.S., Kohorn, E.L., et al. (1988) Borderline ovarian tumors. *Am. J. Obstet. Gynecol.*, **159**, 1088–94.
6. Bell, D.A. and Scully, R.E. (1990) Ovarian serous borderline tumors with stromal microinvasion: a report of 21 cases. *Hum. Path.*, **21**, 397–403.
7. Katsube, Y., Berg, J.W. and Silverberg, S.G. (1982) Epidemiologic pathology of ovarian tumors: a histopathologic review of primary ovarian neoplasms diagnosed in the Denver Standard Metropolitan Statistical area, 1 July–31 December 1969 and 1 July–31

8. Massad, L.S., Hunter, V.J., Szpak, C.A. *et al.* (1991) Epithelial ovarian tumors of low malignant potential. *Obstet. Gynecol.*, **78**, 1027–32.

9. Lim-Tan, S.K., Cajigas, H.E. and Scully, R.E. (1988) Ovarian cystectomy for serous borderline tumors: a follow up study of 35 cases. *Obstet. Gynecol.*, **72**, 775–80.

10. Yazigi, R., Sanstad, J. and Munoz, A.K. (1988) Primary staging in ovarian tumors of low malignant potential. *Gynecol. Oncol.*, **31**, 402–8.

11. Robinson, W.R., Curtin, J.P. and Morrow, C.P. (1992) Operative staging and conservative surgery in the management of low malignant potential ovarian tumors. *Int. J. Gynecol. Cancer*, **2**, 113–18.

12. Russell, P. (1979) The pathological assessment of ovarian neoplasms. I. Introduction to the common epithelial tumors and analysis of benign epithelial tumors. *Pathology*, **11**, 5–26.

13. Buy, J.N., Ghossain, M.A., Sciot, L. *et al.* (1991) Epithelial tumors of the ovary: CT findings and correlation with ultrasound. *Radiology*, **178**, 811–18.

14. Granberg, S., Wikland, M. and Jansson, I. (1989) Macroscopic characterization of ovarian tumors and the relation to the histologic diagnosis: criteria to be used for ultrasound evaluation. *Gynecol. Oncol.*, **35**, 139–44.

15. Bourne, T., Campbell, S., Steer, C. *et al.* (1989) Transvaginal colour flow imaging: a possible new screening technique for ovarian cancer. *Br. Med J.*, **299**, 1367–70.

16. Kurjak, A., Zalud, I., Surkovic, D. *et al.* (1989) Transvaginal color Doppler for the assessment of pelvic circulation. *Acta Obstet. Gynecol. Scand.*, **68**, 131–5.

17. Fleischer, A.C., Rodgers, W.H., Bhaskara, K.R. *et al.* (1991) Assessment of ovarian tumor vascularity with transvaginal colour Doppler sonography. *J. Ultrasound. Med.*, **10**, 563–8.

18. Finkler, N.G., Benacerraf, B., Lavin, R.T. *et al.* (1988) Comparison of serum Ca-125, clinical impression, and ultrasound in the preoperative evaluation of ovarian masses. *Obstet. Gynecol.*, **72**, 659–64.

19. Mogensen, O., Mogensen, B., Jakobsen, A. and Sell, A. (1989) Preoperative measurement of cancer antigen 125 (CA-125) in the differential diagnosis of ovarian tumors. *Acta Oncol.*, **28**, 471–3.

20. Rice, L.W., Berkowitz, R.S., Mark, S.D. *et al.* (1990) Epithelial ovarian tumors of borderline malignancy. *Gynecol. Oncol.*, **39**, 195–8.

21. Tholander, B., Taube, A., Lindgren, A. *et al.* (1990) Pretreatment serum levels of CA-125, carcino embryonic antigen, tissue polypeptide antigen and placental alkaline phosphatase in patients with ovarian carcinoma, borderline tumors, or benign adnexal masses: relevance for differential diagnosis. *Gynecol. Oncol.*, **39**, 16–25.

22. Tasker, M. and Langley, F.A. (1985) The outlook for women with borderline epithelial tumors of the ovary. *Br. J Obstet. Gynecol.*, **92**, 969–73.

23. Navot, D., Fox, J.H., Williams, M. *et al.* (1991) The concept of uterine preservation with ovarian malignancies. *Obstet. Gynecol.*, **78**, 566–8.

24. Andrieu, S.M. and Ochoa-Molina, M.E. (1983) Menstrual cycle, pregnancies and offspring before and after MOPP therapy for Hodgkins disease. *Cancer*, **52**, 435.

25. Bakri, Y.N. and Given, F.T. (1984) Normal pregnancy and delivery following conservative surgery and chemotherapy for ovarian endodermal sinus tumor. *Gynecol. Oncol.*, **16**, 414.

26. Baak, S.P., Langley, F.A., Talerman, A. *et al.* (1987) The prognostic variability of ovarian tumor grading by different pathologists. *Gynecol. Oncol.*, **27**, 166–72.

27. Stalsberg, T.I., Abeler, V., Blom, G.P. *et al.* (1988) Observer variation in histologic classification of malignant and borderline ovarian tumors. *Hum. Pathol.*, **19**, 1030–5.

28. TwaalFhoven, F.A.C., Peters, A.A.W. and Trimbas, S.B. (1991) The accuracy of frozen section diagnosis of ovarian tumors. *Gynecol. Oncol.*, **41**, 189–92.

29. Snider, D.D., Stuart, G.C., Nation, J.G. *et al.* (1991) Evaluation of surgical staging in stage I low malignant potential ovarian tumors. *Gynecol. Oncol.*, **40**, 129–32.

30. Nation, J.G. and Krepart, G.V. (1986) Ovarian carcinoma at low malignant potential: staging and treatment. *Am. J. Obstet. Gynecol.*, **154**, 290–3.

31. Leake, J.F., Rader, R.S., Woodruff, J.D. *et al.* (1991) Retroperitoneal lymphatic involvement

with epithelial ovarian tumors of low malignant potential. *Gynecol. Oncol.*, **42**, 124–30.

32. Nezhat, C., Nezhat, F. and Burrell, M. (1992) Laparoscopically assisted hysterectomy for the management of a borderline ovarian tumor: a case report. *J. Laparoendosc. Surg.*, **2**, 167–9.

33. Cristali, B., Cayol, A., Izard, V. *et al.* (1992) Benefit of operative laparoscopy for ovarian tumors suspected of benignity. *J. Laparendosc. Surg.*, **2**, 69–73.

34. Dembo, A.J., Davy, M., Stenwig, A.E. *et al.* (1990) Prognostic factors in patients with stage I epithelial ovarian cancer. *Obstet. Gynecol.*, **75**, 263–73.

35. Sevelda, P., Dittrich, C. and Salzer, H. (1989) Prognostic value of the rupture of the capsule in stage I epithelial ovarian carcinoma. *Gynecol. Oncol.*, **35**, 321–2.

36. Michael, H. and Roth, L.M. (1986) Invasive and noninvasive implants in ovarian serous tumors of low malignant potential. *Cancer*, **53**, 1240–7.

37. Gershenson, D.M. and Silva, E.G. (1990) Serous ovarian tumors of low malignant potential with peritoneal implants. *Cancer*, **65**, 578–85.

38. Katzenstein, A.A., Mazur, M.T., Morgan, T.E. *et al.* (1978) Proliferative serous tumors of the ovary. Histologic features and prognosis. *Am. J. Surg. Pathol.*, **2**, 339–55.

39. Russell, P. and Merkur, H. (1979) Proliferating ovarian epithelial tumours: a clinical pathological analysis of 144 cases. *Aust. NZ J. Obstet. Gynecol.*, **19**, 45–51.

40. Leake, J.F., Currie, S.L., Rosenshein, N.B. *et al.* (1992) Long term follow-up of serous ovarian tumors of low malignant potential. *Gynecol. Oncol.*, **47**, 150–8.

41. Chien, R., Rehenmaier, M.A., Micha, J.P. *et al.* (1989) Ovarian epithelial tumors of low malignant potential. *Surg. Gynecol. Obstet.*, **169**, 143–6.

42. Fort, G.M., Pierce, V.K., Scigo, P.E. *et al.* (1989) Evidence for the efficacy of adjuvant therapy in epithelial ovarian tumors of low malignant potential. *Gynecol. Oncol.*, **32**, 269–72.

43. Yazig, R., Munoz, A.K., Sandstad, J. *et al.* (1991) Cisplatin based combination chemotherapy in the treatment of stage III ovarian epithelial tumors of low malignant potential. *Eur. J. Gynec. Oncol.*, **6**, 451–5.

44. Sutton, G.P., Bundy, B.N., Omura, G.A. *et al.* (1991) Stage III ovarian tumors of low malignant potential treated with cisplatin combination therapy (a Gynecologic Oncology Group study). *Gynecol. Oncol.*, **41**, 230–3.

45. O'Quinn, A.G. and Hannigan, E.V. (1985) Epithelial ovarian neoplasms of low malignant potential. *Gynecol. Oncol.*, **21**, 177–83.

46. Russell, P. (1984) Borderline epithelial tumors of the ovary: a conceptual dilemma. *Clin. Obstet. Gynecol.*, **11**, 259–76.

47. McCaughey, W.T.E., Kirk, M.E., Lester, W. *et al.* (1984) Peritoneal epithelial lesions associated with proliferative serous tumors of the ovary. *Histopathology*, **8**, 195–208.

48. Hopkins, M.P. and Morley, G.W. (1989) The second look operation and surgical staging in ovarian tumor of low malignant potential. *Obstet. Gynecol.*, **74**, 375–8.

49. Barnhill, D.R., O'Connor, D.M. (1991) Management of ovarian neoplasms of low malignant potential. *Oncology*, **5**, 21–32.

50. Leake, S.F. (1992) Tumors of low malignant potential. *Curr. Opin. Obstet. Gynecol.*, **4**, 81–5.

Chapter 18

Cellular DNA content: the most important prognostic factor in patients with borderline tumors of the ovary. Can it prevent overtreatment?

J. KAERN, C.G. TROPÉ, V. ABELER and E.O. PETTERSEN

18.1 INTRODUCTION

The majority of patients with ovarian borderline tumors and invasive carcinoma stage I have excellent prognosis after surgical removal of the tumor. Nevertheless, nearly all of these patients have received adjuvant treatment, in the absence of prognostic factors to pinpoint the few patients at risk, who might benefit from this treatment. Less extended surgery (than the standard surgery performed) might suffice in many patients, thus allowing young women to remain fertile, if more precise prognostic factors could be identified [1–4].

The classic prognostic parameters such as FIGO stage, histological type and grade, amount of residual tumor after primary surgery, age and performance status are far from sufficient for predicting the prognosis for the individual patient with ovarian cancer. They all have a degree of subjectivity and the reproducibility is too low [5]. In an attempt to improve the predictability of patients' prognosis one must seek more objective and reproducible prognostic variables, such as DNA ploidy and proliferation activity (S-phase fraction).

During the last 10 years several studies have shown nuclear DNA content to be of prognostic value in epithelial ovarian carcinoma. Some of these studies have included borderline tumors, although only a small number of cases [6]. Abnormal DNA content measured by microspectrophotometry of Feulgen stained slides or by flow cytometry (FCM-DNA) has been associated with poor prognosis. A very few borderline tumors show aneuploidy, but aneuploidy has been reported to indicate poor prognosis [7].

The aim of this retrospective study was to analyse the prognostic value of FCM-DNA ploidy in a large group of consecutive borderline tumor patients with long term follow-up treated in one institution, to improve the validity of our pilot study which showed that ploidy determinations might be a helpful tool in identifying the truly malignant borderline tumors.

18.2 MATERIAL AND METHODS

Of 370 patients with ovarian borderline tumors treated at the Norwegian Radium Hospital from 1970 to June 1982, sections from formalin fixed paraffin embedded tissue from the primary tumor were accessible for flow cytometric DNA analysis in 335 cases. The histopathological diagnosis was confirmed by one of us (VA) and sections from the area presenting most cellular atypia of the epithelial cell layers (avoiding inflammatory and necrotic cells) were selected for FCM-DNA. The paraffin method described by Hedley *et al.* was used [8].

A laboratory built high resolution flow cytometer was used for measuring the nuclear DNA content. The use of external standards to perform a zero set of the multi-channel analyser and the ploidy definitions were as described earlier [9]. If only one G0/G1 peak was present the tumor was defined as diploid. If more than one peak, with the exception of the diploid G2 peak were present, the tumor was defined as aneuploid. Because of the relatively poor resolution of the DNA histograms and the many pitfalls in calculation of S-phase using the paraffin technique, we did not perform S-phase analysis in this study. In 14 (4.2%) cases the DNA histograms were not evaluable for ploidy determination ('noise' and coefficient of variation >10%), leaving 321 diploid and aneuploid tumors for final analysis. Histological parameters such as type, cellular atypia, tumor growth on the ovarian surface, tumor size and pseudomyxoma peritonei, together with clinical parameters such as age at diagnosis, stage of disease including ascites, surgical procedure, residual tumor after primary surgery and postoperative treatment, and survival data such as relapse, localization of relapse, relapse-free period, cause of death and survival were documented. Follow-up was complete and August 1991 was selected as the endpoint of the study. The follow-up data were collected from the medical records and the Cancer Registry of Norway.

Table 18.1 Ploidy in relation to classical prognostic factors

	Diploid n = 293	Aneuploid n = 28	p value
Age (years)			
<40	81	7	
40–70	176	14	0.1664
>70	36	7	
Stage			
IA	187	11	
IB	44	2	
IC	19	2	0.0001
IA	2	0	
IIB	13	3	
III	28	10	
Histological type			
Serous	142	7	0.0723
Mucinous	139	17	
Endometrioid	5	1	0.0096
Clear cell	2	0	
Mixed	5	2	
Unclassified	0	1	
Atypia			
Mild	96	7	
Moderate	189	15	<0.0001
Severe	8	6	
Tumor size (cm)			
≤10	120	9	0.4796
>10	173	19	

Table 18.1 *Continued*

	Diploid	Aneuploid n = 293	p value n = 28
Tumor growth on the ovarian surface			
No	236	19	
Yes	48	8	0.2576
?	9	1	
Pseudomyxoma peritonei (mucinous tumor)			
No	119	8	0.0004
Yes	20	9	
Residual tumor			
No	289	26	0.1537
Yes	4	2	
Surgical procedure in patients without residual tumor			
H+BSO+O	227	22	
USO	13	0	
BSO	13	0	0.9170
H+BSO	29	3	
BSO+O	7	1	
Postop. adjuvant treatment in patients without residual tumor			
None	77	2	
External beam	49	7	
Isotope	64	5	
Thiotepa	39	6	0.0575
Ext+Iso	28	3	
Ext+Thio	6	2	
Iso+Thio	26	1	
Relapse			
No	280	11	<0.0001
Yes	13	17	
Survival			
Alive	228	7	
Dead of disease	11	17	<0.0001
Dead of ICD	52	4	

H+BSO+O = Hysterectomy + bilateral salpingo-oophorectomy + omentectomy
USO = Salpingo-oophorectomy (unilateral)
BSO = Salpingo-oophorectomy (bilateral)
H+BSO = Hysterectomy +bilateral salpingo-oophorectomy
BSO+O = Bilateral salpingo-oophorectomy + omentectomy
EXT = External radiotherapy
EXT+ISO = External radiotherapy + isotope
EXT+THIO = External radiotherapy + thiotepa
ISO+THIO = Isotope + thiotepa
ICD = Intercurrent disease

18.3 RESULTS

Patient characteristics in relation to classic prognostic factors are summarized in Table 18.1. The median follow-up was 149 (range 15–83) months. The entire group of 321 patients included 149 serous tumors, 156 mucinous tumors and 16 of other histological types.

Frequency of aneuploidy increased with age, more advanced stage, histological type (different for serous and mucinous), higher degree of atypia and with the presence of pseudomyxoma peritonei. The different surgical procedures and the postoperative treatment modalities, including 'no treatment', were equally distributed between the diploid and aneuploid groups of tumors. Within stage I all patients with an aneuploid tumor had complete surgery and all except one received adjuvant treatment, while only 61% of those with diploid tumors had complete surgery and 34% did not receive adjuvant treatment. Only one of the diploid stage I patients (stage IA) without complete surgery died of disease. Only four (7.8%) of stage IB tumors had macroscopically normal but microscopically diffuse borderline lesions in the contralateral ovary. Within diploid stage I tumors no difference in corrected survival was observed between patients who had received adjuvant treatment and those who had not (98.8% and 98.6%, respectively).

A majority of patients with stage IA diploid tumors survived but only 50% of the patients with stage IA aneuploid tumors survived. By univariate analysis DNA ploidy, stage, histological type, presence of residual tumor, pseudomyxoma peritonei, tumor growth on the ovarian surface, tumor size and age showed prognostic significance (Table 18.2). By Cox multivariate analysis of the 315 tumor-free surgically treated patients, DNA ploidy was by far the strongest prognostic factor for long term survival (Figure 18.1), followed by stage, histological type (non-serous–mucinous) and age. The relative risk

for the individual patient could be calculated and patients could be divided into risk groups for treatment decisions. Patients with aneuploid tumors had a 19 times higher risk of dying of disease than patients with diploid tumors.

18.4 DISCUSSION

The overall corrected survival is very good (91–93%) and extremely good for stage IA patients only (97%). The fertility of patients with stage IA borderline tumors may be reduced due to associated benign intra-abdominal lesions, such as endosalpingiosis, endometriosis, polycystic ovaries and hormonal dysfunction. Also the operative procedure might reduce fertility, especially when wedge biopsy of the remaining ovary is performed. But even manipulation of the remaining ovary might reduce fertility. Another explanation for infertility could be that some patients with a borderline malignant disease become psychologically stressed and do not attempt pregnancy. In our material only 11 patients had the opportunity to become pregnant. Six of these women have been pregnant and given birth to one or more children after unilateral adnexectomy. Our results, although based on small numbers, may indicate that patients without an infertility problem before treatment of their borderline tumor may preserve their fertility, at least if the remaining ovary is not disturbed by large biopsies.

To allow such a conservative approach we must identify the patient at risk. Around 10% of the patients will succumb to disease. Using classic clinical and histopathological criteria, patients with a poor prognosis cannot be selected. Stage of disease is an important prognostic factor but even patients with stage IA died of disease. At the time of diagnosis only a few patients with borderline tumors are at an advanced stage of disease. These patients have a poor prognosis compared to

Table 18.2 Univariate analysis in the group of patients (n=321) with ovarian borderline tumors. 15 years corrected survival

Factor	Chi-square	p value
Ploidy		
Diploid		
Aneuploid	136.4	<0.0001
Stage		
I		
II	71.94	<0.0001
III		
Pseudomyxoma		
No		
Yes	39.15	<0.0001
Residual tumor		
No		
Yes	38.05	<0.0001
Extracapsular growth		
No		
Yes	9.87	0.0017
Histological type		
Serous		
Mucinous	9.92	0.0016
Other		
Age (years)		
<40		
40–70	9.09	0.0029
>70		
Tumor size (cm)		
≤10		
>10	6.57	0.0104
Isotope		
No		
Yes	6.40	0.0114
External irradiation		
No		
Yes	5.06	0.0245
Thiotepa		
No		
Yes	3.32	0.0685

Table 18.2 *Continued*

Factor	Chi-square	P value
Postoperative treatment		
No		
Yes	3.08	0.0793
Surgical procedure		
H+BSO+O		
'less'	2.48	0.1150
Grade of atypia		
Mild		
Moderate	0.26	0.6133
Severe		

Log likelihood = –157.7028
* In 10 patients no information on this parameter
H+BSO+O = Hysterectomy + bilateral salpingo-oophorectomy + omentectomy
'less' = USO, BSO, BSO+H, BSO+O (see Table 18.1)
Postoperative treatment = No or isotope, external irradiation and thiotepa as single therapy or in combination.

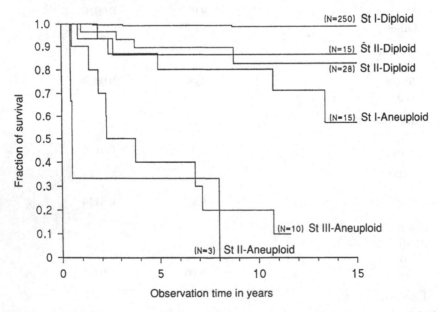

Figure 18.1 Borderline ovarian tumors 1970–1982; 15 year survival rates *vs* stage and ploidy in patients without residual tumor and with adjuvant treatment. St = stage.

stage I patients, but not as poor as patients with advanced stage invasive carcinoma.

DNA ploidy was the most important independent prognostic factor in this study. This is in agreement with most studies in which this technique has been tested, but no study has analysed DNA ploidy in such a large number of patients with complete and long term follow-up. Flow cytometric DNA ploidy has been shown to be of prognostic value in several studies [6,10,11]. All these studies are in agreement, in that the majority of borderline tumors are diploid and the few patients with aneuploid tumors had a poor prognosis. One study by Klemi *et al.* [12] showed no worse prognosis for aneuploid tumors. Comparable studies [13,14] by image cytometry on Feulgen stained material has shown that aneuploid tumors carry a poorer prognosis than diploid tumors. Baak *et al.* [5] have shown that objective morphometric parameters, such as MAI (mitotic activity index) and VPE (volume percentage of epithelium), could identify high risk patients. The use of flow cytometric DNA analysis improves our ability to divide patients into risk groups. But it is not the whole story, as patients with diploid tumors may also succumb. DNA ploidy alone is not sufficient, even with improved technique, as other unknown factors (genetic, tumor–host relationship) may influence the evolution of neoplasia. Morphometric studies of nuclear pattern give additional information different from DNA ploidy regarding prognosis [5]. The morphometric studies support the importance of new additional prognostic information given by quantitative pathology. By combining classic prognostic parameters, DNA cytometry and morphometry the prediction of prognosis for the individual patient might improve considerably. Young patients showed a good prognosis compared to old patients and age was an independent prognostic factor. Within stage I, patients with diploid tumors had extremely good survival independent of adjuvant treatment. Thus,

there is no indication for adjuvant treatment in this group of patients. Benefit from adjuvant treatment may be expected for patients with diploid tumors in advanced stages and in all aneuploid tumors.

18.5 CONCLUSIONS

Independent prognostic factors in patients with epithelial ovarian borderline tumors without residual tumor after primary surgery are DNA ploidy, FIGO stage, histological type and age.

One or preferably two surgical biopsies should be taken from the primary tumor and suspect intra-abdominal lesions for DNA ploidy analysis. Each biopsy should be divided into two parts, one for histopathological examination and one for FCM and ICM analysis.

If paraffin embedded tumor material is used for DNA ploidy measurement the tissue is selected by the pathologist from the part of the tumor demonstrating the highest degree of nuclear atypia and containing largely 'pure' tumor cells (avoiding necrotic cells and stromal tissue).

Standard surgery in patients over 40 years of age should include collection of peritoneal washings, bilateral adnexectomy, omentectomy and total hysterectomy. Retroperitoneal lymph node sampling is not indicated.

Conservative surgery in patients of fertile age is recommended and includes unilateral adnexectomy and omentectomy. Peritoneal washings should be done. Biopsy of the contralateral ovary is not indicated if the macroscopic appearance is normal.

Conservative surgery is also indicated in young fertile women who have not completed their family and who have a diploid stage IA tumor. As intraoperative DNA ploidy analysis is impossible at present, repeat laparotomy is necessary if the DNA analysis yields an aneuploidy result, or if the histological examination reveals disseminated disease.

Postoperative adjuvant therapy is not indicated in patients with diploid stage I tumors.

Whether the high risk patients (all aneuploid tumors and diploid tumors in advanced stages) will benefit from adjuvant treatment remains to be proven.

A prospective randomized study of high risk borderline tumor patients to determine survival benefit from cisplatin/ carboplatin as single or combination regimens is difficult to contrive, because of the relatively few high risk patients.

Follow-up should be life long, with patients seen at three monthly intervals for the first two years, then every six months. The tests include gynecological examination, ultrasound and serum CA125 (although the prognostic significance of CA125 in borderline tumors is not so important as for invasive carcinoma).

REFERENCES

1. Dembo, A.J., Davy, M., Stenwig, A.E. *et al.* (1990) Prognostic factors in patients with stage I epithelial ovarian cancer. *Obstet. Gynecol.*, **75**, 263–73.
2. Berek, J.S. (1990) Adjuvant therapy for early-stage ovarian cancer. *N. Engl. J. Med.*, **322**, 1076–8.
3. Young, R.C., Walton, L.A., Ellenberg, S.S. *et al.* (1990) Adjuvant therapy in stage I and stage II epithelial ovarian cancer. *N. Engl. J. Med.*, **322**, 1021–7.
4. Finn, C.B., Luesley, D.M., Buxton, E.J. *et al.* (1992) Is stage I epithelial ovarian cancer overtreated both surgically and systemically? Results of a five-year cancer registry review. *Br. J. Obstet. Gynecol.*, **99**, 54–8.
5. Baak, J.P.A., Langley, F.A., Talerman, A. *et al.* (1987) The prognostic variability of ovarian tumor grading by different pathologists. *Gynecol. Oncol.*, **27**, 166–72.
6. Friedlander, M.L., Russell, P., Taylor, I.W. *et al.* (1984) Flow cytometric analysis of cellular DNA content as an adjunct to the diagnosis of ovarian tumours of borderline malignancy. *Pathology*, **16**, 301–6.
7. Kaern, J., Tropé, C., Kjørstad, K.E. *et al.* (1990) Cellular DNA content as a new prognostic tool in patients with borderline tumors of the ovary. *Gynecol. Oncol.*, **38**, 452–7.
8. Hedley, D.W., Friedlander, M.L., Taylor, I.W. *et al.* (1983) Method for analysis of cellular DNA content of paraffin-embedded pathological material using flow cytometry. *J. Histochem. Cytochem.*, **31**, 1333–5.
9. Fosså, S.D., Berner, A., Heiden, T. *et al.* (1992) DNA ploidy in cell nuclei from paraffin-embedded material – comparison of results from two laboratories. *Cytometry*, **13**, 395–403.
10. Iversen, O.E., Skaarland, E. (1987) Ploidy assessment of benign and malignant ovarian tumors by flow cytometry. A clinicopathologic study. *Cancer*, **60**, 82–7.
11. Kühn, W., Kaufmann, M., Feichter, G.E. *et al.* (1989) DNA flow cytometry, clinical and morphological parameters as prognostic factors for advanced malignant and borderline ovarian tumors. *Gynecol. Oncol.*, **33**, 360–7.
12. Klemi, P.J., Joensuu, H., Mäenpää, J. *et al.* (1990) Influence of cellular DNA content on survival in ovarian carcinoma. *Obstet. Gynecol.*, **65**, 200–4.
13. Erhardt, K., Auser, G., Björkholm, E. *et al.* (1984) prognostic significance of nuclear DNA content in serous ovarian tumors. *Cancer Res.*, **44**, 2198–202.
14. Dietel, M., Arps, H., Rohlff, A. *et al.* (1986) Nuclear DNA content of borderline tumors of the ovary: correlation with histology and significance for prognosis. *Virchows Arch. (Pathol. Anat.)*, **409**, 829–36.

Chapter 19

Complementary and coordinate markers for detection of epithelial ovarian cancers

R.C. BAST JR., F. XU, R.P. WOOLAS, Y. YU, M. CONAWAY, K. O'BRIANT,
L. DALY, D.H. ORAM, A. BERCHUCK, D.L. CLARKE-PEARSON, J.T. SOPER,
G. RODRIGUEZ and I.J. JACOBS

Early detection of ovarian cancer might substantially improve results of therapy. After careful surgical staging, 90% of patients with stage I disease and 70% of patients with stage II disease can be cured with currently available therapy. Epithelial ovarian cancer may be one of the malignancies that lends itself to early detection with a blood test. Antigens shed from the ovarian surface into the peritoneal cavity are taken up by diaphragmatic lymphatics and pass through the alternative thoracic duct into the venous circulation. In early work by Knauf and Urbach [1] the OCA antigen could be detected in 70% of patients with early stage disease. OCA was also found in approximately 10% of healthy individuals, precluding its use in screening. This observation did, however, suggest that shed tumor products could be found in the circulation in an early stage of disease.

CA-125 has been evaluated for early detection of ovarian cancer. Shortly after the development of the CA-125 assay [2], it was possible to study, in retrospect, a single patient from whom multiple specimens of serum had been saved prior to the presentation of epithelial ovarian cancer [3]. Some 10–12 months lead time was observed between the first elevation of CA-125 and the clinical presentation of her disease. In a larger study utilizing the JANUS serum bank in Oslo, Norway, Zurawski *et al.* [4] had found elevations of CA-125 in half of patients ranging up to 18 months prior to diagnosis. Even five years prior to diagnosis 24% of patients destined to develop epithelial ovarian cancer had more than 30 units of CA-125 per ml of serum, compared to 7% of age matched controls. Whether elevation of CA-125 levels several years prior to diagnosis reflected very slow tumor growth or preneoplastic disease remains to be resolved.

To be effective in screening, a marker must not only provide lead time over conventional diagnostic techniques but also be extraordinarily sensitive and specific. With regard to sensitivity, CA-125 has been elevated in approximately 50% of patients with stage I disease and 90% of patients with stage II disease [5]. Taken together, some 60% of patients with early stage disease have had an elevation of the marker. While this is reasonably sensitive for a serum marker, it falls substantially short of that observed with transvaginal sonography.

With regard to specificity, CA-125 is remarkably specific when observed over time and when combined with sonography. In a

189

trial of 5550 apparently healthy women over 40 years of age, Einhorn *et al.* observed an elevated CA-125 in 175 patients [6]. An additional 175 controls with normal CA-125 were followed by the investigators. All 350 patients were evaluated with quarterly CA-125 determinations, semiannual pelvic examinations and transabdominal sonography. If only women over 50 years of age were considered, 2% had more than 30 U ml^{-1} of CA-125. Consequently, CA-125 proved sufficiently specific to provide a cost-effective trigger for transabdominal ultrasound in this study. Six cases of epithelial ovarian cancer were detected, four of which were early stage. There were, however, three cases that were not detected by the screen and subsequently found in the Swedish Tumor Registry, consistent with the suboptimal sensitivity of CA-125.

Given the importance of sensitivity for early detection of disease, we have asked whether multiple complementary markers would provide a more sensitive test for ovarian cancer. Over the last decade a number of potential markers have been developed using the monoclonal technology to detect tumor associated antigens in serum or in urine (Table 19.1). We have reported results using macrophage colony stimulating factor as a marker [7,8]. Xu *et al.* had found that approximately 68% of patients with clinically evident disease would have an elevated M-CSF level in serum [8]. When 25 sera were evaluated from women with clinically evident disease despite CA-125 <35 U ml^{-1}, 56% had an elevation of M-CSF. In addition, when 29 patients with positive second looks despite CA-125 <35 U ml^{-1} were tested, 31% had an elevated M-CSF. Consequently, there appeared to be complementarity between CA-125 and M-CSF.

OVX1 antigen has provided another marker that appeared complementary to CA-125 [9,10]. This determinant is recognized by a murine monoclonal IgM antibody that was

Table 19.1 Antigenic markers for epithelial ovarian cancer

CA125
Carcinoembryonic antigen
CA19-9
CA15-3
TAG 72
HMFG2
Placental alkaline phosphatase
Tissue peptide antigen
Lipid associated sialic acid
NB70K
Urinary gonadotrophin fragment

raised by sequential immunization of mice with different ovarian cancer cell lines [9]. The OVX1 antigen is distinct from 10 previously described ovarian associated antigens and appears to be a modified Lewis X determinant. Multiple OVX1 epitopes are present on a high molecular weight mucin. Consequently, a double determinant immunoradiometric assay has been developed [10]. Although OVX1 was elevated in only 45% of patients with epithelial ovarian cancer, the antigen detected disease in 67% of patients who had clinically evident ovarian cancer despite serum CA-125 <35 U ml^{-1}. In addition, 27% of 45 patients with residual disease and a normal CA-125 had elevated OVX1 levels.

Given the complementarity observed between CA-125, OVX1 and M-CSF, all three markers have been used to evaluate sera from patients with stage I epithelial ovarian cancer. One of the three markers was elevated in 98% of 46 sera from patients with stage I disease obtained at the Royal London Hospital and at Duke University Medical Center [11]. In addition to epithelial ovarian cancers, borderline tumors and non-epithelial malignances were detected. Given this encouraging result, we attempted to utilize M-CSF and OVX1 to detect preclinical disease. In a study of 22 000 women in the UK, CA-125 (>30 U ml^{-1}) was used to trigger transabdominal ultrasound [12]. Among 340 women with abnormal CA-125 levels, 40 ultrasounds were also abnormal, prompting laparotomy. Eleven cases of epithelial ovarian cancer were detected and several were early stage. A retrospective analysis of serum samples from 18 asymptomatic women who participated in this study with CA-125 <30 U ml^{-1} and developed ovarian cancer within 24 months of venepuncture revealed that eight (44%) had an elevated level of M-CSF or OVX1 prior to diagnosis. Thus, a panel of CA-125, OVX1 and M-CSF appeared to have sensitivity that approaches what one might expect to achieve with transvaginal sonography.

The three marker panel has a more modest specificity. One of the three assays would be elevated in 11% of 204 patients who had been screened and subsequently failed to develop a neoplasm within two years [11]. A specificity of 89% would not be sufficient to prompt laparotomy based on an abnormal blood test alone but could be used to trigger the performance of transvaginal sonography (TVS). The strategy would eliminate approximately 90% of potentially costly transvaginal sonograms. In addition, the three marker panel can distinguish malignant from benign masses with a specificity of approximately 50%. Although this is not impressive in itself, when used as a trigger for TVS, at least half of benign lesions would never be examined and consequently would avoid the performance of unnecessary laparotomies for false positive results.

If the specificity for distinguishing benign from malignant lesions could be improved, the cost efficacy of this strategy might be increased. Consequently, we have examined whether additional markers could improve the specificity for discriminating benign from malignant pelvic masses [13]. Eight different markers have been used to assay sera from 429 patients who underwent laparotomy for a pelvic mass (Woolas *et al.*, in preparation).

Among these individuals, 192 had malignant disease and 273 benign conditions. Markers included CA-125 (>35 U ml^{-1}), M-CSF (>3.1 ng ml^{-1}), OVX1 (>12.1 U ml^{-1}), LASA (>200 mg ml^{-1}), CA-15-3 (>32 U ml^{-1}), CA-72.4 (>3.8 U ml^{-1}), CA-19-9 (>39 U ml^{-1}) and CA-54-61 (>20 U ml^{-1}). Among these eight markers, CA-125 exhibited the greatest sensitivity (Table 19.2). Several methods of analysis were utilized in an attempt to improve upon the sensitivity of 78% and specificity of 77% associated with CA-125. Elevation in two of five markers from a panel that included CA-125, OVX1, LASA, CA-15-3 and CA-72.4 produced a sensitivity of 83% and a specificity of 84%. Logistic regression analysis of all eight markers produced a similar sensitivity and specificity of 85% and 83% respectively. An apparent improvement in analysis was obtained with classification and regression tree analysis for five markers yielding a sensitivity of 92% and a specificity of 93%. When prospective studies are performed, the sensitivity and specificity of this particular CART analysis will almost certainly decrease, but it appears at least equal and quite possibly superior to other techniques. Thus, with several different methods of analysis, the use of multiple markers not only improved the specificity but also the sensitivity of CA-125 alone in distinguishing malignant from benign pelvic masses.

Table 19.2 Sensitivities and specificities of individual tumor markers

Marker	Threshold	Sensitivity %	Specificity %
CA125	35 U ml^{-1}	78.1	76.8
M-CSF	3.1 ng ml^{-1}	66.2	76.0
OVX 1	12.1 U ml^{-1}	40.1	82.7
LASA	200 mg ml^{-1}	52.1	87.8
CA15-3	32 U ml^{-1}	62.5	86.5
CA72-4	3.8 U ml^{-1}	54.2	91.6
CA19-9	39 U ml^{-1}	24.0	88.2
CA54-61	20 U ml^{-1}	52.1	88.2

The use of multiple markers in this setting might not only improve screening, but also might be used in the clinical management of premenopausal patients with a pelvic mass. In the past, we have placed very little significance upon a normal CA-125, recommending that the clinician manage a patient with a pelvic mass and a normal CA-125 in exactly the same fashion as if the CA-125 value were not known. If sensitivity and specificity exceed 90%, however, greater emphasis might be placed on serum markers that were consistent with benign disease. In premenopausal patients, 90% of pelvic masses will be benign. In this setting the negative predictive value of CART analysis should approach 99%. Consequently, careful observation of a patient with a pelvic mass and a benign CART analysis might be justified.

In the future, urine markers may prove even more useful in providing a cost-effective screen for early stage cancer. At the present time, our group is exploring 2-D gel analysis of proteins found in the urine of patients with ovarian cancer and of healthy controls. In addition, we are utilizing subtraction cloning to detect the mRNAs for prevalent low molecular weight proteins that would be expressed in cancer cells, but in few normal tissues. Proteins of low molecular weight might find their way into the urine in the absence of specific tubular reabsorption.

REFERENCES

1. Knauf, S. and Urbach, G.I. (1980) A study of ovarian cancer patients using a radioimmunoassay for human ovarian tumor-associated antigen OCA. *Am. J. Obstet. Gynecol.*, **138**, 1222–3.
2. Bast, R.C. Jr., Klug, T.L., St John, E. *et al.* (1983) A radioimmunoassay using a monoclonal antibody to monitor the course of epithelial ovarian cancer. *N. Engl. J. Med.*, **309**, 883–7.
3. Bast, R.C. Jr., Siegal, F.P., Runowicz, C. *et al.* (1985) Elevation of serum CA 125 prior to diagnosis of epithelial ovarian carcinoma. *Gynecol. Oncol.*, **22**, 115–20.
4. Zurawski, V.R. Jr., Orjaseter, H., Andersen, A. and Jellum, E. (1988) Elevated serum CA 125 levels prior to diagnosis of ovarian neoplasia: relevance for early detection of ovarian cancer. *Int. J. Cancer*, **42**, 677–80.
5. Jacobs, I. and Bast, R.C. Jr. (1989) The CA 125 tumour-associated antigen: a review of the literature. *Hum. Reprod.*, **4**, 1–12.
6. Einhorn, N., Sjovall, K., Knapp, R.C. *et al.* (1992) Prospective evaluation of serum CA 125 levels for early detection of ovarian cancer. *Obstet. Gynecol.*, **80**, 14–18.
7. Ramakrishnan, S., Xu, F.J., Brandt, S.J. *et al.* (1989) Constitutive production of macrophage colony-stimulating factor by human ovarian and breast cancer cell lines. *J. Clin. Invest.*, **83**, 921–6.
8. Xu, F.J., Ramakrishnan, S., Daly, L. *et al.* (1991) Increased serum levels of macrophage colony-stimulating factor in ovarian cancer. *Am. J. Obstet. Gynecol.*, **165**, 1356–62.
9. Xu, F.J., Yu, Y.H., Li, B.Y. *et al.* (1991) Development of two new monoclonal antibodies reactive to a surface antigen present on human ovarian epithelial cancer cells. *Cancer Res.*, **51**, 4012–19.
10. Xu, F.J., Yu, Y.A., Daly, L. *et al.* (1993) The OVX1 radioimmunoassay complements CA 125 for predicting the presence of residual ovarian carcinoma at second look surgical surveillance procedures. *J. Clin. Oncol.*, **11**, 1506–10.
11. Woolas, R.P., Xu, F.J., Jacobs, I.J. *et al.* (1993) Elevation of multiple serum markers in stage I ovarian cancer. *J. Natl. Cancer Inst.*, in press.
12. Jacobs, I., Prys Davies, A. and Oram, D. (1992) Role of CA-125 in screening for ovarian cancer. In *Ovarian Cancer 2: Biology, Diagnosis and Management*, (eds F. Sharp, W.P. Mason and W. Creasman), Chapman & Hall, London, pp. 265–76.
13. Woolas, R., Jacobs, I.J., Xu, F.J. *et al.* (1993) Serum levels of CA 125, M-CSF and OVX1 in stage I and preclinical ovarian cancer. *Proc. Am. Soc. Clin. Oncol.*, **12**, 110.

Part Four
Chemotherapy, Radiotherapy and Ethics

Chapter 20

Chemotherapy options in ovarian carcinoma – a dose intensity perspective

L. LEVIN

20.1 INTRODUCTION

Ovarian carcinoma is a moderately chemo-sensitive tumour and since most patients present with advanced disease, attention continues to be focused on new systematic treatment initiatives. Comparisons between clinical trial outcomes in ovarian carcinoma have in the past been made difficult as a result of differences between populations studied, variations in sample size which has affected the statistical power to compare two or more treatment arms, and inattention or inability to account for variations in drug doses between studies.

The meta-analysis reported by Levin and Hryniuk in 1987 [1] addressed many of these issues by pooling data sets from advanced ovarian carcinoma randomized studies in which known prognostic variables were kept as constant as possible between studies by clearly defining criteria for inclusion of studies into the analysis. This allowed for an investigation of the impact of dose intensity (mg m^{-2} week^{-1}) of each drug (relative dose intensity or RDI) and of the regimen as a whole (average dose intensity or ADI) by comparing regimens containing one or more of the drugs cyclophosphamide (C), hexamethylmelamine (H), doxorubicin (A) and cisplatin (P) with a standard regimen. Details of

the methodology for calculating RDI and ADI have been previously published [1]. This analysis allowed a comparison to be made from a pooled population of 3108 patients and the main findings were:

1. Average dose intensity and RDI for P (P-RDI) correlated significantly with clinical response and with median survival time;
2. There was a distinct advantage for multi-agent regimens over single alkylating agents, especially when the former contained cisplatin;
3. The contribution of P-RDI to outcome was disproportionate to RDI for C, H or A. It was possible to reach this conclusion by applying a refinement to the dose intensity analysis by calculating RDI which allowed drug equivalencies (or non-equivalencies) within multiagent regimens to be tested in a meta-analysis for the first time. This finding was not surprising, since it followed the important observation by Ozols *et al.* [2] that 33% of patients who relapsed on standard doses of P subsequently responded to higher doses of this drug.

These findings may have been partly responsible for a more appropriate dose of platinum-containing drug regimens to be used in treating advanced ovarian cancer.

Whereas, in the original dose intensity analysis [1], 50% of studies had incorporated cisplatin at an RDI of <1.0, none of 16 treatment arms in eight randomized studies published since 1986 which would have fitted the criteria for selection into the original analysis used cisplatin or carboplatin at an RDI <1.0. However, the disproportionate contribution of P to outcome may have been misinterpreted to imply that other drugs should not necessarily be used in combination with P.

In this chapter, the optimal use of P alone and in combination within multiagent regimens will be reviewed together with the relative contribution of ADI and RDI to outcome as evaluated by prospective trials and meta-analyses aimed at testing the original dose intensity hypothesis.

20.2 PROSPECTIVE TRIALS ADDRESSING THE CONTRIBUTION OF P-RDI TO OUTCOME

In five studies published between 1989–1992, the P-RDI was doubled in one treatment arm [3–7] and in two out of three studies which incorporated C, the RDI for this drug was kept constant [3–4] (Table 20.1). In two of the three studies which have matured sufficiently to allow for statistical comparisons to be made between the treatment arms [3,4], there was a significant improvement in the clinical response and survival in the high P-RDI *vs* the low P-RDI arm. In the third study [5], there was no improvement in clinical response or survival comparing the high P-RDI and low PRDI arms. Differences in the number of patients who underwent optimal surgical debulking is unlikely to account for these discrepant results, since the study of Kaye *et al.* [4] found a significant difference between high and low P-RDIs even when the amount of residual disease prior to chemotherapy was adjusted for. The study design by McGuire

et al. [5], however, kept the total dose of chemotherapy delivered constant between the two treatment arms, whereas that of Kaye *et al.* [4] did not. In order to keep the total dose received by patients in each treatment arm constant, in the study reported by McGuire *et al.* [5] the number of cycles in the high dose intensity arm was only four, while patients in the low dose intensity arm received eight cycles. It is questionable whether four cycles of chemotherapy was sufficient to eradicate all disease in patients, all of whom had been suboptimally surgically debulked. This and selection factors may be responsible for the fact that the high dose intensity arm of this GOG study does not fit within the general population of studies included in the dose intensity analysis (Figure 20.1). The relative contribution to outcome of total dose received, dose intensity and number of cycles given is therefore still not clear.

It is important to interpret with caution the studies presented in Table 20.1 which were designed to test the impact of P-RDI on outcome. While in the original dose intensity analysis [1] the range of P-RDI within multi-agent regimens was 0.33 to 1.67, the ranges tested prospectively (Table 20.1) in each study were 1.3 *vs* 2.7 [3] and 1.1 *vs* 2.2 [4,5]. These studies did not, therefore, test the original P-RDI range. The data, as presented in Figure 20.1, demonstrate that the fairly steep P-RDI slope does not necessarily hold out beyond a P-RDI of 1.6 (approximately 25 mg m^{-2} week^{-1}) for multiagent regimens and 1.8 (approximately 30 mg m^{-2} week^{-1}) for single agent regimens. Nevertheless, the P-RDI curve does not necessarily plateau beyond these values and it is not possible to interpret the extent to which higher P-RDIs will impact on long term survival.

It is interesting to note that clinical responses reported from prospective randomized studies published since the orginal dose intensity analysis all fit well on the original P-RDI *vs* clinical response curve (Figure 20.1),

Table 20.1 Randomized trials testing two doses of cisplatin alone or with other drug doses fixed

| Authors | n | RDI | | | Average MST | | | CR/PR |
		C	H	A	P	DI	(MO)	
Ngan *et al.* [3] (Hong Kong Ovarian Carcinoma Study Group)	44	1.1	–	–	2.7	1.0	60% 3 year	85%
		1.1	–	–	1.3	0.6	30% 3 year	54% [*p*<0.02]
Kaye *et al.* [4] (Scottish Gynaecological Cancer Study Group)	159	1.4	–	–	2.2	0.9	31	61%
		1.4	–	–	1.1	0.6	17	34% [*p* 0.005]
McGuire *et al.* [5] (Gynecologic Oncology Group)	485	1.9	–	–	2.2	1.0	21	45%
		0.9	–	–	1.1	0.5	24	53%
Boni *et al.* [6]	101	–	–	–	4.0	1.0	34	69%
		–	–	–	2.2	0.5	28	52%
Colombo *et al.* [7]	68	–	–	–	3.3	0.8	–	86%
		–	–	–	1.7	0.4	–	72%

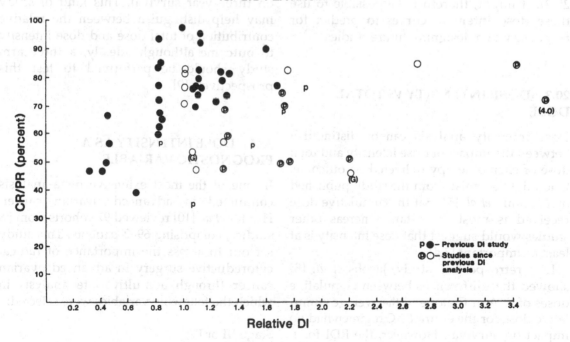

Figure 20.1 Dose intensity (DI) *vs* clinical response (CR/PR) for cisplatinum.

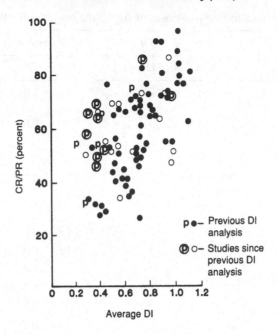

Figure 20.2 Average dose intensity (DI) *vs* clinical response (CR/PR).

as do ADI *vs* clinical response data (Figure 20.2). It might, therefore, be possible to use these dose intensity curves to predict for response when designing future studies.

20.3 DOSE INTENSITY *VS* TOTAL DOSE

Dose intensity analysis cannot distinguish between the impact of dose intensity and total dose of chemotherapy delivered on outcome. One might surmise from the study published by McGuire *et al.* [5] that the cumulative dose received is most important whereas other studies would suggest that dose intensity is at least as important [3,4].

In a retrospective study, Jacobs *et al.* [8] showed that differences between cumulative doses of P, A or C alone or the average cumulative dose for the entire PAC regimen had no impact on survival. However, the RDI for P and A and the average dose intensity for the

PAC regimen did have a significant impact on three year survival. This kind of study may help distinguish between the relative contribution of total dose and dose intensity to outcome although, ideally, a three arm study should be performed to test this prospectively [9].

20.4 DOSE INTENSITY AS A PROGNOSTIC VARIABLE

In one of the most extensive meta-analysis conducted in advanced ovarian cancer, Hunter *et al.* [10] reviewed 97 cohorts from 58 studies, comprising 6962 patients. This study set out to assess the importance of radical cytoreductive surgery in advanced ovarian cancer through a multivariate analysis in which the following variables were selected:

Stage III or IV;
Percentage maximum cytoreductive surgery;

198

Dose intensity of chemotherapy;
Presence or absence of cisplatin.

In a univariate analysis, each 10 point increase in percent maximum cytoreductive surgery was associated with a 16.3% increase in median survival time ($p < 0.001$). However, in a multiple linear regression model which included percent stage IV, dose intensity and the use of platinum, the impact of maximum cytoreductive surgery on median survival time became insignificant so that each 10 point increase in percentage maximum cytoreductive surgery was only associated with a 4.1% increase in median survival time. In this model, each increase of 0.2 units in dose intensity was associated with an 11.1% increase in median survival time ($p < 0.001$) and the presence of platinum was associated with a 53% increase in median survival time ($p < 0.001$).

The study reported by Hunter *et al.* [10] examined the importance of dose intensity within the context of other prognostic variables and infers that the contribution of optimal cytoreductive surgery on outcome might not be as important as hitherto accepted, provided that patients receive dose intensive platinum based chemotherapy.

20.5 SINGLE AGENT *VS* MULTIAGENT P-CONTAINING REGIMENS

A regression analysis [11] performed on randomized studies incorporating P, CAP and CHAP provided retrospective evidence that CAP and CHAP combinations produced greater response rates than P alone for a fixed, planned RDI for P ($p < 0.01$). The lower range of doses of C and A used in multiagent regimens than have been found to be effective as single agents may have contributed to the failure to demonstrate an impact of C-RDI on the outcome in multiagent regimens. Despite this, however, there was a significant

improvement in outcome associated with an increase in A-RDI. In 84% of multiagent regimens studied, A was used at an RDI of less than 15 mg m^{-2} week^{-1} and in 47% of studies, the drug was used at an RDI of less than 10 mg m^{-2} week^{-1}. When one considers that a dose intensity for A of 25 mg m^{-2} week^{-1} produces a clinical response rate of 40% when used as a single agent in previously untreated patients with ovarian carcinoma, it is possible that higher RDIs for this drug within multiagent regimens may have shown a significant relationship between RDI for A and response.

In a meta-analysis performed by the Ovarian Cancer Meta-Analysis Project [12], four randomized trials comparing CP with CAP were studied and the survival benefit found for CAP ($p = 0.02$).

One of the problems in comparing various P-containing trials is the intertrial variation in P-RDI, especially when the P-RDI is less than 1.1 – this being a steep part of the P-RDI *vs* response curve. The meta-analysis comparing P, CAP and CHAP [6] was able to adjust for variations in P-RDI. However, individual studies in which multiagent P-containing *vs* single agent P were compared but P-RDI was not fixed in the treatment arms being compared [13,14,15], are open to criticism in this respect.

One of the largest prospective randomized studies in which P was compared with CP and CAP was reported by Gruppo Interegionale Cooperativo Oncologico Ginecologia [16] in a three arm study of 565 patients. The study design ensured that P-RDI was fixed in each arm, as was the C-RDI in the two arms incorporating this drug. Clinical response rates increased with the addition of C and A to P (49% for P, 56% for CP and 66% for CAP [$p=0.009$]). In a smaller study [17] in which P-RDI was fixed in two arms and P compared to AP, the clinical response was 31% for P and 66% for AP, again demonstrating an advantage in adding another drug to P.

These studies have demonstrated the importance of adding A or C to P and the necessity to keep the P-RDI constant in all treatment arms if this question is being addressed in a prospective randomized study.

20.6 CONCLUSION

Most meta-analyses and prospective randomized studies performed since the original dose intensity analysis and hypothesis was published [1] have supported the use of P at 25 mg m^{-2} week^{-1} when used within multiagent regimens and at 30 mg m^{-2} week^{-1} when used as a single agent. While the curve beyond these data points does not necessarily plateau, it is very much shallower than the curves generated up to these points. Nevertheless, the impact on long term survival when using doses of P beyond these levels is unknown. The updated dose intensity analysis demonstrates clearly that adding C and A (and possibly H) to P improves the response for any fixed dose of P and that there is a linear relationship between A-RDI and outcome. Doses of C and A within multiagent regimens consistent beyond those used historically with those found to be effective when used as single agents may further enhance responses and raise important questions for future prospective randomized studies.

REFERENCES

1. Levin, L. and Hryniuk, W.M. (1987) Dose intensity analysis of chemotherapy regimens in ovarian carcinoma. *J. Clin. Oncol.*, **5**, 756–67.
2. Ozols, R.F., Corden, B.J., Jacob, J. *et al.* (1984) High dose cisplatinum in hypertonic saline. *Ann. Intern. Med.*, **100**, 19–24.
3. Ngan, H.Y.S., Choo, Y.C., Cheung, M. *et al.* (1989) A randomized study of high dose *vs* low-dose cisplatinum combined with cyclophosphamide in the treatment of advanced ovarian cancer. *Chemotherapy*, **35**, 221–7.
4. Kaye, S.B., Lewis, C.R., Paul, J. *et al.* (1992) Randomized study of two doses of cisplatin with cyclophosphamide in epithelial ovarian cancer. *Lancet*, **340**, 329–33.
5. McGuire, W.P., Hoskins, W.J., Brady, M.F. *et al.* (1992) A phase III trial of dose intense (DI) *vs* standard dose (DS) cisplatin (CDDP) and cytoxan (CTX) in advanced ovarian cancer (AOC). Proc. *Am. Soc. Clin. Oncol.*, **11**, A718.
6. Boni, C., Cocconi, G., Lottici, R. *et al.* (1990) Conventional *vs* high dose intensity cisplatin in advanced ovarian cancer. Preliminary report of a randomized trial. *Proc. Am. Soc. Clin. Oncol.*, **9**, A651.
7. Colombo, N., Pittelli, M.R., Marzola, M. *et al.* (1990) Randomized study of two cisplatin (P) dose intensity regimens in patients with stage III/IV epithelial ovarian cancer (EOC). *Proc. Am. Soc. Clin. Oncol.*, **9**, A619.
8. Jacobs, A.J., Sommers, G.M., Homan, S.M. *et al.* (1988) Therapy of ovarian carcinoma: the relationship of dose level and treatment intensity to survival. *Gynecol. Oncol.*, **31**, 233–45.
9. Levin, L. (1993) Dose intensity in the treatment of ovarian carcinoma. In *Cancer of the Ovary* (eds M. Markman and W.J. Hoskins), Raven Press, New York, pp. 251–60.
10. Hunter, R.W., Alexander, N.D.E. and Soutter, W.P. (1992) Meta-analysis of surgery in advanced ovarian carcinoma: is maximum cytoreductive surgery an independent determinant of prognosis? *Am. J. Obstet. Gynecol.*, **166**, 504–11.
11. Levin, L., Simon, R. and Hryniuk, W.M. (1993) The importance of multiagent chemotherapy regimens in ovarian carcinoma – dose intensity analysis. *J. Natl. Cancer Inst.*, **85**, 1732–42.
12. Ovarian Cancer Meta-Analysis Project (1991) Cyclophosphamide plus cisplatin *vs* cyclophosphamide, doxorubicin, and cisplatin chemotherapy in ovarian carcinoma: a meta-analysis. *J. Clin. Oncol.*, **9**, 1668–74.
13. Kankipati, S.R. and Wiltshaw, E. (1981) A prospective randomized study of cisplatinum as a single agent and in combination with chlorambucil in advanced ovarian carcinoma. *Br. J. Cancer.*, **44**, 289.

14. Tomirotti, M., Perrone, S., Gie, P. *et al.* (1988) Cisplatin (P) *vs* cyclophosphamide, adriamycin and cisplatin (CAP) for stage III/IV epithelial ovarian carcinoma: a prospective randomized trial. *Tumori*, **74**, 573–7.

15. Wiltshaw, E., Evans, B., Rustin, G. *et al.* (1986) A prospective randomized trial comparing high dose cisplatin with low dose cisplatin and chlorambucil in advanced ovarian carcinoma. *J. Clin. Oncol.*, **4**, 722–9.

16. Gruppo Interegionale Cooperativo Oncologico Ginecologia (1987) Randomized comparison of cisplatin with cyclophosphamide/cisplatin and with cyclophosphamide/doxorubicin/cisplatin in advanced ovarian cancer. *Lancet*, ii, 353–9.

17. Bruckner, H.W., Cohen, C.J., Goldberg, J.D. *et al.* (1981) Improved chemotherapy for ovarian cancer with cis-diammine dichloroplatinum and adriamycin. *Cancer*, **47**, 2288–94.

Chapter 21

Drug resistance in ovarian cancer and potential for its reversal

T.C. HAMILTON, S.W. JOHNSON, A.K. GODWIN, M.A. BOOKMAN,
P.J. O'DWYER, K. HAMAGUCHI, K. JACKSON and R.F. OZOLS

Ovarian cancer is characterized as a disease responsive to chemotherapy and current medical treatment strategies are based on the use of a platinum containing anticancer drug, either cisplatin or carboplatin, as the cornerstone of post surgical treatment [1,2]. Unfortunately, the majority of patients with stage III or IV disease are not cured by platinum containing combination chemotherapy and when ovarian cancers recur, especially after short disease-free intervals, they are generally refractory to a variety of other unrelated chemotherapeutic agents [1,3]. It is clear that our understanding of this aspect of ovarian cancer biology could have substantial clinical impact if approaches to reverse the failure of therapy or prevent treatment failure could be discovered.

One possibility is that treatment failure occurs due to altered host pharmacology but it is more likely that it results from either the outgrowth of small subpopulations of intrinsically drug resistant tumor cells or that repeated cyclic exposure to anticancer drugs induces changes within tumor cells which render them refractory to killing by the drugs. Irrespective of which of these possible processes yields drug resistant tumors, it is important to ascertain the mechanisms responsible.

Our approach to identify the mechanisms of drug resistance in ovarian cancer is to develop ovarian cancer cell lines with high levels of cisplatin resistance and cross resistance to other drugs used for the treatment of this disease. We have chosen to examine cells with primary cisplatin resistance since this drug has made the greatest impact on the treatment of ovarian cancer during the last decade [2]. It is our belief that cell lines with high levels of primary cisplatin resistance are a relevant starting point for defining the fullest possible repertoire of mechanisms that contribute to primary cisplatin resistance and the cross resistance characteristic of clinical ovarian cancer. We have based this approach on two points:

1. If one examines multiple unrelated ovarian cancer cell lines, their range in cisplatin sensitivities is greater than 100-fold [4,5];
2. The use of models with high levels of resistance to natural products and methotrexate has yielded mechanisms of resistance to these drugs which have been subsequently shown to be of clinical relevance [6,7].

In order to develop cell lines with high levels of cisplatin resistance, we have exposed a relatively cisplatin sensitive ovarian cancer

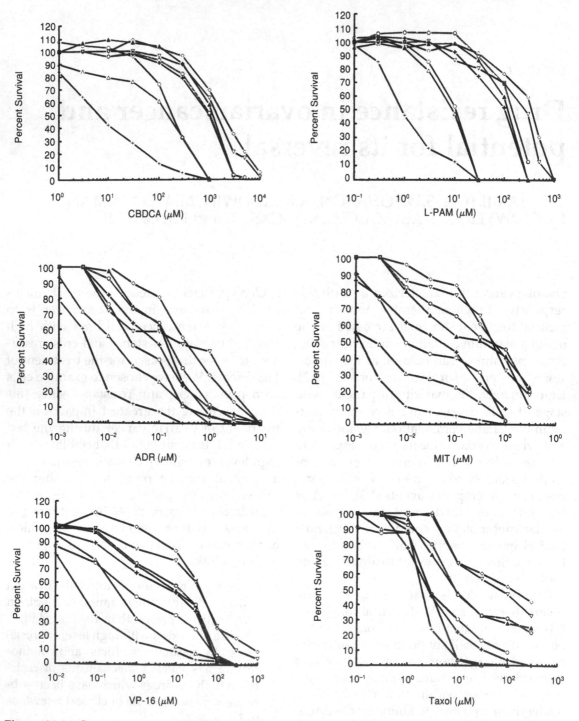

Figure 21.1 Cross resistance of CDDP resistant human ovarian cancer cell lines: A2780 (+), CP20 (Δ), CP70 (o), C30 (+), C50 (▲), C80 (•), C100 (▽) and C200 (♦) to various drugs. Cytotoxicity was determined by the MTT assay after continuous exposure to a range of drug concentrations for three days. Points, mean of three independent experiments; CBDCA, carboplatin; L-PAM, melphalan; ADR, adriamycin; MIT, mitoxantrone; VP-16, etoposide.

cell line (A2780) derived from the ovarian tumor of an untreated patient to increasing concentrations of cisplatin over a six year period. This has enabled us to develop cell lines with a range of cisplatin sensitivities by removing the cells from drug exposure at various intervals during dose escalation. This approach has yielded cell lines with primary cisplatin resistance ranging from a few fold to greater than 400-fold (Figure 21.1). Furthermore, these cell lines show cross resistance to diverse anticancer drugs including the cisplatin analogue carboplatin, the classic alkylating agent melphalan and natural products including adriamycin, VP-16, mitoxantrone and Taxol [8]. Cross resistance to Taxol only developed in cell lines with high levels of primary cisplatin resistance (i.e. >200-fold). This is consistent with the clinical observation of Taxol use as salvage therapy in some drug refractory ovarian cancer patients [2].

Although the primary focus of our drug resistance work is on platinum resistance, the substantial cross resistance observed with natural product drugs was of obvious interest since mechanisms of drug resistance may be inferred from the known pharmacologic properties of these agents. Thus, we examined these cell lines for increased expression of the MDR-1 (multidrug resistance) and MRP (multidrug resistance protein) genes as well as altered adriamycin accumulation and the effect of verapamil on cytotoxicity. These studies provided no evidence that classic natural product resistance was operative in these cell lines [8].

In efforts to define at a functional level the mechanisms responsible for resistance to cisplatin, it is necessary to evaluate at least three broad categories of potential resistance mechanisms:

1. Decrease in cell associated drug;
2. Increased cellular inactivation of drug;
3. Alterations in DNA damage and repair.

Various molecular biological approaches are then required to define the bases for these functional changes and to uncover any unanticipated changes which may contribute to resistance.

We have measured total cell associated cisplatin by atomic absorption spectrometry in the panel of *in vitro* selected cisplatin resistant cell lines (A2780/C series). Our results indicate that accumulation is non-saturable and approximately linear with increasing cisplatin concentration, up to 200 μM. Cisplatin accumulation is approximately 7-fold higher in the cisplatin sensitive A2780 cell line as compared to the highly resistant C200 cell

Table 21.1 Relationship between cisplatin cytotoxicity, cisplatin accumulation and DNA platination in cisplatin sensitive and resistant ovarian cancer cell lines

Cell line	Cisplatin IC50*	Fold resistant	Accumulation ng Pt 10^{-6} cells**	DNA platination pg Pt μg^{-1} DNA**
A2780	0.35	1	79	106
CP70	5.5	16	39	46
C30	98	280	11	18
C80	144	411	12	14
C200	147	418	12	16

* Cytotoxicity was determined by cisplatin treatment for 72 h with assay using 3-(4,5-dimethylthiazol-2-yl)-2,5-diphenyltetrazolium bromide (MTT). The IC50 is the concentration (μM) which inhibited growth by 50%. The IC50 values were measured in triplicate in two independent experiments
** Cells were incubated with 200 μM cisplatin for 2 h at 37°C

line. Decreased accumulation is also apparent in cell lines with relatively modest cisplatin resistance. Accumulation decreases with increasing resistance but appears to plateau in the more highly resistant cell lines (i.e. C30, C50, C80 and C200; Table 21.1). Differences in cisplatin sensitivity were apparent among this group of resistant cell lines. These data suggest that decreased accumulation may be one change which contributes significantly to cisplatin resistance.

Total DNA platination was also measured using atomic absorption spectrometry. This analysis revealed that DNA platination increased linearly with respect to cisplatin dose (Figure 21.2A). We also observed that the amount of platinum bound to genomic DNA was decreased in the drug resistant variants (Figure 21.2A). In this panel of cell lines, the DNA platination showed a near linear relationship with cisplatin accumulation (Figure 21.2B) such that those cells which had

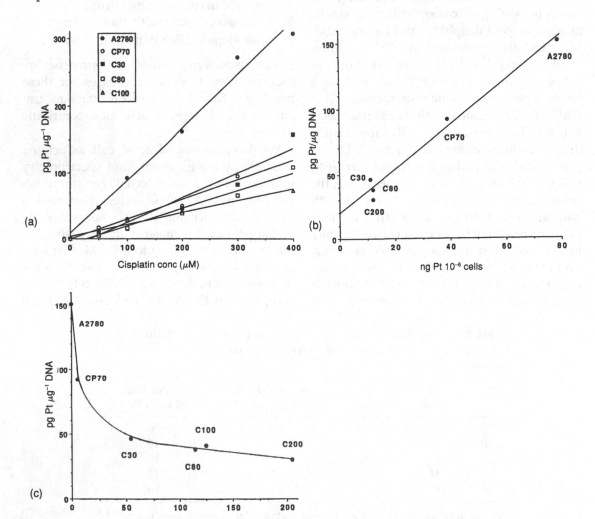

Figure 21.2 Relationship between total DNA platination and cisplatin concentration (a), cellular cisplatin accumulation (b) and cytotoxicity (c). In (b) and (c), cells were treated with 200 μM cisplatin for two hours at 37°C.

decreased platinum accumulation exhibited decreases in DNA bound platinum. Consistent with the clustering of platinum dose dependent accumulation patterns in C30–C200 cells, we observed similar levels of DNA platination in these variants, which at the time of analysis exhibited a wide range of sensitivities to cisplatin. Therefore, in this group of cells with moderate to high levels of cisplatin resistance, DNA platination showed no linear relationship to cytotoxicity (Figure 21.2C). Other mechanisms including alterations in DNA damage and repair may intervene to increase the resistance in these latter cell lines.

When studying the role of repair of cisplatin induced DNA damage in drug resistance, it is very important to consider the choice of drug exposure conditions. Under conditions in which individual cell lines were treated with cisplatin doses that yielded similar total platinum–DNA adduct levels (0.77–1.02 Pt adducts/10 kb) there was a clear relationship between the ability to remove platinum from DNA and the degree of resistance (Figure 21.3). This finding in several related cell lines expands our initial observation of increased DNA repair as monitored by unscheduled DNA synthesis in CP70 cells [9–11]. We have speculated that DNA repair could be a mechanism of cisplatin resistance distinct from a process which would influence the innate sensitivity of cells to cisplatin. This view was based on the observation that inhibition of cisplatin induced DNA repair by aphidicolin, an inhibitor of DNA polymerase α, influenced the cytotoxicity of cisplatin in the moderately cisplatin resistant CP70 cells but not in the parental A2780 cells from which they were derived [9]. The present data further support this hypothesis. When the relationship between % total platinum–DNA adduct removal and IC50 of cisplatin is examined, it is noteworthy that the inclusion of A2780 weakens a near perfect linear relationship (Figure 21.3) among CP70, C30, C80 and C200 (r=0.998).

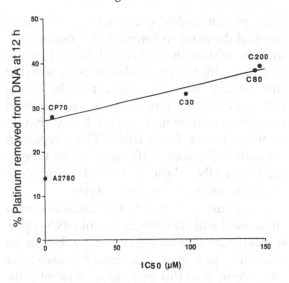

Figure 21.3 The relationship between platinum removal at 12 hours and cisplatin cytotoxicity for cisplatin sensitive and resistant ovarian cancer cell lines.

Consistent with our finding of a relationship between total platinum–DNA adduct removal and degree of cisplatin resistance, we observed increased DNA sequence specific removal of cisplatin–interstrand crosslinks in resistant *vs* sensitive cells at four hours post-treatment. Two categories of DNA sequences were examined, one which contains actively transcribed genes (17 kb *Hind*III restriction fragment of the 28S ribosomal RNA gene) and one which contains non-transcribed, non-gene encoding sequences (23 kb *Hind*III restriction fragment of a variable number tandem repeat (VNTR) region on chromosome 17). The increased repair was more apparent when the transcribed sequences were examined [12].

In addition to the results supporting a role for total DNA repair and DNA sequence specific interstrand crosslink removal in cisplatin resistance, our data suggest other important possibilities as to cisplatin resistance mechanisms which have not previously been described. It was of particular interest that in the presence of near equivalent amounts of total platinum–DNA damage, there was a marked decrease in interstrand crosslink formation within the ribosomal RNA gene as resistance increased. It should be noted that this pattern was not apparent when total DNA interstrand crosslinks were measured [13]. Hence, it would appear likely that in addition to the direct role of DNA repair in cisplatin resistance, differences in the type of platinum–DNA lesions formed could contribute to the resistance phenotype.

Based on our functional measurements showing the likely contribution of DNA repair to cisplatin resistance, we have begun to examine potential molecular bases for enhancement of this process in resistant cells. It is likely that nucleotide excision repair is the major mechanism responsible for removal of cisplatin damage. What is known concerning this complex process in mammalian cells has been reviewed in detail [14,15]. It is clear that numerous enzymes, many yet to be identified, participate in the multiple steps which comprise this process including: damage recognition, removal of damaged nucleotides, resynthesis and ligation. We have examined the steady-state mRNA levels for several enzymes involved in DNA repair including:

DNA polymerase α, DNA polymerase β ERCCI (excision repair cross complementing) and ERCC2. In the case of DNA polymerase α and β and ERCC2, we observed no alteration of expression. We did, however, observe increases in steady-state mRNA levels for ERCC1 (Figure 21.4). This is of particular interest in view of recent data indicating a relationship between ERCC1 expression in white blood cells and response to platinum therapy [16]. Ongoing investigations include transfection of a full length cDNA for ERCC1 into the relatively cisplatin sensitive A2780 cells in order to determine if increased ERCC1 expression in the absence of other changes alters cellular sensitivity to cisplatin.

If enhanced ability to repair DNA damage is in fact a contributor to cisplatin resistance, it is important to consider clinically relevant approaches to inhibit this process. To this end, we have utilized aphidicolin and its water soluble derivative, aphidicolin glycinate, in *in vitro* and *in vivo* studies to determine if inhibition of DNA repair increases the activity of cisplatin [17]. *in vivo* we have observed that aphidicolin glycinate (q3hx4 on day 4 post-tumor implantation and q3hx2 on day 5 at 30 mg kg^{-1} per dose) increases the median sur-

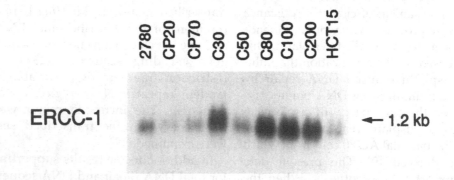

Figure 21.4 ERCC-1 steady-state mRNA expression in cisplatin resistant ovarian cancer cell lines. RNA gels were routinely stained with ethidium bromide and visualized to ensure that equivalent amounts of total RNA were analysed in each case. Standard Northern blotting was performed and the blots hybridized with a ^{32}P labeled 1.2kb full-length cDNA probe isolated from a human λ-Zap-II library using a partial clone kindly provided by Marcel van Duin. After hybridization the blot was washed and radioactivity visualized by autoradiography.

vival of nude mice bearing the OVCAR3 human ovarian cancer cell line from 85 days for cisplatin alone (5 mg kg⁻¹) to greater than 130 days for the combination of aphidicolin glycinate and cisplatin [17]. These data in combination with European Phase I clinical trial data on aphidicolin glycinate [18] suggest that a strategy of using aphidicolin glycinate and cisplatin has potential clinical merit.

The observation described above, indicating that in the presence of similar levels of total DNA platination there were decreases in sequence specific interstrand crosslink formation, suggests that either DNA secondary or tertiary structural modifications or inactivation by glutathione (GSH) contributes to the cisplatin resistance phenotype. Both protein and non-protein sulfhydryl molecules have been implicated in this process. The most prominent non-protein sulfhydryl molecule is glutathione (GSH) and we and others have developed a substantial body of evidence which suggests that it plays an important role in cisplatin and classical alkylating agent resistance [5,19–21]. Based on these data, we have preclinically evaluated several strategies to lower cellular GSH. The most clinically applicable approach has been to utilize buthionine sulfoximine (BSO), a synthetic amino acid analogue developed in Alton Meister's laboratory [22]. BSO irreversibly binds γ-glutamylcysteine synthetase (γ-GCS), the rate limiting enzyme in GSH synthesis, and hence reduces cellular GSH levels. We and others have shown *in vitro* and *in vivo* that this strategy to lower GSH increases the efficacy of classic alkylating agents and platinum drugs [23,24]. Based on these studies, BSO was developed as a clinical chemotherapeutic agent sensitizer and Phase I clinical trials of BSO and melphalan have been initiated at our institution [25]. The goals of this trial were, first, to determine the concentration and treatment scheme necessary to decrease tumor cell and white blood cell (as a surrogate tissue) GSH to ~10% of control

values and, secondly, to determine if the combination of BSO and melphalan could be safely administered. BSO was given at 12 hour intervals ×6 with melphalan (15 mg m⁻²) given at the time of the fifth BSO dose. The starting dose for BSO of 1500 mg m⁻² did not reproducibly lower cellular GSH and dose escalation was instituted. It was determined that BSO at a dose of 13 g m⁻² was necessary to achieve our goal of decreasing cellular GSH to ~10% control in >90% of patients. The effect of 13 g m⁻² BSO on tumor cell and leukocyte GSH levels of a representative patient are shown in Figure 21.5. This level of GSH depletion necessitated decreasing the melphalan dose to 10 mg m⁻² in this heavily pretreated group of patients. Future clinical trials at our institution include:

1. A phase II trial of BSO and melphalan to determine efficacy;
2. A Phase I trial of BSO and carboplatin;
3. In the long term, potentially combining BSO, aphidicolin glycinate and carboplatin.

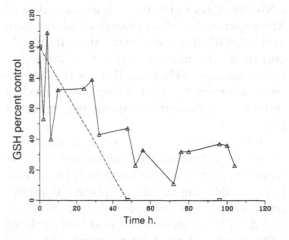

Figure 21.5 Effect of BSO treatment on tumor and leukocyte GSH content. A patient with colon cancer was treated with BSO 13 g m⁻² as described in the text. At the time points shown, leukocytes (Δ) and tumor biopsies (☐) were obtained and assessed for GSH content.

Substitution of carboplatin for cisplatin in the treatment of advanced ovarian cancer has achieved equivalent response rates and long term survival with a significant reduction in non-hematologic toxicity. Several strategies have been proposed to optimize carboplatin based therapy, including increased dose intensity, combinations with taxol or other reagents for reversal of drug resistance.

Clinical trials of dose intense therapy with carboplatin have been limited by hematologic toxicity, particularly thrombocytopenia. The use of first generation hematopoietic growth factors (i.e. G-CSF, GM-CSF) has failed to consistently reduce the magnitude of thrombocytopenia. Interleukin-1 (IL-1) is a 17 kd cytokine produced by monocyte/macrophages with diverse effects mediated through an 80 kd transmembrane receptor expressed on T lymphocytes, vascular endothelium, hepatocytes, keratinocytes, fibroblasts, chondrocytes and synovium. In animal models, IL-1 has been shown to protect against radiation and chemotherapy induced myelosuppression through induction of secondary cytokines, including IL-3, IL-6, IL-7, IL-11, G-CSF and GM-CSF. Other effects, such as induction of Mn-superoxide dismutase, ceruloplasmin and metallothionein may also indirectly contribute to marrow protection following chemotherapy. When rhuIL-1α was administered after single-agent carboplatin, a modest reduction in thrombocytopenia was reported [26].

The use of rhuIL-1α was evaluated at Fox Chase in untreated ovarian cancer patients receiving a dose intense regimen (CPC) of carboplatin (600 mg m^{-2} d1), cisplatin (50 mg m^{-2} d8 and d15), and cyclophosphamide (250 mg m^{-2} d1) [27]. Patients received one cycle of CPC alone followed by a second and third cycle with the addition of rhuIL-1α (Immunex Corporation, Seattle, WA) by subcutaneous injection d2-d5 at dose levels of 0.3, 1.0, 3.0 or 10 μg m^{-2}. The degree of myelosuppression was compared for each patient between cycles 1 and 2. Dose modifications of CPC were not permitted for reversible myelosuppression, although subsequent cycles could be delayed for as long as two weeks to allow for marrow recovery. If the dose of carboplatin is converted to an equivalent dose of cisplatin, each cycle of CPC achieves a dose intensity of 250 mg m^{-2}, compared to standard dose cisplatin at 75 mg m^{-2}.

A total of 17 patients were enrolled on the study with a median age of 56 (range 20–73). Two patients never received rhuIL-1α due to early cisplatin induced nephrotoxicity. Three patients with late ototoxicity had one or two doses of cisplatin omitted from cycle 3. In addition, six patients received only cycles 1 and 2, due to prolonged myelosuppression after cycle 2 resulting in greater than a two week delay. Dose limiting reversible hypotension occurred in 1/3 patients at 10 μg m^{-2} rhuIL-1α. Dose related fever and chills occurred following each dose of rhuIL-1α at all levels.

There was no definite improvement in either the degree or duration of thrombocytopenia or neutropenia during cycle 2 with rhuIL-1α compared to cycle 1 without rhuIL-1α. Prophylactic or therapeutic platelet transfusions were given to 41% (7/17) of patients during cycle 1, 53% (8/15) during cycle 2 and 62% (5/8) during cycle 3. In addition, one patient developed life-threatening gastrointestinal bleeding during cycle 3 in the setting of prolonged but reversible thrombocytopenia that was refractory to platelet transfusion. Analysis of platelet counts tended to show prolongation of nadirs for each cycle, in spite of administration of rhuIL-1α (Figure 21.6).

Lack of efficacy in this study may relate to the inclusion of d8 and d15 cisplatin or suboptimal scheduling of rhuIL-1α. It remains to be determined whether including rhuIL-1α will reduce the need for platelet transfusions and/or permit the safe delivery of increased carboplatin dosage.

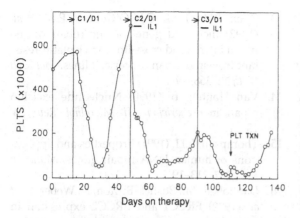

Figure 21.6 Serial platelet counts for a patient with stage IV ovarian cancer treated with CPC and rhuIL-1α. CPC was administered at full dosage without modification for each of the three cycles and there was no measurable change in renal function as determined by serum creatinine and 24 hour creatinine clearance. The dose of rhuIL-1α during cycle 2 was 10 μg m^{-2}, but this was reduced to 3 μg m^{-2} due to transient hypotension that required pressor support. Note the more rapid onset and prolonged platelet nadir during cycle 2 (post-rhuIL-1α) and the prolonged nadir with platelet transfusion during cycle 3.

Use of a targeted area under the curve (AUC) dosing schema based on calculated or measured GFR [28] has resulted in more uniform and predictable platelet toxicity, and allowed for safer delivery of more dose intense therapy. Ongoing studies at Fox Chase have included targeted AUC dosing in conjunction with peripheral blood progenitor cell support for untreated patients with advanced ovarian cancer. Following optimized recruitment and recovery of progenitor cells, patients receive two consecutive cycles of high dose carboplatin (AUC $\geq$12 mg × min × ml^{-1}) and Taxol (250 mg m^{-2}), with administration of cryopreserved progenitor cells after each cycle.

Preliminary data from the Gynecologic Oncology Group (GOG) suggest that the combination of cisplatin and Taxol may have greater efficacy than cisplatin and cyclophosphamide [29]. There has been considerable interest in developing effective and safe combinations of carboplatin with Taxol. A dose escalating pilot study (GOG-9202) of carboplatin (AUC 5–10 mg × min × ml^{-1}) and Taxol (135–225 mg m^{-2} over 24 hours) in untreated patients with advanced ovarian cancer is in progress [30]. Neutropenia was dose limiting, but partially abrogated using G-CSF without the frequent occurrence of hospitalizations for febrile neutropenia. Patients could safely receive six complete cycles of carboplatin (AUC 7.5) and Taxol (135 mg m^{-2}) without excessive cumulative toxicity and Taxol dosage is being escalated to determine the MTD with AUC 7.5 carboplatin. Thus far, thrombocytopenia requiring platelet transfusion has been uncommon (2/19 patients). Modification to use a three hour Taxol infusion could permit outpatient therapy with reduced myelosuppression, depending on the relative antitumor efficacy of Taxol using a 3 hour *vs* 24 hour infusion.

We have reached several interim conclusions based on the investigations described. It is clearly possible to develop cell lines with high levels of cisplatin resistance and the cross resistance characteristic of cisplatin refractory clinical ovarian cancer. Even in these relatively simple *in vitro* models of drug resistance, multiple mechanisms contribute to the resistance phenotype. Based on identification of mechanisms of resistance including increased DNA repair and increased drug inactivation by GSH, it has been possible to develop clinically relevant strategies for the reversal of resistance. Ongoing and future investigations will determine whether these strategies will have an impact on disease-free survival, quality of life and/or overall survival.

REFERENCES

1. Ozols, R.F., O'Dwyer, P.J. and Hamilton, T.C. (1993) Drug resistance in ovarian cancer. In *Cancer of the Ovary*, (eds M. Markman and

W. Hoskins), W.B. Saunders, Philadelphia, pp. 261–76.

2. Ozols, R.F. (1992) Ovarian cancer. Part II: Treatment. *Curr. Probl. Cancer*, **XVI**, 67–126.

3. Ozols, R.F. and Young, R.C. (1991) Chemotherapy of ovarian cancer. *Semin. Oncol.*, **18**, 222–32.

4. Perez, R.P., O'Dwyer, P.J., Handel, L.M. *et al.* (1991) Comparative cytotoxicity of CI-973, cisplatin, carboplatin and tetraplatin in human ovarian cell lines. *Int. J. Cancer*, **48**, 265–9.

5. Mistry, P., Kelland, L.R., Abel, G. *et al.* (1991) The relationships between glutathione, glutathione-S-transferase and cytotoxicity of platinum drugs and melphalan in eight human ovarian carcinoma cell lines. *Br. J. Cancer*, **64**, 215–20.

6. Fojo, A., Hamilton, T.C., Young, R.C. *et al.* (1987) Multidrug resistance in ovarian cancer. *Cancer*, **60**, 2075–80.

7. Cowan, K.H., Goldsmith, M.E., Levine, R.M. *et al.* (1982) Dihydrofolate reductase gene amplification and possible rearrangement in estrogen-responsive methotrexate-resistant human breast cancer cells. *J. Biol. Chem.*, **257**, 15079–84.

8. Hamaguchi, K., Godwin, A.K., Yakushiji, M. *et al.* (1993) Cross-resistance to diverse drugs is associated with primary cisplatin resistance in ovarian cancer cell lines. *Cancer Res.*, **53**, 5225–32.

9. Masuda, H., Ozols, R.F., Lai, G-M. *et al.* (1988) Increased DNA repair as a mechanism of acquired resistance to cis-diamminedichloroplatinum (II) in human ovarian cancer cell lines. *Cancer Res.*, **48**, 5713–16.

10. Lai, G-M., Ozols, R.F., Smyth, J.F. *et al.* (1988) Enhanced DNA repair and resistance to cisplatin in human ovarian cancer. *Biochem. Pharmacol.*, **37**, 4597–600.

11. Lai, G-M., Ozols, R.F. and Hamilton, T.C. (1989) Role of glutathione on DNA repair in cisplatin resistant human ovarian cancer cell lines. *J. Natl. Cancer Inst.*, **81**, 535–9.

12. Johnson, S.W., Perez, R.P., Godwin, A.K. *et al.* (1994) Role of platinum–DNA adduct formation and removal in cisplatin resistance in human ovarian cancer cell lines. *Biochem. Pharm.*, **47**, 689–97.

13. Zhen, W.P., Link, C.J., O'Connor, P.M. *et al.* (1992) Increased gene-specific repair of cisplatin interstrand cross-links in cisplatin-resistant human ovarian cancer cell lines. *Mol. Cell Biol.*, **12**, 3689–98.

14. Van Houten, B. (1990) Nucleotide excision repair in *Escherichia coli*. *Microbiol. Rev.*, **54**, 18–51.

15. Thompson, L.H. (1991) Properties and applications of human DNA repair genes. *Mutation Res.*, **247**, 213–19.

16. Dabholkar, M., Bostick-Bruton, F., Weber, C. *et al.* (1992) ERCC1 and ERCC2 expression in malignant tissues from ovarian cancer patients. *J. Natl. Cancer Inst.*, **84**, 1512–17.

17. O'Dwyer, P.J., Moyer, J.D., Suffness, M. *et al.* (1994) Antitumor activity and biochemical effects of aphidicolin glycinate (NSC 303812) alone and in combination with cisplatin *in vivo*. *Cancer Res.*, **54**, 724–9.

18. Sessa, C., Zucchetti, M., Davoli, E. *et al.* (1991) Phase I and clinical pharmacological evaluation of aphidicolin glycinate. *J. Natl. Cancer Inst.*, **83**, 1160–4.

19. Godwin, A.K., Meister, A., O'Dwyer, P.J. *et al.* (1992) High resistance to cisplatin in human ovarian cancer cell lines is associated with marked increase in glutathione synthesis. *Proc. Natl. Acad. Sci. USA*, **89**, 3070–4.

20. Hosking, L.K., Whelan, R.D.H., Shellard, S.A. *et al.* (1990) An evaluation of the role of glutathione and its associated enzymes in the expression of differential sensitivities to antitumor agents shown by a range of human tumor cell lines. *Biochem. Pharmacol.*, **40**, 1833–42.

21. Meijer, C., Mulder, N.H., Timmer-Bosscha, H. *et al.* (1992) Relationship of cellular glutathione to the cytotoxicity and resistance of seven platinum compounds. *Cancer Res.*, **52**, 6885–9.

22. Meister, A. and Anderson, M.E. (1993) Glutathione. *Ann. Rev. Biochem.*, **52**, 711–60.

23. Hamilton, T.C., Winker, M.A., Louie, K.G. *et al.* (1985) Augmentation of adriamycin, melphalan and cisplatin cytotoxicity in drug-resistant and -sensitive human ovarian cancer cell lines by buthionine sulfoximine mediated glutathione depletion. *Biochem. Pharmacol.*, **34**, 2583–6.

212

24. Ozols, R.F., Louie, K.G., Plowman, J. *et al.* (1987) Enhanced melphalan cytotoxicity in human ovarian cancer *in vitro* and in tumor bearing nude mice by buthionine sulfoximine depletion of glutathione. *Biochem. Pharmacol.*, **36**, 147–53.

25. O'Dwyer, P.J., Hamilton, T.C., Young, R.C. *et al.* (1992) Depletion of glutathione in normal and malignant human cells *in vivo* by buthionine sulfoximine: clinical and biochemical results. *J. Natl. Cancer Inst.*, **84**, 264–7.

26. Smith, J.W., Longo,D.L., Alvord, W.G. *et al.* (1993) The effects of treatment with interleukin-α on platelet recovery after high-dose carboplatin. *N. Engl. J. Med.*, **328**, 756–61.

27. Bookman, M.A, Caron, D.A., Hogan, W.M. *et al.* (1993) Phase-1 evaluation of dose-intense chemotherapy with interleukin-1α (IL1-α) for gynecologic malignancies. *Proc. ASCO*, **12**, A868.

28. Calvert, A.H., Newell, D.R., Gumbrell, L.A. *et al.* (1989) Carboplatin dosage: prospective evaluation of a simple formula based on renal function. *J. Clin. Oncol.*, **7**, 1748–56.

29. McGuire, W.P., Hoskins, W.J., Brady, M.F. *et al.* (1993) A Phase III trial comparing cisplatin/cytoxan (PC) and cisplatin/taxol (PT) in advanced ovarian cancer (AOC). *Proc. ASCO*, **12**, A808.

30. Ozols, R.F., Kilpatrick, D., O'Dwyer, P. *et al.* (1993) Phase I and pharmacokinetic study of taxol (T) and carboplatin (C) in previously untreated patients (PTS) with advanced epithelial ovarian cancer (OC): a pilot study of the Gynecologic Oncology Group. *Proc. ASCO*, **12**, A824.

Chapter 22

Taxol and Taxotere: new drugs of interest in the treatment of advanced ovarian cancer

M.J. PICCART

22.1 TAXOL

Taxol was identified 22 years ago as the active substance of the bark of the Pacific yew, *Taxus brevifolia* [1].

The NCI developed an interest in this drug when S. Horwitz's group identified its unique mechanism of action: namely inhibition of microtubule depolymerization [2,3].

Taxol underwent a slow clinical development in the 1980s, due to problems of drug supply – which have since been solved – and due to drug induced hypersensitivity reactions which have been largely overcome by the use of prolonged 24 hour infusions and steroid based prophylaxis [4].

Taxol was approved by the FDA in late 1992 for patients with platinum refractory ovarian cancer. Individual studies and a collaborative group trial by the Gynecological Oncology Group (GOG) found a consistent response rate of about 30% (Table 22.1) [5–8]. This response rate was not restricted to patients having a platinum-free interval and was superior to that achieved by the chemotherapeutic agents commonly used on patients not responding to cisplatin or carboplatin.

The Gynecological Oncology Group took the next logical step by incorporating Taxol into

Table 22.1 Taxol studies in advanced and refractory ovarian cancer

Group (ref)	No. of patients	Complete responses	Partial responses	% response	95% confidence interval
JH [5]	46	1	9	22	11–37
AE [6]	32	2	4	19	8–37
GOG [7]	46	5	9	30	18–46
NCI [8]	15	2	4	40	17–67
NCI [8]	50	1	17	36	23–51
Total	189	11	43		25–39

JH = John Hopkins
AE = Albert Einstein
GOG = Gynecologic Oncology Group
NCI = National Cancer Institute

chemotherapy regimens for advanced ovarian cancer for bulky residual disease (>1 cm): results of a randomized trial comparing the classic regimen cisplatin–cyclophosphamide to a cisplatin–Taxol combination were presented at the 1993 meeting of the American Society of Clinical Oncology. An ongoing GOG study is trying to define the role of Taxol, as well as the role of platinum dose intensity, in optimally debulked ovarian cancer patients.

Future directions for Taxol in advanced ovarian cancer include intraperitoneal administration for small volume disease or consolidation of pathological complete responses, Taxol as a radiosensitizer and Taxol in combination with other active drugs in the treatment of ovarian cancer.

The rationale for the search for semisynthetic rather than natural taxoids includes the following:

1. Taxol, due to its poor solubility in water, is prepared and administered in a vehicle containing Cremophor EL, a polyoxyethylated castor oil, and ethanol in a 50:50 ratio. This vehicle is toxic and can induce lethal hypotension in dogs [9,10];
2. Although neutropenia is the main toxic effect of Taxol, other side effects complicate its clinical use. These include cardiac and neurological toxicity [4,11–14] and hypersensitivity reactions, even after preventive treatment with steroids, antihistamines and H2 blockers;
3. Resistance to Taxol can develop and at least two mechanisms have been identified: (over)expression of multidrug resistant genes and overproduction of tubulin [15,16].

22.2 TAXOTERE

Taxotere is the first semisynthetic taxoid compound to have entered clinical trials. Its precursor is 10-deacetyl baccatin III – a compound isolated from the leaves of the

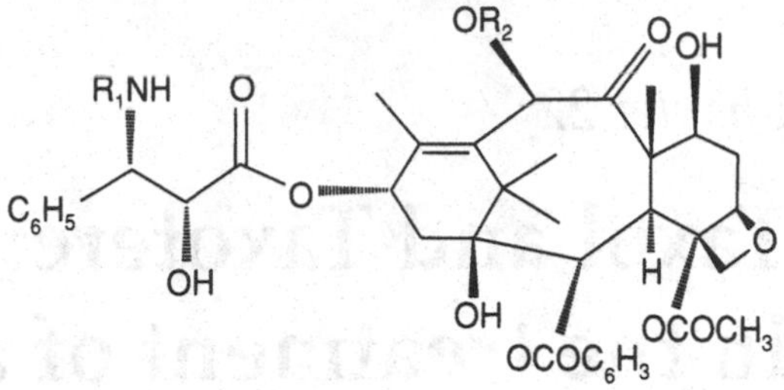

Taxotere: R_1 = COOC(CH$_3$): R_2 = H
Taxol: R_1 = COC$_6$H$_5$; R_2 = COCH$_3$

Figure 22.1 Chemical structure of Taxol and Taxotere.

European yew, *Taxus baccata*. The important side chain in the 13-position of the taxane ring is made by total synthesis (Figure 22.1) [17–19]. There are only two differences between the chemical structures of Taxol and Taxotere: the first is on the side chain, at the level of the 3' amino substituent, the second is on the taxane ring, at position 10, where a hydroxy group replaces an acetyl group. These changes result in a 25% enhanced water solubility of Taxotere in comparison with Taxol.

Studies to define structure/activity relationships have shown that the binding of Taxol and Taxotere to tubulin is quite sensitive to the conformation of the side chain and to the presence of two distinct domains: a hydrophilic area including the oxygenated functions at position 7–9–10 of the taxane ring and a hydrophobic area involving the benzoate group at C2 and the substituent at C3 of the side chain.

Taxotere was first formulated in polysorbate 80 and ethanol (50/50 : u/u). This formulation was used for the initial preclinical safety evaluation and for the treatment of 90% of the patients enrolled in phase I clinical trials. Later on, a second formulation became available, consisting of 100% polysorbate 80. This second formulation has been selected for all ongoing phase II trials.

Taxotere retains the unique mechanism of action of Taxol at the microtubule level. Microtubules are essential components of eukaryotic cells: they are responsible for cellular mobility and chromosome movements during mitosis and they play a role in hormone secretion and granule transportation as well as regulation of cell shape. Microtubules are assembled from tubulin, a protein which comprises two 50 kd subunits, α and β. Microtubule assembly or disassembly is under complex biochemical regulation and can be altered by several drugs.

Unlike other plant derived antimicrotubule agents such as colchicine, podophyllotoxin and the vinca alkaloids, which inhibit microtubule assembly, Taxol promotes the assembly of tubulin and stabilizes the microtubules so formed against depolymerization by calcium ions and low temperature [2,20]. Taxotere behaves similarly but appears approximately 2.5 times more potent than Taxol using a tubulin depolymerization *in vitro* assay [2, 20–22]. Taxotere does not alter the number of protofilaments in normal microtubules, which is 13, while Taxol induces the formation of 12 protofilaments in microtubules [23]. In addition, Taxotere seems to alter certain classes of microtubules – especially tau-dependent microtubules – in a different way when compared to Taxol [24].

The antiproliferative properties of Taxotere have been evaluated against murine and human tumor cell lines grown in liquid medium, using a continuous drug exposure for four days. As shown in Table 22.2, IC50 values of Taxotere range from 4 to 35 ng/ml and the drug is more potent (1.9–9 fold) than the first generation compound, Taxol [25].

The cytotoxicity of Taxotere has also been studied by cloning experiments in soft agar of freshly obtained human tumor specimens and has been observed in ovarian, breast, lung, renal and colorectal cancer and melanoma [26–29]. On a concentration basis Taxotere was often found to be more cytotoxic than Taxol. Of special interest was the observation of incomplete cross resistance between the two drugs [26,28,29], as well as a higher frequency of antitumor efficacy of Taxotere on doxorubicin resistant biopsies.

Taxotere has a good spectrum of efficacy *in vivo* against a panel of murine transplantable tumors. Ten of the 12 models used responded to intravenous Taxotere [30]. More specifically, Taxotere cures early stage colon C38 and pancreatic P03 adenocarcinomas. The

Table 22.2 Cytotoxicity of Taxotere and Taxol against murine and human cancer cell lines

Cell line	IC50 ng/ml Taxotere	Taxol	IC50 Taxol/ IC50 Taxotere
P388 murine leukemia	35	180	5
P388/DOX (resistant to doxorubicin)	750	–	–
SV ras murine fibrosarcoma	35	300	9
Calc18 human breast adenocarcinoma	5	30	6
Calc18/AMSA (resistant to amsacrine)	5.5	–	–
HCT 116 human colon adenocarcinoma	7	9	1
T24 human bladder carcinoma	4	8	2
KE human epidermoid carcinoma	8	75	9
KE[1] human epidermoid carcinoma	300	20000	67
N417[1] human small cell lung carcinoma	150	2000	13

drug is also able to induce complete remissions of these two tumors at an advanced stage.

A 2.7 higher log cell kill in B16 melanoma is observed with Taxotere as compared to Taxol and this striking antitumor activity has been confirmed with the new Taxotere formulation. Therapeutic responses of human tumor xenografts to Taxotere have also been observed, with long term tumor-free survivors reported for the MX-1 mammary carcinoma and the OVCAR-3 carcinoma [31]. Of note, both Taxol and Taxotere display higher antitumor activity than cisplatin against human ovarian carcinoma xenografts [32].

Taxotere is considered as a schedule independent drug: antitumor activity correlates with the total dosage administered and dose fractionation does not appreciably change the efficacy.

Taxotere has shown moderate to marked synergism with vincristine [33], etoposide, cyclophosphamide and 5-fluorouracil (data not yet published) which is different from what is known for Taxol [34].

In vitro, Taxotere is inactive against the P388 cell line resistant to doxorubicin (P388/Dox), a cell line expressing the multidrug resistance (MDR) phenotype [35]. However, sublines expressing the MDR phenotype are sometimes sensitive to Taxotere [36]. On the other hand, no cross resistance is observed in the human breast carcinoma cell line Calc 18, resistant to Amsacrine (Calc 18/AM), a cell line with no detectable expression of MDR but bearing modifications on topoisomerase II [36]. *In vivo*, Taxotere is inactive on several resistant tumors including P388/Dox, P388/VCR, L1210/cisDDP and L1210/BCNU [30].

Additional studies are needed to clarify the mechanisms conferring resistance of cancer cells to Taxotere as well as to verify in clinical models the partial non-crossresistance between Taxol and Taxotere.

Preclinical toxicology studies of Taxotere, formulated in polysorbate 80 and ethanol, have been carried out in dogs and mice using NCI protocols [37]. No change in the acute drug toxicity profile in mice has been observed with the new formulation. Toxic effects of Taxotere are most evident in tissues with a high cell turnover or in those where microtubules play an important functional role: they consist mainly in myelosuppression and lymphoid organ depletion associated with peripheral leucopenia in both species, hair loss in both species, severe intestinal toxicity in dogs and peripheral neurotoxicity in mice. These toxicities are dose dependent and appear to be cumulative over a five day treatment.

In a specific cardiovascular study performed in dogs, the hypotensive effect of polysorbate 80 was well documented and shown to be prevented or reversed by antihistamines.

The starting dose for phase I clinical trials was 5 mg m^{-2} or one third of the toxic dose low determined in dogs, which was the most sensitive species.

Phase I clinical trials of Taxotere have been conducted in Europe and the United States (Table 22.3): different schedules of intravenous administration have been used, including a day 1 + 8 schedule never tested for Taxol.

238 patients have been treated with Taxotere (including 25 with the new formulation) at doses ranging from 5 to 115 mg m^{-2} per course. Throughout the five dosing schedules, the major dose limiting toxicity is neutropenia, which is dose dependent and generally of brief duration (< 1 week) with complete recovery usually by day 21. Available data show it to be schedule independent and not cumulative in contrast to what is observed with Taxol. When it occurs, grade 4 neutropenia (<500 mm^{-3}) results in very low morbidity, except when oral mucositis complicates more prolonged (6–24

Table 22.3 Phase I studies of Taxotere

Institution (ref)	Schedule	Dose levels mg m^{-2} (#)	# Pts	MTD mg m^{-2}	Dose limiting toxicity	Other significant toxicities
St. Louis/CLB [38]	1 to 2-h q2 to 3w	5–115 (10)	56 + 9*	115	Neutropenia	Skin
J. Bordet [39]	1-h d1 + 8 q3w	20–110 (6)	33 + 6*	110	Neutropenia	Asthenia
UTHSC [40]	6-h q3w	5–100 (7)	40	100	Febrile neutropenia	Stomatitis
	2-h q3w	100–115 (2)	15	115	Neutropenia	Skin
Univ. of Glasgow [41]	24-h q3w	10–90 (6)	30	90	Neutropenia	Stomatitis
M.D. Anderson [42]	1-h x 5d q3w	5–80 (6)	39	80	Febrile neutropenia	Stomatitis
Geneva, Switzerland	1-h q3w	70–100 (2)	10*	32	Neutropenia	Skin

Total = 238 patients/720 courses

* Second formulation without ethanol

hours) or repeated (d1–5) infusion schedules. Thrombocytopenia is rare.

Nausea, vomiting and diarrhea, usually of mild to moderate intensity (grade 1–2), were encountered in less than 30% of patients. The overall incidence of hypersensitivity reactions in phase I trials was 18% with 4% being qualified as 'severe' and consisting of any of the following: bronchospasm, hypotension (<80 mmHg systolic blood pressure), generalized urticaria, angioedema. These reactions resolve with discontinuation of the infusion and treatment with steroids and antihistamines. Restarting the infusion after the symptoms have resolved is seldom accompanied by a further hypersensitivity reaction. As with Taxol, these reactions can develop within minutes of starting the Taxotere infusion and are seen mostly during the first or second drug administration. None of the phase I investigators has recommended routine prophylaxis for phase II studies.

Miscellaneous toxicities reported in the phase I trials are alopecia (49%), reversible paresthesias (17%) mainly in patients pretreated with cisplatin and/or vinca alkaloids, phlebitis (9%), conjunctivitis (7%), headache (6%) and liver function test alterations not clearly related to Taxotere (6%).

Of interest is the lack of any sign of cardiac toxicity, further supported by routine Holter monitoring in some phase I patients who show neither significant bradycardia nor significant arrhythmias during Taxotere infusion [39]. On the other hand, the short infusion schedules of Taxotere have been associated with the development of skin toxicity not reported for Taxol [38,39]. This toxicity is mainly observed within one week of doses ≥65 mg m^{-2} and can consist of localized erythema, mainly palmoplantar, with mild or severe desquamation (epidermolysis), maculopapular eruption and nail changes (discoloration with or without erosion). These skin 'toxic' effects are reversible. They have been reported in 18/32 patients receiving ≥85 mg m^{-2} in the 1–2 hour schedule (with three severe cases) and in 10/25 patients receiving ≥65 mg m^{-2} in the 1 hour d1 + 8 schedule (two severe cases). The underlying mechanisms are still unknown; skin biopsies suggest toxic dermatitis.

Finally, another peculiar and unexpected side effect of Taxotere, noted by the investigators of the day 1+8 schedule, has been the appearance of peripheral edema in 9/32 patients after a median number of six Taxotere infusions (i.e. three day 1+8 courses) with a completely reversible weight gain in six of them, ranging from 2% to 15% of body weight [39]. An associated phenomenon was the appearance of or increase in pre-existing pleural changes (thickening or effusion). A few of these patients were actually responding to the drug and investigations seemed to rule out etiologic factors such as significant hypoalbuminemia, proteinuria, congestive heart failure or thyroid dysfunction.

Throughout all phase I studies [36–39,43] response to treatment of ovarian carcinoma has been defined as a significant (>50%) and sustained decline in CA-125 levels; two clinical partial responses have been observed [17].

The recommended dose for all European and US phase II studies is 100 mg m^{-2} given as a short IV infusion repeated every three weeks. The choice of this schedule for phase II is based on giving the highest possible dose intensity with an acceptable profile of side effects. With a short infusion peak plasma levels were higher and in the range of those observed in successfully treated tumor bearing mice. The intermittent q 3 weeks short IV infusion administration schedule was also chosen because of the relatively low incidence of stomatitis, the ease of outpatient treatment and the prospect of combination with other drugs.

A broad phase II program has been initiated to define antitumor activity in several tumor types and to confirm the safety profile of RP 56976. Currently more than 500 patients have been enrolled in phase II studies in Europe and the US. With the exception of one ongoing breast cancer trial using the day 1+8 schedule, all studies use the one hour schedule every three weeks at the initial dose of 100 mg m^{-2}. The toxicity profile of the drug, as obtained from the phase I trials, has essentially been confirmed. Neutropenia is the main toxic effect: grade 4 neutropenia was seen in 68% of the patients (n = 208 evaluable patients) with 18% being accompanied by fever requiring antibiotics. Three deaths due to toxicity have so far been reported in more than 500 patients.

Hair loss is almost universal, while digestive toxicity and neurotoxicity are rarely a problem. Skin toxicity is confirmed. Peripheral edema generally accompanied by weight gain is also seen mostly in patients who are responding and have had four or more courses of treatment. Toxicity may be disabling and can lead to premature discontinuation of treatment. Preventive measures need to be found. Initial phase II studies have not used routine prophylaxis with antihistamine and corticosteroids.

Although the overall incidence of hypersensitivity reactions has very slightly increased in comparison with the phase I experience (24% in comparison with 18%) and 'severe' reactions have remained in the same range (4%), there is a consensus on both sides of the Atlantic that giving the drug without premedication is 'stressful' to medical and nursing staff and requires a very close patient monitoring which may be difficult to organize. Future phase II trials will therefore incorporate some form of premedication and the 'optimal' regimen needs to be defined.

The Early Clinical Trials Group of the EORTC is conducting a large, multicentric phase II trial of Taxotere in platinum pretreated ovarian cancer patients. Three groups of patients have been prospectively defined:

group I includes patients deteriorating within four months of a platinum containing regimen (cisplatin ≥ 75 mg m^{-2} and/or carboplatin ≥ 300 mg m^{-2}), group II consists of patients having a 'platinum-free interval' of between four and 12 months and group III includes patients with a platinum-free interval of >12 months. The minimum response rates for these three groups were defined as 20%, 30% and 40%, respectively.

Preliminary data of an interim analysis [44] show an encouraging response rate in groups I and II of 25% in 75 evaluable patients (95% confidence limits: 15–36%).

In conclusion, the taxoid family shows promise for the treatment of advanced ovarian cancer. Taxotere is superior to Taxol in terms of supply and cardiac toxicity. On the other hand Taxotere frequently induces troublesome skin toxicity and peripheral edema. Data are too preliminary to make any valuable comparison for hypersensitivity, neurotoxicity or antitumor activity.

In an event, Taxol and Taxotere should not be viewed as competitive drugs: they represent significant discoveries in the field of naturally occurring anticancer agents.

REFERENCES

1. Wani, M.C., Taylor, H.L., Wall, M.E. *et al.* (1971) Plant antitumor agents. VI. The isolation and structure of Taxol, a novel antileukemic and antitumor agent from *Taxus brevifolia. J. Am. Chem. Soc.*, **93**, 2325–7.

2. Schiff, P.B., Fant, J. and Horwitz, S.B. (1979) Promotion of microtubule assembly *in vitro* by Taxol. *Nature*, **22**, 665–7.

3. Schiff, P.B. and Horwitz, S.B. (1980) Taxol stabilizes microtubules in mouse fibroblast cells. *Proc. Natl. Acad. Sci. USA*, **77**, 1561–5.

4. Rowinsky, E.K., Cazenave, L.A. and Donehower, R.C. (1990) Taxol: a novel investigational antimicrotubule agent. *J. Natl. Cancer Inst.*, 1247–59.

5. McGuire, W.P., Rowinsky, E.K., Rosenhein, N.B. *et al.* (1989) Taxol: a unique antineoplastic agent with significant activity in advanced ovarian epithelial neoplasms. *Ann. Intern. Med.*, **111**, 273–9.

6. Einzig, A.I., Wiernik, P., Sasloff, J. *et al.* (1990) Phase II study of Taxol in patients with advanced ovarian cancer. *Proc. Am. Soc. Clin. Oncol.*, **31**, 1114.

7. Thigpen, T., Blessing, J., Ball, H. *et al.* (1990) Phase II trial of Taxol as second-line therapy for ovarian carcinoma: a gynecologic oncology group study. *Proc. Am. Soc. Clin. Oncol.*, **9**, 604.

8. Sarosy, G., Kohn, E., Link, C. *et al.* (1992) Taxol dose intensification in patients with recurrent ovarian cancer. *Proc. Am. Soc. Cancer. Res.*, **11**, 226.

9. Lorenz, W., Reichmann, H.J., Schmal, A. *et al.* (1977) Histamine release in dogs by Cremophor EL and its derivatives: oxethylated oleic acid is the most effective constituent. *Agents and Actions*, **7**, 63–7.

10. *Taxol Investigator's Brochure* (1991) National Cancer Institute, Bethesda, MD.

11. Chabner, B.A. (1991) Taxol. *Principles Practice Oncol. Updates*, **5**, 1–9.

12. Weiss, R.B., Donehower, R.C., Wiernik, P.H. *et al.* (1990) Hypersensitivity reactions from Taxol. *J. Clin. Oncol.*, **8**, 1263–8.

13. New, P., Barohn, R., Gales, T. *et al.* (1991) Taxol neuropathy after long term administration. *Proc. Am. Assoc. Cancer Res.*, **32**, 1226.

14. Rowinsky, E.K., McGuire, W.P., Guarnieri, T. *et al.* (1991) Cardiac disturbances during the administration of Taxol. *J. Clin. Oncol.*, **9**, 1704–12.

15. Horwitz, S.B. (1992) *Mechanisms of Taxol Resistance.* Proceedings of the Second National Cancer Institute Workshop on Taxol and Taxus, September 23–24, Alexandria, VA.

16. Kirschner, L.S., Greenberger, L.M., Hsu, S.I.H. *et al.* (1992) Biochemical and genetic characterization of the multidrug resistance (MDR) phenotype in murine macrophage-like J774.2 cells. *Biochem. Pharmacol.*, **43**, 77.

17. Denis, J.N., Greene, A.E., Guénard, D. *et al.* (1988) A highly efficient, practical approach to natural Taxol. *J. Am. Chem. Soc.*, **110**, 5917–19.

18. Mangatal, L., Adeline, M.I., Guénard, D. *et al.* (1989) Application of the vicinal oxyamination

reaction with asymmetric induction to the hemisynthesis of Taxol and analogues. *Tetrahedron*, **45**, 4177–90.

19. Denis, J.N., Correa, A. and Greene, A.E. (1990) An improved synthesis of the Taxol side chain and of RP 56976. *J. Organ. Chem.*, **55**, 1957–9.

20. Kumar, N. (1981) Taxol-induced polymerization of purified tubulin. Mechanism of action. *J. Biol. Chem.*, **256**, 10435–41.

21. Ringel, I. and Horwitz, S.B. (1991) Studies with RP 56976 (Taxotere): a semi-synthetic analog of Taxol. *J. Natl. Cancer Inst.*, **83**, 288–91.

22. Guéritte-Voegelein, F., Guénard, D., Lavelle, F. *et al.* (1991) Relationships between the structure of Taxol analogues and their antimitotic activity. *J. Med. Chem.*, **34**, 992–8.

23. Peyrot, V., Briand, C., Diaz, J.F. and Andreu, J.M. (1992) Biophysical characterization of the assembly of purified tubulin induced by Taxol and Taxotere (RP56976). *Proceedings of the Second Interface Clinical and Laboratory Responses to Anticancer drugs: Drugs and Microtubules*, 24 April, Marseille.

24. Fromes, Y., Goumon, P., Bissery, M.C. and Fellous, A. (1992) Differential effects of Taxol and Taxotere (RP 56976, NSC 628503) on tau and MAP2 containing microtubules. *Proc. Am. Assoc. Cancer Res.*, **33**, 3055.

25. Riou, J.F., Naudin, A., Lavelle, F. (1992) Effects of Taxotere on murine and human cell lines. *Biochem. Biophys. Res. Comm.*, **187**, 164–70.

26. Hanauske, A.R., Degen, D., Hilsenbeck, S.G. *et al.* (1992) Effects of Taxotere and Taxol on *in vitro* colony formation of freshly explanted human tumor cells. *Anticancer Drugs*, **3**, 121–4.

27. Alberts, D.S., Garcia, D., Fanta, P. *et al.* (1992) Comparative cytotoxicities of Taxol and Taxotere *in vitro* against fresh human ovarian cancers. *Proc. Am. Soc. Clin. Oncol.*, **11**, 719.

28. Aapro, M., Braakhuis, B., Dietel, M. *et al.* (1992) Superior activity of Taxotere (Ter) over Taxol (Tol) *in vitro*. *Proc. Am. Soc. Clin. Oncol.*, **33**, 3086.

29. Vogel, M.M., Danhauser-Riedl, S., Block, T. *et al.* (1992) Preclinical activity of Taxotere (RP 56976) and Taxol against human tumor colony forming units. *Proc. Am. Soc. Clin. Oncol.*, **33**, 3115.

30. Bissery, M.C., Guénard, D., Guéritte-Voegelein, F. and Lavelle, F. (1991) Experimental activity of Taxotere (RP 56976, NSC 628 503), a Taxol analogue. *Cancer Res.*, **51**, 4845–52.

31. Harrison, S.D., Dykes, D.J., Shepherd, R.V., *et al.* (1992) Response of human tumor xenographs to Taxotere. *Proc. Am. Soc. Clin. Oncol.*, **33**, 3144.

32. Nicoletti, M.I., Massazza, G., Abbott, B.J. *et al.* (1992) Taxol and Taxotere antitumor activity on human ovarian carcinoma xenografts. *Proc. Am. Soc. Clin. Oncol.*, **33**, 3101.

33. Bissery, M.C., Vrignaud, P., Bayssas, M. and Lavelle, F. (1992) *In vivo* evaluation of Taxotere (RP 56976, NSC 628 503) in combination with cisplatinum, doxorubicin, or vincristine. *Proc. Am. Assoc. Cancer Res.*, **33**, 443.

34. Rose, W.C. (1992) Taxol-based combination chemotherapy and other *in vivo* preclinical antitumor studies. *Second National Cancer Institute Workshop on Taxol and Taxus*, 23–24 September, Alexandria.

35. Johnson, R.K., Chitnis, M.P., Embrey, W.M. and Gregory, E.B. (1978) *In vivo* characteristics of resistance and cross-resistance of an adriamycin-resistant subline of P388. *Cancer Treat. Rep.*, **62**, 1535–47.

36. Hill, B.T., Whelan, R.D.H., Shellard, S.A., *et al.* (1992) Differential cytotoxic effects of Taxotere in a range of mammalian tumor cell lines *in vitro*. *7th NCI-EORTC Symposium on New Drugs in Cancer Therapy*, 17–20 March, Amsterdam.

37. Lowe, M.C. and Davis, R.D. (1987) The current toxicology protocol of the National Cancer Institute. In *Principles of Cancer Chemotherapy*, (eds. S.K. Carter and K. Hellman) McGraw Hill, New York, pp. 228–35.

38. Extra, J.M., Rousseau, F., Bruno, R. *et al.* (1993) Phase I and pharmacokinetic study of Taxotere (RP 56976; NSC 628503) given as a short I.V. infusion, every 21 days. *Cancer Res.*, **53**, 1037–42.

39. Tomiak, E., Piccart, M.J., Kerger, J. *et al.* (1991) A phase I study of Taxotere (RP 56976, NSC 628503) administered as a one hour intravenous (iv) infusion on a weekly basis. *Eur. J. Cancer*, **27** (Suppl. 2), 1184.

40. Burris, H., Irvin, R., Kuhn, J. *et al.* (1992) A phase I clinical trial of Taxotere as a 6 hour infusion repeated every 21 days in patients with refractory solid tumors. *Proc. Am. Soc. Oncol.*, **11**, 369.

41. Bissett, D., Cassidy, J., Setanolans, A. *et al.* (1992) Phase I study of Taxotere (RP 56976) administered as a 24 hour infusion. *Proc. Am. Assoc. Cancer Res.*, **33**, 3145.

42. Pazdur, R., Newman, R.A., Newman, B.M. *et al.* (1992) Phase I trial of Taxotere: five-day schedule. *Cancer Inst.*, **84**, 1781–8.

43. Lefevre, D., Riou, J.F., Zhou, D. *et al.* (1991) Study of molecular markers of resistance to m-AMSA in a human breast cancer cell line: decrease of topoisomerase II and increase of both topoisomerase I and acidic glutathione S transferase. *Biochem. Pharmacol.*, **41**, 1967–79.

44. Piccart, M.J., Gore, M., Ten Bokkel Huinink, W. *et al.* (1993) Taxotere (RP56976, NSC628503): an active new drug for the treatment of advanced ovarian cancer (OVCA). *Proc. Am. Soc. Clin. Oncol.*, **12**, 258.

Chapter 23

The European–Canadian study of paclitaxel in ovarian cancer. High *vs* low dose; long *vs* short infusion

K.D. SWENERTON and E.A. EISENHAUER

23.1 INTRODUCTION

Paclitaxel (Taxol) has demonstrated activity in platinum pretreated ovarian cancer [1–3]. Because of severe hypersensitivity reactions seen early in the evaluation of the drug, treatment protocols were developed which gave paclitaxel over 24 hours together with anti-allergic premedication. This maneuver resulted in a decrease in the frequency of severe reactions, although many patients continued to experience mild symptoms [4]. Shorter outpatient infusions with premedication had not been evaluated and the question of their safety remained unknown.

A second question which arose out of the early development of the drug was whether it exhibited a dose–response effect. It had been recognized that granulocytopenia was the major dose limiting effect of paclitaxel and phase II studies (done without growth factors) suggested this agent produced clinical responses when given in doses ranging from 135–250 mg m^{-2}. Thus, before proceeding to dose–response studies in which expensive growth factors were used, it seemed reasonable to first ask the question comparing doses of the drug which could be administered without the need for growth factors.

These two questions, the safety of short infusions with premedication and paclitaxel dose–response, led to the design of a randomized trial coordinated by the NCI Canada Clinical Trials Group which was carried out in 34 European and Canadian institutions and sponsored by Bristol-Myers Squibb.

23.2 STUDY DESIGN

23.2.1 ELIGIBILITY

Patients were required to have invasive epithelial ovarian cancer and to have undergone one or two prior courses of therapy; each regimen had to include a platinum analogue (cisplatin or carboplatin). Patients were further required to have measurable disease, an ECOG performance status of ≤2 and adequate hematologic, renal and hepatic function. The interval since prior therapy had to be more than four weeks.

23.2.2 TRIAL DESIGN

Patients were randomized in a bifactorial design to a higher *vs* a lower dose (175 or 135 mg m^{-2}) and also randomized between two infusion schedules (24 hours *vs* three hours). Patients were further stratified according to the participating centre and the preceding intertreatment interval (greater or less than 90 days).

The original planned sample size of 300 patients would permit the detection of a difference of 15% in response rates between doses or schedules with a power of 80% and a two-sided alpha of 0.05. The sample size would also permit detection of a >10% increase in the rate of serious hypersensitivity reactions in the short infusion arm (assuming a rate of 8% in the long infusion arm) with a one-sided alpha of 0.05 and a power of 80%. Early stopping rules were established to permit termination of accrual to the three hour infusion arm should a specified number of serious hypersensitivity reactions have been seen after 30, 60, 90 or 120 patients had been entered.

23.2.3 TRIAL THERAPY

All patients were premedicated with dexamethasone 20 mg po given both 12 and six hours prior to paclitaxel and diphenhydramine 50 mg, plus ranitidine 50 mg both IV 30 minutes prior to paclitaxel. Alternative compounds from the same classes could be used.

Treatment cycles were repeated every three weeks and assessment for response according to WHO criteria [5] repeated every two cycles. Those achieving an objective response continued to receive the drug until progression or until four cycles beyond maximum response; those with disease stability continued to a maximum of 10 cycles; those with disease progression were removed from study therapy. Weekly hemograms were obtained in all patients and assessment for other toxic effects was carried out prior to each cycle.

23.3 RESULTS

23.3.1 PATIENTS

Between July 1991 and March 1992, a total of 407 patients was randomized (Table 23.1). 3.4% of patients were ineligible, leaving 393

Table 23.1 Accrual

# Patients:		
	Randomized	407
	Eligible	393
	Evaluable for toxicity	393
	Evaluable for responses	384

Table 23.2 Patient characteristics (%)

	Dose (mg m^{-2})		Infusion (h)	
	175 (n = 194)	135 (n = 199)	24 (n = 206)	3 (n = 187)
Performance status				
ECOG 0,1	86	80	83	83
2	14	19	17	17
Prior regimens				
one	56	54	51	58
two	44	46	49	42
Serous histology	55	58	60	53
Maximum diameter				
>5 cm	68	70	68	70
Progression on last chemo	27	29	23	34
Intertreatment interval				
<6 months	61	57	58	59

(96.6%) of patients evaluable for toxicity. 384 (94.3%) of patients were evaluable for response and at the time of this analysis a total of 2331 cycles of treatment had been given and median follow-up is 16 months.

The characteristics of the patients and disease are shown in Table 23.2; the arms appear to be well balanced with regard to these factors.

23.3.2 TOXICITY

Minor hypersensitivity reactions (usually dermal flushing) were common, but severe reactions (one or more of: angioedema, respiratory distress requiring treatment, hypotension or generalized urticaria) occurred in only 1.5% of patients (Table 23.3). There appeared to be no difference between the treatment arms with respect to the frequency or severity of these reactions. In the vast majority of patients, symptoms required no intervention and infusions were completed without interruption.

Non-hematologic toxicity is shown in Table 23.4. A syndrome of arthralgia/ myalgia was commonly seen with an onset two to three days after treatment and resolu-

Table 23.3 Hypersensitivity reactions (% patients)

	Dose (mg m^{-2})		Infusion (h)	
	175 (n = 194)	135 (n = 199)	24 (n = 206)	3 (n = 187)
Minor reaction	43	40	44	39
Severe reaction	1.5	1.5	1.0	2.1

Table 23.4 Non-hematological toxicity (% patients)

	Dose (mg m^{-2})		Infusion (h)	
	175 (n = 194)	135 (n = 199)	24 (n = 206)	3 (n = 187)
Artharalgia/myalgia				
any	66	54	57	63
≥ grade 3	7	4	5	5
*Neurosensory				
any	51	36	40	48
≥ grade 3	1	–	0.5	0.5
Stomatitis				
any	27	26	31	21
≥ grade 3	1.5	0.5	1.9	–
Hair loss	89	86	87	89
Nausea/vomiting				
≥ grade 3	7	9	7	9
Cardiovascular				
≥ grade 3 dysrhythmia	<1	<1	<1	<1

*Pts normal at baseline

Table 23.5 Hematological toxicity (% patient)

	Dose (mg m^{-2})		Infusion (h)	
	175 (n = 194)	135 (n = 199)	24 (n = 206)	3 (n = 187)
Granulocytes grade 4	51	42	72	19
Febrile neutropenia	7	6	12	0
Platelets grade 4	4	1	3	1

tion within several more days. These symptoms, although rarely severe, were troublesome. Their frequently and severity appear to be more a function of dose than infusion time.

A sensory neuropathy, described as a burning paresthesia by most, was common but rarely severe. The frequency of this seemed affected by dose but not by infusion duration.

Mild stomatitis was seen in less than one third of the patients and was slightly more frequent in those receiving the longer infusion. Hair loss was common and its frequency unaffected by study parameters. Similarly, nausea and vomiting, rarely severe, appeared unaffected by dose or schedule.

Importantly, significant cardiovascular toxicity was rare – in only three cases was the infusion interrupted and/or additional intravenous fluids administered because of bradycardia or hypotension. Patients were asymptomatic in all instances.

Hematologic toxicity (Table 23.5) was as expected, with marked neutropenia being frequent. What was not expected was that infusion time, rather than dose, was the most important determinant of the severity of neutropenia. Severe neutropenia was four times more common in the patients receiving the 24 hour infusion and febrile neutropenia was seen only in this group. Thrombocytopenia was rarely severe.

23.3.3 EFFICACY

Efficacy was assessed using clinical response rates, time to progression and survival. At the time of this report, the data are too immature to allow for survival comparisons. WHO criteria for response have been utilized and an external review of clinical response has been completed in all Canadian patients.

The overall clinical response rate is 19% (74/384). A multivariate analysis found that favourable prognostic factors for response include a smaller tumor diameter, a longer intertreatment interval, serous histology and fewer disease sites. The response rate in platinum resistant patients (those progressing on their most recent platinum regimen) is 12% (13/109) and 22% (61/275) in the remainder.

23.4 CONCLUSION

In summary, patients receiving the higher dose (175 mg m^{-2}) experienced more neurosensory toxicity and arthromyalgia. Those randomized to the three hour infusion demonstrated significantly less hematologic toxicity (particularly neutropenia and infection) without an increase in hypersensitivity reactions. The best toxicity index appears to be achieved with the shorter infusion. That paclitaxel can be given safely in an outpatient setting will reduce the costs and inconvenience of treatment.

While the overall response rate is modest, a proportion of those with truly platinum resistant tumors will respond, indicating a potentially important degree of therapeutic non-cross resistance.

ACKNOWLEDGEMENT

We are grateful to those many individuals involved in this study. Our particular thanks to Kaniza Ishmail for her assistance.

REFERENCES

1. Thigpen, T., Blessing, J., Ball, H. *et al.* (1990) Phase II trial of taxol as second-line therapy for ovarian cancer: A Gynecologic Oncology Group Study. *Proc. Am. Soc. Clin. Oncol.*, **9**, 156.

2. McGuire, W.P., Rowinsky, E.K., Rosenhein, N.B. *et al.* (1989) Taxol, a unique antineoplastic agent with significant activity in advanced ovarian epithelial neoplasms. *Ann. Intern. Med.*, **111**, 273.

3. Einzig, A.L., Wiernik, P.H., Sasloff, J. *et al.* (1992) Phase II study and long term follow-up of patients treated with taxol for advanced ovarian cancer. *J. Clin. Oncol.*, **10**, 1748–53.

4. Weiss, R.B., Donehower, R.C., Wiernik, P.H. *et al.* (1990) Hypersensitivity reactions from taxol. *J. Clin. Oncol.*, **8**, 1263.

5. Miller, A.B., Hoogstraten, B., Staquet, M. *et al.* (1981) Reporting results of cancer treatment. *Cancer*, **47**, 207–14.

Chapter 24

Intraperitoneal recombinant interferon-gamma in ovarian cancer patients with residual disease at second look laparotomy

E. PUJADE-LAURAINE, J.P. GUASTALLA, N. COLOMBO, E. FRANCOIS,
P. FUMOLEAU, A. MONNIER, M.A. NOOY, L. MIGNOT, R. BUGAT,
C.M.D. OLIVEIRA, M. MOUSSEAU, G. NETTER, F. MALOISEL,
S. LARBAOUI, P. DEVILLIER and M. BRANDELY

24.1 INTRODUCTION

Despite the improved overall response rate of debulking surgery and combination chemotherapy in advanced epithelial ovarian cancer, 60–70% of the patients have persistent disease at second look laparotomy [1,2].

Since ovarian cancer, even in its advanced stages, tends to remain confined to the abdominal cavity, 'salvage' intraperitoneal (IP) administration of antitumor agents has been advocated [3–7]. Recombinant cytokines, like interferons (IFNs) and interleukin-2 (IL-2), are attractive for the treatment of refractory residual disease as chemoresistant tumor cell lines have been reported to be sensitive to these agents [8]. Clinical trials have indeed demonstrated that IP administration of IFN-α and IL-2 can achieve complete surgically documented responses in patients with residual advanced ovarian cancer [9,10].

IFN-γ is a natural lymphokine secreted by T lymphocytes in response to specific antigenic or mitogenic stimuli. IFN-γ shares pleiotropic actions with the other IFNs but interacts through a distinct cell surface receptor from the receptor for IFN-α/β. IFN-γ is a cytokine of particular interest in ovarian cancer in view of its antiproliferative and immunomodulatory activities [11]. Direct antiproliferative activity of IFN-γ has been experimentally demonstrated in human ovarian cancer both *in vitro* on tumor cell lines and *in vivo* in a model of ovarian xenograft in nude mice [12–14]. Although the IFN-γ mediated growth inhibitory effect is not fully understood, IFN-γ has been reported to modulate the expression of several oncogenes and in particular to reduce the overexpression of the proto-oncogene c-*erb*B-2, an important indicator for bad prognosis in ovarian cancer [15]. IFN-γ also induces a marked increase of HLA antigen expression in human ovarian malignant cells which may impact on their growth, metastatic capability and sensitivity to the cytotoxic activity of class II specific T lymphocytes [16–19].

In addition to these direct effects on malignant cells, IFN-γ, also called the immune

231

interferon, has a complex modulatory activity on host defense mechanisms. Particularly relevant to its antitumor activity, IFN-γ is a potent activator of macrophage cytotoxicity [20] against tumor cells *in vitro*, including ovarian carcinoma cells [21]. *In vivo*, intraperitoneal rIFN-γ has been reported to activate *in situ* effector cells including macrophages in patients with recurrent ascitic ovarian carcinoma [19] or minimal residual tumor after chemotherapy [22]. A potential antitumor activity of intravenously administered rIFN-γ in patients with ovarian cancer has been suggested by Welander *et al.* [23].

In this chapter, we report the results of a European multicenter phase II trial of human rIFN-γ administered IP in 108 patients with persistent residual ovarian tumor at second look laparotomy after conventional first line chemotherapy.

24.2 MATERIALS AND METHODS

24.2.1 PATIENT ELIGIBILITY

Patients eligible for entry into this trial had a histologically confirmed ovarian epithelial cancer, FIGO stage IIb, IIc or III and persistent microscopic or macroscopic peritoneal residual disease documented at second look laparotomy after first line platinum based chemotherapy.

Additional eligibility criteria included age less than 75 years, performance status of $\geq 60\%$ (Karnofsky scale), estimated life expectancy of at least six months, no concomitant severe cardiovascular disease or second malignancy, white blood cell count > 3000 cells μl^{-1}, platelet count > 100000 cells μl^{-1}, serum creatinine ≤ 110 $\mu mol\, l^{-1}$ and total bilirubin ≤ 25 $\mu mol\, l^{-1}$.

In addition, patients had no prior radiotherapy, no systemic or IP chemotherapy after the second look laparotomy and no multiple abdominal adhesions documented after the second look laparotomy.

24.2.2 TREATMENT

The IP therapy was administered via percutaneous injections or an implanted peritoneal catheter. In the latter case, a peritoneal catheter with a subcutaneous delivery device (Port-a-Cath, Pharmacia, Uppsala, Sweden) or a Tenckoff catheter (Davol Inc., Grandon, RI) was placed during the second look laparotomy. Intraperitoneal rIFN-γ treatment started within four weeks of this surgical procedure after having assessed the distribution of fluid throughout the abdominal cavity. The human rIFN-γ (RU 42369) was provided by Roussel Uclaf (Romainville, France). Specific activity was $\geq 20 \times 10^6$ IU mg^{-1} protein, based on antiviral activity measured by inhibition of infection of human Wish cells by vesicular stomatitis virus using NIH standard as reference. The final purity was >95% as determined by sodium dodecyl sulfate-polyacrylamide gel electrophoresis. Absence of pyrogenicity was assessed by classic tests.

The rIFN-γ was provided as sterile lyophilized powder in glass vials stored at 4°C and reconstituted with sterile water immediately prior to injection. The reconstituted drug diluted in 250 ml 0.9% saline solution was administered after infusion of 1–2 l warm dialysis fluid. No attempt to drain the fluid was made. The duration of rIFN-γ infusion given in an outpatient setting lasted no more than two hours. rIFN-γ was delivered at a dose of 20×10^6 IU m^{-2} twice a week for 3–4 months. At each infusion, acetaminophen was given every four hours for 24 hours. Corticosteroids were contra-indicated.

24.2.3 STUDY DESIGN

Every four weeks, physical examination, including recording of body temperature before and six hours after the rIFN-γ injection, was performed as well as complete blood count, chemistry, urinalysis and serum CA 125 level determination.

Adverse reactions were recorded using the World Health Organization (WHO) toxicity scale. In the event of a grade 3 adverse reaction, the treatment was discontinued until recovery and renewed at 50% of the scheduled dose. If the treatment was delayed by ≥ 3 weeks or in the presence of unacceptable toxicity, the patient was withdrawn from the study.

Tumor response was evaluated 1–4 weeks after completion of the rIFN-γ therapy unless disease progression occurred during treatment. In the absence of clinical evidence of disease, patients underwent a third look laparotomy with multiple biopsies including node sampling and collection of cytology specimens. Laparoscopy was performed only in patients who declined laparotomy.

A complete response (CR) was defined as the disappearance of all macroscopic and microscopic disease with negative IP cytology. Partial response (PR) included the regression of macroscopic disease by at least 50% of the product of the largest diameter and its perpendicular measurement, in the absence of any new lesion; or the presence of positive cytology at completion of therapy only in those patients who had had macroscopic disease. Any response less than PR was considered to be no response. All data were reviewed by a panel of three investigators prior to final analysis.

24.2.4 STATISTICAL ANALYSIS

Prognostic factors for tumor response to rIFN-γ were determined by univariate analysis with Fisher tests completed by a multivariate analysis using a stepwise logistic regression. Progression-free survival and survival were calculated from the date of inclusion using a stepwise Cox model. The tumor response was logged as a time dependent covariate, the other covariates being the variables introduced in the logistic regression. All

analyses were performed on an IBM 9121 computer using the SAS statistical software, version 6.06 (SAS Institute Inc., SAS Circle, Box 8000, Cary, NC, USA).

24.3 RESULTS

24.3.1 PATIENT CHARACTERISTICS

A total of 108 patients were entered in this trial. Patient and tumor characteristics are summarized in Table 24.1. Median age was 56 (range 28–74). Seventy-eight patients (72%) had serous or papillary carcinomas and 87 (81%) had grade 2 or 3 tumors. One hundred and one patients (94%) were FIGO stage III and 90 (87%) FIGO stage IIIc; 67 (62%) had ascites and first surgery was optimal (postsurgical residual tumors <2 cm) in 32 (30%). All patients were treated with first line platinum based chemotherapy with a median of six cycles (range 4–13). At the time of the second look laparotomy, 15 (14%) had microscopic residual disease and 25 (23%), 31 (28%), 37 (35%) respectively <5 mm, 5 mm–2 cm, ≥2 cm residual disease. Performance status (Karnofsky scale) was >80 in 82% patients and between 70–80 in 18%.

24.3.2 RESPONSE

Ninety-eight patients were evaluable for tumor response. Six patients were ineligible: one patient had a borderline tumor, two patients had a FIGO stage IV disease and three patients had no residual disease at the second look laparotomy. Four additional patients were excluded as they were not reassessed for response: one patient died suddenly from pulmonary embolism and three patients stopped their treatment prematurely after one injection in two patients and five injections in one patient.

The response was assessed by laparotomy in 62 patients, laparoscopy in nine patients and clinical investigations (physical examination,

233

Table 24.1 Patient characteristics

No. entered	108
Medium age (yr) (range)	56 (28–74)
FIGO stage	
II B–C	5
III A–B	11
III C	90
IV *	2
Histology	
Serous or papillary	78
Endometrioid	8
Clear cell	2
Mixed	4
Mucinous	4
Undifferentiated	11
Borderline *	1
Grade	
1	11
2	55
3	32
Unknown	10
Ascites	67
Optimal surgery	32
First line chemotherapy	
Regimen	
PAC	19
PC	54
Other P-based regimen	35
No. courses (mean) (range)	6 (4–13)
Response	
PR	50
SD + Pg	51
Unknown	7
Size of residual cancer	
Microscopic	15
< 5 mm	25
< 2 cm (≥ 5 mm)	31
≥ 2 cm	37

Abbreviations:
PAC, cisplatin, adriamycin (doxorubicin) cyclophosphamide; P, cisplatin; C, cyclophosphamide; Pg, progression; SD, stationary disease; PR, partial response
*Ineligible

CA 125 level, peritoneal cytology, CT scan or ultrasound examination) in 27 patients.

Of the 98 evaluable patients treated by IP rIFN-γ, 31 patients (31%, 95% confidence interval, 23%–42%) experienced a response, 23 patients achieved a CR and eight patients a PR. Of the 23 patients with a CR, 20 patients were assessed with a third look laparotomy and three patients with a laparoscopy with respectively 19, 17 and 15 peritoneal biopsies including diaphragmatic. Three additional patients were considered as clinically free of disease at the end of the treatment but were not classified as responders as they refused surgical restaging.

In the univariate analysis, factors predicting tumor response to rIFN-γ were tumor size at second look laparotomy ($p = 0.004$), age ($p = 0.006$), FIGO stage ($p = 0.01$), optimal first surgery ($p = 0.02$) and neutropenia ($p = 0.04$).

The multivariate analysis showed that age and tumor size were the only two independent factors influencing IP rIFN-γ response (Table 24.2). Older patients (≥60 years) had a 16% response rate (95% CI: 6–31%) compared to 42% (95% CI: 29–52%) in younger patients (<60 years). Similarly, patients with tumor size ≥2 cm had an 11% response rate (95% CI: 3–27%) compared to 43% (95% CI: 30–53%) in patients with residual disease < 2 cm.

This analysis identified a subpopulation of patients with a high probability of response to IP rIFN-γ, that is women less than 60 years and with a residual tumor size less than 2 cm. 41 (41%) patients in the series had these criteria. Their global response rate is 54% (95% CI: 37–69%) with 17 (41%) patients achieving a CR.

Conversely, the probability of response to rIFN-γ was found to be independent of previous response to first line chemotherapy (Table 24.3). Neither the inclusion of anthracycline in the combination regimen nor the dose intensity of platinum significantly influenced the efficacy of the subsequent treatment with IP rIFN-γ. In addition, cell type

Table 24.2 Surgically defined responses to IP IFN-γ: influence of tumour size and patient age

	No. of patients	CR	PR	CR + PR (%)	p
Total	98	23	8	31	
Tumour size					
Microscopic	10	6	—	60	
<5 mm	23	8	2	43	
<2 cm (≥ 5 mm)	30	6	5	37	
≥2 cm	35	3	1	11	0.004
Age (years)					
< 50	23	8	4	52	
50–59	37	11	2	35	
≥60	38	4	2	16	0.006
Tumour size < 2 cm and age < 60 years	41	17	5	54	

Abbreviations: CR = complete response; PR = partial response

Table 24.3 Response to IFN-γ *vs* response to first-line chemotherapy, the inclusion of adriamycin in the combination and the dose-intensity of platinum.

First line chemotherapy	No. of patients	Response to IFN-γ n (%)	p
Response			
PR	46	14 (30)	
SD + Pg	45	15 (33)	NS
Adriamycin			
Yes	28	9 (32)	
No	67	22 (33)	NS
Dose intensity of platinum (mg m^{-2} week^{-1})			
< 20	32	14 (44)	
≥ 20 and < 25	29	8 (28)	
> 25	34	9 (26)	NS

Abbreviations: see Table 24.1

and histological grade were not found to be relevant to rIFN-γ activity.

24.3.3 TOXICITY

All 108 patients entered in the trial were analysed for toxicity. The most common clinical adverse event related to rIFN-γ was fever (94%) (Table 24.4). The mean body temperature measured six hours after rIFN-γ delivery was 38.2 ± 0.9°C and fever never exceeded WHO grade 2 (≤40°C) with the prophylactic administration of acetaminophen.

A significant flu-like syndrome was the reason for interruption of treatment in three patients (3%) and for reduction of rIFN-γ dose in six patients (5%). Other clinical side effects related to rIFN-γ included headache (9%), nausea and vomiting (7%), diarrhoea (5%), abdominopelvic pain (13%) and insufficient peritoneal fluid resorption (8%). 6% of patients complained of paraesthesia which may have been related to previous cisplatin treatment.

Most of the serious clinical adverse events observed during the trial were secondary to the intraperitoneal mode of rIFN-γ delivery (Table 24.5). Peritoneal infections were documented in 18 patients: *Staphylococcus aureus* and *Staphylococcus epidermidis* were the most

Table 24.4 Adverse events related to IFN-γ

Clinical	
Fever	98 (94%)
Flu-like syndrome	9 (8%)
Headache	10 (9%)
Abdominopelvic pain	14 (13%)
Nausea/vomiting	8 (7%)
Diarrhoea	6 (5%)
Ascites (non-malignant)	9 (8%)
Paraesthesia	7 (6%)
Biological	
Anaemia	25 (23%)
Neutropenia	44 (41%)
Liver enzymes increase	36 (33%)

Table 24.5 Clinical adverse events related to the technique of IP administration

Injection technical problems	19 (18%)
Peritoneal infections	18 (17%)
Injection site reactions	6 (6%)
Abdominal wall complications	5 (5%)
Pseudocyst	4 (4%)
Ileus	3 (3%)
Bowel perforation	1 (1%)
Hemoperitoneum	1 (1%)

common pathogens (50%) followed by gram-negative bacteria (21%) and *Streptococcus* (15%).

Technical problems were encountered in 19 patients and included catheter leakage or obstruction, dislodgement of the catheter and diffusion of the fluid into the abdominal wall. Injection site reactions (six patients) consisted of local pain, eruption or inflammation, and abdominal wall complications (five patients) included eventration and hematoma. Transitory intestinal ileus was noted in three patients and two additional patients underwent a surgical procedure for a bowel perforation and a hemoperitoneum respectively. Overall, 14 patients (13%) were prematurely withdrawn due to the onset of adverse events related to the IP route of administration.

The occurrence of peritoneal adhesions and fibrosis was carefully assessed in the 71 patients who had a third look laparotomy or laparoscopy. Peritoneal adhesions which were not present at second look were observed in 10 patients (14%), with four patients developing pseudocysts around the tip of the peritoneal catheter. Histological examination of the peritoneal samples, however, showed the appearance of fibrosis in a single patient.

Neutropenia was the most common biological adverse event (Table 24.4). 44 patients (41%) experienced neutropenia which resulted in reduction of rIFN-γ dose in nine. Other biological adverse events included anemia (23%), transaminase increase (33%) and alkaline phosphatase increase (19%).

24.3.4 SURVIVAL

The median follow-up is 24 months. The 102 eligible patients had a median survival of 21 months. The median survival of patients with ≥2 cm, 5 mm–2 cm and <5 mm residual disease is 10, 21 and 27 months respectively and is not yet reached for patients with residual microscopic disease.

The median duration of response to rIFN-γ is 21 months. The median survival of responder patients is not yet reached. The projected two year survival of responder patients is 86% (95% CI: 64–95%).

The following parameters have been included in the multivariate analysis of survival: cell type, histological grade, FIGO stage, ascites, optimal first surgery, response to first line chemotherapy, dose intensity of platinum, inclusion of anthracycline in the combination, size of residual tumor at second look laparotomy, debulking surgery, performance status at inclusion and response to rIFN-γ as a time dependent covariable. Response to IP rIFN-γ was the most significant predictive variable ($p < 0.001$). Other prognostic factors included size of residual tumors at second look laparotomy ($p < 0.001$), debulking surgery ($p = 0.002$), performance status at inclusion ($p = 0.006$) and cell type ($p = 0.009$).

Debulking surgery was defined as a surgery at second laparotomy which achieved a significant decrease of tumor size within the four categories ≥2 cm, 5 mm–2 cm, <5 mm and microscopic. The cell type variable separated serous vs non-serous ovarian carcinoma with a better clinical outcome for serous tumors.

24.4 DISCUSSION

This is the first report demonstrating the efficacy of IP administration of rIFN-γ in patients with residual ovarian carcinoma after first line chemotherapy. Characteristics of the 108 patients included in the trial are mostly those associated with poor prognosis in ovarian carcinoma: 87% had FIGO stage IIIc, 62% ascites, 70% tumors greater than 2 cm after first surgery and 86% had macroscopic residual disease with peritoneal nodules greater than 2 cm in 34% at second look laparotomy. Among the 98 evaluable patients, 23 achieved a surgical CR to IP rIFN-γ and eight additional patients a PR for a global response rate of 31% (95% CI: 23–42%). Responses are long-lasting with a median duration of 21 months.

These favorable results of IP rIFN-γ are, however in disparity with those reported by D'Acquisto *et al.* [24]. These authors treated 27 patients with advanced ovarian cancer in a phase I trial with escalating doses of IP rIFN-γ ranging from 0.05–8.0 × 10⁶ U m⁻² week⁻¹. The maximum tolerated dose of rIFN-γ was not reached and no evidence of response was observed with particular reference to five surgically re-evaluated patients, three of whom had residual disease <5 mm before therapy. The higher rIFN-γ dosage (20 × 10⁶ U m⁻²

twice a week) and the longer duration of therapy in our trial may account for the difference in the results between the two studies. *In vitro* and *in vivo* experimental studies have pointed out the dose dependency of IFN-γ antiproliferative activity [12–14]. In this setting, a clearcut advantage of the IP rIFN-γ administration compared to the systemic route has been demonstrated *in vivo* in mice [25]. The IP administration not only enables a direct contact between rIFN-γ and the malignant target but also exposes the peritoneal cavity to high concentrations of drugs [26] with a ratio of rIFN-γ mean peak levels of peritoneal fluid to serum up to 550:1 [24].

Tumor burden before therapy appears a critical factor for response to IP rIFN-γ. Global and complete response rates to rIFN-γ were respectively 60%, 43%, 37%, 11% and 60%, 35%, 20%, 9% in patients with microscopic, <5 mm, ≥5 mm but <2 cm, ≥2 cm residual tumors (Table 24.2).

Correlation between size of residual tumors after first line chemotherapy and response to

Table 24.6 Complete pathological responses IP chemotherapy and interferon alpha *vs* interferon gamma

Treatment	Tumor size (cm)		
	≤ 0.5	0.5–2	≥ 2
1. Multiagent chemotherapy			
Markman *et al.* [5]	10/25	0/15	2/17
Piver *et al.* [6]	5/17	0/7	0/6
Markman *et al.* [28]	6/19	1/17	0/8
Total chemotherapy	22/61 (34%)	1/39 (2%)	2/31 (6%)
2. IFN-α			
Berek *et al.* [9]	4/7	0/1	0/6
Willemse *et al.* [29]	5/11	0/6	–
Nardi *et al.* [30]*	7/14	–	–
Berek *et al.* [31]*	2/6	0/4	0/7
Total IFN-α	18/38 (47%)	0/11 (0%)	0/13 (0%)
3. IFN-γ	14/33 (42%)	6/30 (20%)	3/35 (9%)

* IFN-α plus cisplatin

'salvage' therapy has been repeatedly reported in previous trials using either IP chemotherapy [3–6] or immunotherapy [9,27]. The great majority of surgical complete responses showed both by polychemotherapy and rIFN-α have been observed in patients with minimal residual disease less than 5 mm (Table 24.6). rIFN-γ compares favourably with these IP therapies. When tumor size ranges from 5 mm to 2 cm, rIFN-γ still achieves a significant 20% complete response rate whereas CR are scarce with either rIFN-α or polychemotherapy.

The activity of the first line therapy and the factors which modulate this activity are important to consider in the analysis of the efficacy of subsequent 'salvage' treatment. The dose intensity of platinum [32] and the inclusion of anthracycline in the platinum based regimen [33] are the two most significant factors which are known to determine the response rate to first line chemotherapy in ovarian cancer. How these two factors influence the activity of IP chemotherapy is not yet known. However, the response rate of this latter IP treatment is closely correlated with previous response to first line chemotherapy [34]. In contrast, IP rIFN-γ activity was found independent of first line chemotherapy response rate. In addition, neither the dose intensity of platinum nor the association of anthracyclines in the combination influence tumor response to rIFN-γ. This equivalent clinical activity in chemoresistant and in chemosensitive ovarian cancer underlines the unique mechanism of antitumor action of rIFN-γ and its potential value as adjuvant treatment to chemotherapy in ovarian cancer.

Age, together with tumor burden, were found to be the most significant predictive factors of rIFN-γ response. Response rates were 52%, 35% and 16% in patients respectively less than 50 years, between 50 and 59 years and more than 60 years old. The ability of younger patients to respond better suggests that the immunocompetence which

decreases with age may be of importance for rIFN-γ activity. With the IP delivery the cytokine comes into direct contact with the peritoneal immunocompetent cells surrounding malignant tumors. IP rIFN-γ has been shown to effectively activate *in situ* effector cells including NK cells and macrophages in patients with ovarian carcinoma [19,22]. However, a correlation between the immunomodulatory and the antitumor activity of rIFN-γ is still lacking [22].

Despite its potential advantages in terms of efficacy, the IP route was associated in this trial with a certain number of adverse events which accounted for premature cessation of treatment in 13% of the cases. The incidence of local complications was closely correlated with the experience of the different centers in the management of IP therapy. However, the risk of peritoneal infection (17% of cases) was underestimated at the initiation of this trial. The greater risk of peritoneal infections compared to other forms of IP therapies [3–6, 9,35] may be related to the greater number of IP injections and should be prevented by the strict application of aseptic and antiseptic technique. On the other hand, rIFN-γ seems devoid of irritant local effects. The occurrence of abdominal pain was much less frequent than that reported with IP chemotherapy [3–6, 28, 35]. In addition only one patient had peritoneal fibrosis. Peritoneal fibrosis is a common side effect of IP cytokines such as IFN-α, IFN-β or IL-2 [9,36,37] which can preclude continuation of therapy. The lack of fibroplastic peritoneal response to repeated high doses of rIFN-γ may be related to its well documented *in vitro* and *in vivo* antifibrotic activity [38–41]. On the whole, clinical and biological toxicities of rIFN-γ were tolerable and included moderate fever and flu-like syndrome, neutropenia and increase in liver enzymes.

Responders to rIFN-γ have an 86% (95% CI: 64–95%) two year survival despite the fact that most patients (86%) had macroscopic residual disease at second look laparotomy which is usually associated with a poor clinical outcome. Controlled prospective trials only will determine if IP rIFN-γ leads to a prolongation of survival in the whole population or, more likely, a subset of ovarian cancer patients. In the multivariate analysis of survival, however, response to rIFN-γ was found to be the most significant predictive criterion of patient survival, even before the size of residual tumor, a well established pre-eminent prognostic factor [42–44]. Unexpectedly, debulking surgery at second laparotomy was significantly associated with a good prognosis. The role of second debulking surgery remains controversial [45]. The capacity of IP rIFN-γ to complete surgical secondary cytoreduction in a fraction of the patients with residual cancer may render this procedure again valuable. This could be the case in patients who are more likely to respond to IP rIFN-γ, that is patients less than 60 years old and with residual lesions less than 2 cm, where complete and global response rates of respectively 41% and 54% are expected.

Finally, there is experimental evidence that rIFN-γ acts synergistically with cytotoxic drugs [46] and with other cytokines such as TNF-α [47] and IL-2 [48,49]. Therefore, there is a rationale for the use of rIFN-γ in combination to optimize antitumor therapies in ovarian cancer.

REFERENCES

1. Piver, M.S. (ed.) (1987) *Ovarian Malignancies: Diagnostic and Therapeutic Advances,* Churchill Livingstone, London, pp. 109–128.
2. Louie, K.G., Ozols, R.F., Myers, C.E. *et al.* (1986) Long term results of a cis-platin containing combination chemotherapy regimen (Chex-up) for the treatment of advanced ovarian carcinoma. *J. Clin. Oncol.,* **4**, 1579–85.
3. Howell, W.B., Pleifle, C.E., Wung, W.E. *et al.* (1983) Intraperitoneal cis-diaminedichloroplatinum with systemic thiosulfate protection. *Cancer Res.,* **43**, 1426–31.
4. Ten Bokkel Huinink, W.W., Dubbelman, R., Franklin, A. *et al.* (1985) Experimental and clinical results with intraperitoneal cisplatin. *Semin. Oncol.,* **12**, 43–6.
5. Markman, M., Cleary, S., Lucas, W. *et al.* (1986) IP chemotherapy employing a regimen of cisplatin, cytarabine and bleomycin. *Cancer Treat. Rep.,* **70**, 755–60.
6. Piver, M.S., Lele, S.B., Marchetti, D.L. *et al.* (1988) Surgically documented response to intraperitoneal cisplatin, cytarabine and bleomycin after intravenous cisplatin-based chemotherapy in advanced ovarian adenocarcinoma. *J. Clin. Oncol.,* **6**, 1679–84.
7. Oldham, R.K. (1984) Biologicals and biological response modifiers: fourth modality of cancer treatment. *Cancer Treat Rep.,* **68**, 221–3.
8. Allavena, P., Grandi, M., D'Incalci, M. *et al.* (1987) Human tumor cell lines with pleiotropic drug resistance are efficiently killed by interleukin 2 activated killer cells and by activated monocytes. *Int. J. Cancer,* **40**, 104–7.
9. Berek, J.S., Hacker, N.F., Lichtenstein, A. *et al.* (1985) Intraperitoneal recombinant alpha-interferon for 'salvage' immunotherapy in stage III epithelial ovarian cancer. *Cancer Res.,* **45**, 4447–53.
10. Lembersby, B., Baldisseri, M., Kunscher, A. *et al.* (1989) Phase I–II study of intraperitoneal (IP) low dose of interleukin-2 (IL-2) in refractory stage III ovarian cancer (OC). *Proc. Am. Soc. Clin. Oncol.,* **8**, 636.
11. Bonnem, E.M. and Oldham, R.K. (1987) Gamma-interferon: physiology and speculation on its role in medicine. *J. Biol. Response Modif.,* **6**, 275–83.
12. Saito, T., Berens, M.E. and Welander, C.E. (1984) Direct and indirect effects of human recombinant gamma-interferon on tumor cells in a clonogenic assay. *Cancer Res.,* **46**, 1142–7.
13. Balkwill, F., Ward, B., Moodie, E. and Fiers, W. (1987) Therapeutic potential of tumor factor-α and γ-interferon in experimental human ovarian cancer. *Cancer Res.,* **47**, 4755–8.
14. Malik, S.T.A., Knowles, R.G., East, N. *et al.* (1991) Antitumor activity of gamma-interferon in ascitic and solid models of human ovarian cancer. *Cancer Res.,* **51**, 6643–9.
15. Marth, C., Müller-Holzner, E., Greiter, E. *et al.* (1990) Gamma interferon reduces expression

of the protooncogene c-*erb*B-2 in human ovarian carcinoma cells. *Cancer Res.*, **50**, 7037–41.

16. Wallich, R., Bulbuc, N., Hammerling, G.J. *et al.* (1985) Abrogation of metastatic properties of tumor cells by *de novo* expression of H-2K antigens following H-2 gene transfection. *Nature*, **315**, 301–3.

17. Tanaka, K., Hayashi, H., Hamada, C. *et al.* (1986) Expression of major histocompatibility complex class I antigens as a strategy for the potentiation of recognition of tumor cells. *Proc. Natl. Acad. Sci. USA*, **83**, 8723–7.

18. Weber, J., Jay, G., Tanaka, K. *et al.* (1987) Immunotherapy of a murine tumor with interleukin-2 increased sensitivity after MHC class I gene transfection. *J. Exp. Med.*, **166**, 1716–33.

19. Allavena, P., Peccatori, F., Maggioni, D. *et al.* (1990) Intraperitoneal recombinant γ-interferon in patients with recurrent ascitic ovarian carcinoma: modulation of cytotoxicity and cytokine production in tumor-associated effectors and of major histocompatibility antigen expression on tumor cells. *Cancer Res.*, **50**, 7318–23.

20. Mannel, D.N. and Falk, W. (1983) Interferon-gamma is required in activation of macrophages for cytotoxicity. *Cell. Immunol.*, **79**, 396–402.

21. Saito, T., Berens, M.E. and Welander, C.E. (1987) Characterisation of the indirect antitumor effects of γ-interferon using ascites-associated macrophages in a human tumor clonogenic assay. *Cancer Res.*, **47**, 673–9.

22. Colombo, N., Peccatori, F., Paganin, C. *et al.* (1992) Antitumor and immunomodulatory activity of intraperitoneal interferon-gamma in ovarian carcinoma patients with minimal residual tumor after the chemotherapy. *Int. J. Cancer*, **51**, 42–6.

23. Welander, C.E., Homesley, H.D., Reich, S.D. *et al.* (1988) A Phase II study of the efficacy of recombinant interferon gamma in relapsing ovarian adenocarcinoma. *Am. J. Clin. Oncol.*, **II**, 455–60.

24. D'Acquisto, R., Markman, M., Hakes, T. *et al.* (1988) A phase I trial of intraperitoneal recombinant gamma-interferon in advanced ovarian carcinoma. *J. Clin. Oncol.*, **6**, 689–95.

25. Belardelli, F., Greser, I., Maury, C. and Maunoury, M.T. (1982) Antitumor effects of interferon in mice injected with interferon-sensitive and interferon-resistant friend leukemia cells. *Int. J. Cancer*, **30**, 813–20.

26. Markman, M., Reichmann, B., Hakes, T. *et al.* (1993) Intraperitoneal chemotherapy in the management of ovarian cancer. *Cancer*, **71**, 1465–70.

27. Berek, J.S., Hacker, N., Lichtenstein, A. *et al.* (1985) Intraperitoneal immunotherapy of epithelial ovarian cancer with *Corynebacterium parvum*. *Am. J. Obstet. Gynecol.*, **152**, 1003–9.

28. Markman, M., Hakes, T., Reichman, B. *et al.* (1991) Intraperitoneal cisplatin and cytarabine in the treatment of refractory or recurrent ovarian carcinoma. *J. Clin. Oncol.*, **9**, 204–10.

29. Willemse, P., de Vries, E., Mulder, N. *et al.* (1990) Intraperitoneal human recombinant interferon alpha 2b in minimal residual disease ovarian cancer. *Eur. J. Cancer*, **26**, 353–8.

30. Nardi, M., Cognetti, F., Pollera, C.F. *et al.* (1990) Intraperitoneal recombinant alpha-2-interferon alternating with cisplatin as salvage therapy for minimal residual disease ovarian cancer. *J. Clin. Oncol.*, **8**, 1036–41.

31. Berek, J.S., Welander, C., Schink, J. C. *et al.* (1991) A Phase I–II trial of intraperitoneal cisplatin and α-interferon in patients with persistent epithelial ovarian cancer. *Gynecol. Oncol.*, **40**, 237–43.

32. Markman, M., Cleary, S., Lucas, W.E. *et al.* (1986) Intraperitoneal chemotherapy employing a regimen of cisplatin, cytarabine and bleomycin. *Cancer Treat. Rep.*, **70**, 755–60.

33. Ovarian Cancer Meta-Analysis Project (1991) Cyclophosphamide plus cisplatin versus cyclophosphamide, doxorubicin, and cisplatin chemotherapy of ovarian carcinoma: a meta-analysis. *J. Clin. Oncol.*, **9**, 1668–74.

34. Markman, M., Reichman, B., Hakes, T. *et al.* (1991) Responses to second-line cisplatin-based intraperitoneal therapy in ovarian cancer: influence of prior response to intravenous cisplatin. *J. Clin. Oncol.*, **9**, 1801–5.

35. Piccart, M., Speyer, J.L., Markman, M. *et al.* (1985) Intraperitoneal chemotherapy: technical experiences at five institutions. *Semin. Oncol.*, **8**, 1618–29.

36. Lotze, M.T., Custer, M.C. and Rosenberg, S.A. (1986) Intraperitoneal administration of interleukin-2 in patients with cancer. *Arch. Surg.*, **121**, 1373–9.

37. Rambaldi, A., Introna, M., Colotta, F. *et al.* (1985) Intraperitoneal administration of interferon β in ovarian cancer patients. *Cancer*, **56**, 294–301.

38. Elias, J. A., Jimenez, S.A. and Freundlich, B. (1987) Recombinant gamma, alpha, and beta interferons regulation of human lung fibroblast proliferation. *Am. Rev. Respir. Dis.*, **135**, 62–5.

39. Kähäri, V.M., Heino, J., Vuorio, T. and Vuorio, E. (1988) Interferon-α and interferon-gamma reduce excessive collagen synthesis and procollagen mRNA levels of scleroderma fibroblasts in culture. *Biochem. Biophys. Acta*, **968**, 45–50.

40. Giri, S. N., Hyde, D.M. and Marafin, B.J. (1986) Ameliorating effect of murine gamma-interferon on bleomycin-induced lung collagen fibrosis in mice. *Biochem. Med. Meth. Biol.*, **36**, 194–7.

41. Granstein, R.D., Murphy, F.G., Margolis, R.G. *et al.* (1987) Gamma interferon inhibits collagen synthesis *in vivo* in the mouse *J. Clin. Invest.*, **79**, 1254–8.

42. Björkholm, E., Petersson, F., Einhorn, N. *et al.* (1982) Long term follow-up and prognostic factors in ovarian carcinoma: the Radiumhemmet series 1958–1973. *Acta Radiol. Oncol. Radiat. Phys. Biol.*, **21**, 413–19.

43. Lippman, S.M., Alberts, D.S. Slymen, D.J. *et al.* (1988) Second look laparotomy in epithelial ovarian carcinoma. *Cancer*, **61**, 2571–7.

44. De Gramont, A., Drolet, Y., Varette, C. *et al.* (1989) Survival after second look laparotomy in advanced epithelial cancer. *Eur. J. Cancer Clin. Oncol.*, **25**, 251–7.

45. Chambers, S.K., Chambers, J.T., Kohorn, E.I. *et al.* (1988) Evaluation of the role of second look surgery in ovarian cancer. *Obstet. Gynecol.*, **72**, 404–8.

46. Saito, T., Berens, M.E. and Welander, C.E. (1987) Interferon gamma and cytotoxic agents studied in combination using a soft agarose human tumor clonogenic assay. *Cancer Chemother. Pharmacol.*, **19**, 233–9.

47. Mutch, D.G., Massard, S.L., Kao, M.S. and Collins, J.L. (1990) Proliferative and antiproliferative effects of interferon-γ and tumor necrosis factor-α on cell lines derived from cervical and ovarian malignancies. *Am. J. Obstet. Gynecol.*, **163**, 1920–4.

48. Maekawa, R., Kitagawa, T., Hojok, R. *et al.* (1988) Differential efficacies of recombinant interferon γ and recombinant human interleukin-2 against EL4-bearing mice. *J. Interferon Res.*, **8**, 241–9.

49. Silagi, S., Dutkowski, R. Schaeger, A. *et al.* (1988) Eradication of mouse melanoma by combined treatment with recombinant human interleukin-2 and recombinant murine interferon gamma. *Int. J. Cancer.* **41**, 315–22.

References

Chapter 25

Matrix metalloproteinases and their role in ovarian cancer

B. DAVIES, M.S. NAYLOR and F.R. BALKWILL

25.1 INTRODUCTION

25.1.1 BASEMENT MEMBRANE INTEGRITY AND METASTASIS

Basement membrane is a dense condensation of connective tissue found at the basal surface of all normal epithelial cells. It is a physically and chemically tough structure consisting of a lattice of type IV collagen around which other components such as proteoglycan and laminin are arranged. If a primary epithelial tumour is to metastasize to distant sites it is necessary for it to breach the basement membrane into the underlying mesothelium. Non-invasive carcinoma *in situ* is surrounded by a complete basement membrane, whilst this structure is absent from truly invasive carcinomas [1].

25.1.2 MATRIX METALLOPROTEINASES

The capacity of epithelial tumours to degrade basement membrane probably determines their metastatic competence. Basement membrane can be destroyed by the activity of matrix metalloproteinases (MMPs). MMPs comprise a gene family with certain common features. All have a highly conserved active site of 15 amino acids which binds a zinc atom essential for catalysis and they are all secreted as inactive precursors. Activation results from cleavage of a short sequence from the N-terminus of the molecule which contains a cysteine residue which interacts with zinc at the active site in the inactive molecule [2]. Members of the MMP family differ from each other in their substrate specificities. For example, stromelysin (MMP-3) degrades proteoglycan [3,4] and interstitial collagenase (MMP-1) degrades type I collagen [5]. There are two members of the MMP family which are capable of efficient degradation of the basement membrane component type IV collagen, namely 72 kd type IV collagenase (MMP-2) [6] and 92 kd type IV collagenase (MMP-9) [7]. Expression and activation of these enzymes is probably necessary if a fully metastatic phenotype is to develop. Activation of the 72 kd enzyme is mediated by a fibroblast cell surface bound proteolytic activity. This is probably an MMP because it is inhibited by compounds which inhibit other members of the MMP family [8]. Activation of the 92 kd enzyme can be achieved *in vitro* with other proteases including trypsin and stromelysin but the mechanism of activation *in vivo* remains unclear [9].

In addition to transcriptional, post-transcriptional and post-translational control of MMP activity, there exists a further element of complexity: two natural inhibitors of MMPs. Tissue inhibitors of metalloproteinase (TIMP-1, TIMP-2) have been characterized. These are small (28.5 and 21 kd respectively) peptides which are frequently cosecreted with MMPs [2].

Although some continuous cell lines derived from epithelial cell lines can secrete MMPs [6,10] and early histochemical studies showed tumour cell to be immunoreactive for type IV collagenase, recent *in situ* hybridization studies of a wide variety of tumour types including breast [10], colon [12], skin [13] and bladder (Davies, unpublished observations) have shown that *in vivo* it is not the tumour cells which express MMPs but associated stromal cells. Immunohistochemical studies showing the presence of tumour cell bound MMPs probably identify enzyme secreted by the stromal cells bound to cell surface receptors [14]. Tissue culture studies have shown that the 72 kd type IV collagenase is secreted chiefly by fibroblasts [15,16] whilst the 92 kd enzyme is a product of cells of the mononuclear phagocyte lineage [7, 17]. Fibroblasts and macrophages present in the tumour stroma are probably responsible for the type IV collagenase activity associated with tumours. Since normal tissues may contain fibroblasts and/or macrophages but do not express type IV collagenases, there must be specific factors expressed by the tumour cells which activate stromal cells to express active MMPs.

In this chapter we investigate the distribution of type IV collagenases in primary ovarian tumours using gel substrate analysis (zymography) and *in situ* hybridization of mRNA for collagenases and TIMPs-1 and 2. Typically, ovarian carcinoma is invasive locally and metastases throughout the peritoneal cavity are very common. We have also studied the action of a synthetic inhibitor of MMPs in human ovarian cancer xenografts growing in nude mice.

25.2 ANALYSIS OF TYPE IV COLLAGENASE EXPRESSION IN HUMAN OVARIAN TUMOURS BY GEL SUBSTRATE ANALYSIS (ZYMOGRAPHY)

Various investigators have attempted to measure type IV collagenase activity in tumours by release of soluble products from radiolabelled type IV collagen by tumour homogenates. These assays are, however, very insensitive, are affected by the presence of TIMPS and cannot detect proforms of the enzymes. Consequently there is little published information concerning type IV collagenase expression in solid tumours and their progression. We have examined type IV collagenase expression in ovarian tumour biopsies using gel substrate analysis (zymography). Unlike conventional assays of type IV collagenase using radiolabelled substrate, this method is sufficiently sensitive to enable detection and quantification of type IV collagenases from as little as 10 μg of biopsy material. Practically, this has enabled measurements to be made from a single 5 μm thick cryostat section. Adjacent sections were analysed for protein to standardize the results or stained for histological examination. Zymography has additional advantages over conventional assays in that it can distinguish between 92 kd and 72 kd type IV collagenases, it can detect inactive proforms and is unaffected by the presence of TIMPS [10].

Tumour biopsies were homogenized in SDS/glycerol sample buffer and applied to SDS/polyacrylamide gels impregnated with gelatin and subjected to electrophoresis under non-reducing conditions. Following electrophoresis, SDS was washed from gels to enable enzyme renaturation. Gels were then incubated overnight in a low salt buffer during which period renatured type IV collagenases digest incorporated gelatin. Following staining with Coomassie blue, bands of type IV collagenase activity were visualized as clear areas on the gel (Figure 25.1)

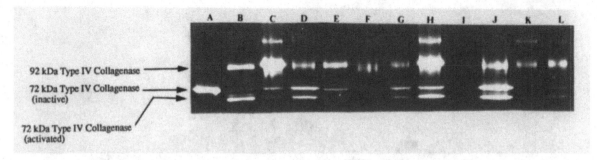

Figure 25.1 Zymography of ovarian tumour biopsies. Lane A = RPMI 7951 supernatant showing 72 kd type IV collagenase. Lane B = TPA stimulated HT-1080 supernatant showing 92 kd type IV collagenase, 72 kd type IV collagenase and its activated form. Lanes C–L = ovarian carcinoma biopsies.

The 72 kd enzyme appears on the zymogram as a doublet (proenzyme and activated species) but the human 92 kd enzyme appears as a single band because the proforms and active forms are not resolved due to their similarity of size and the presence of differently glycosylated forms. Linear densitometric scanning of gels could not be used to quantify the levels of type IV collagenolytic activity from the gels, because the level of enzyme affects not only the intensity but also the width of the band. However, the integrated density of each band (determined by computer assisted image analysis) was found to be proportional to the level of enzyme [18]. Using this method we have quantified the levels of 92 kd and 72 kd type IV collagenases in ovarian tumours. In a preliminary study with 25 cases of ovarian cancer we detected the 92 kd type IV collagenase in all specimens, the inactive proform of 72 type IV collagenase in 23/25 cases and the active form of this enzyme in 21/25 cases. There was no significant difference in distribution of any of these species between grades (Table 25.1). We intend to expand this study using a greater number of tumours because of the relatively low numbers of grade I and II biopsies in our study.

The results in Table 25.1 clearly show that ovarian carcinomas do express type IV collagenases and that these enzymes may be

Table 25.1 Levels of type IV collagenases in epithelial ovarian tumours

Enzyme	Grade		
	I (n=3)	II (n=6)	III (n=16)
92 kd type IV collagenase	41.0*±12.4	77.8±58.1	49±15.0
72 kd type IV collagenase (inactive)	39.1±24.4	6.4 ± 2.4	7.2±1.9
72 kd type IV collagenase (active)	8.2±3.6	1.5±0.7	6.1±3.4

*units/10 μg protein

involved in the pathology of the disease. Ovarian cancer is highly locally invasive and this may be because of the relatively high expression of MMPs. We have performed similar studies on breast and bladder tumours and in each case we have observed a strong correlation between histological grade and 1) high expression of 92 kd enzyme and 2) high levels of activated 72 kd enzyme ([11] and Davies *et al.* in preparation). Breast and bladder carcinomas are not as locally invasive as are ovarian tumours and it may be significant that it was only the high grade tumours which contained high MMP activities.

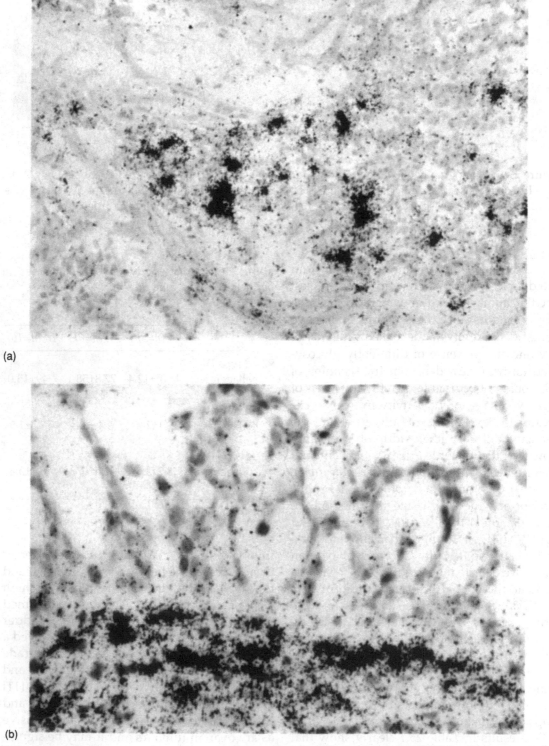

(a)

(b)

Figure 25.2 *In situ* hybridization of mRNAs for type IV collagenases and TIMPS in ovarian carcinoma biopsies. (a) 92 kd type IV collagenase. (b) 72 kd type IV collagenase. (c) TIMP-1. (d) TIMP-2.

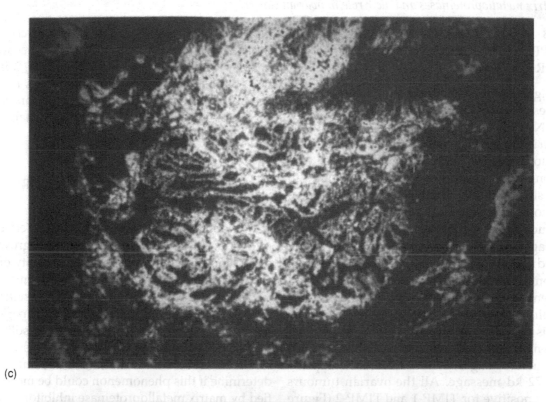

(c)

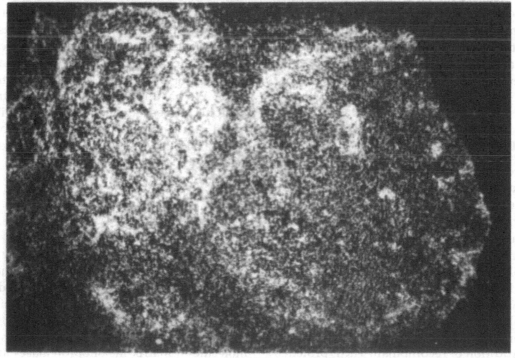

(d)

Figure 25.2 *(contd)*

25.3 LOCALIZATION OF MMP EXPRESSION IN OVARIAN CARCINOMAS

In agreement with studies on other tumour types, Figure 25.2 shows the localization of mRNA for MMPs in ovarian cancer to be restricted to the stromal elements of the tumour rather than epithelial areas. The strongest concentration of mRNA is found in the stroma immediately adjacent to epithelial tumour cells, suggesting that the tumour cells induce the stromal cells to generate type IV collagenases either by cell–cell contact or by production of a soluble factor. The exact stromal cell types expressing the type IV collagenase genes are difficult to define on morphological grounds alone. However, on the basis of *in vitro* studies, the 92 kd type IV collagenase positive cells are probably infiltrating macrophages, whilst fibroblasts express the 72 kd message. All the ovarian tumours were positive for TIMP-1 and TIMP-2 (Figure 25.2 c,d) and so it is unclear if the type IV collagenases would be active within the tumour environment. The mRNA for TIMP-1 and -2 was also located in the stromal areas and not the epithelial tumour cells.

25.4 MMPs AS TARGETS FOR DRUG INTERVENTION

There is now substantial evidence that MMPs are involved in metastasis formation and thus strategies to block the activity of these enzymes could be used therapeutically. Suitable approaches include:

1. Blocking transcriptional activation of MMP genes;
2. Activating transcription of TIMP genes;
3. Blocking *in vivo* activation of inactive proenzymes;
4. Addition of recombinant TIMP proteins;
5. Addition of synthetic inhibitors.

Not enough is known about the transcriptional activation of MMP and TIMP genes to enable 1 and 2 to be practical. Similarly, 3 is not possible. Use of recombinant TIMPs is a possibility but use of synthetic inhibitors is preferable due to lower cost, increased stability and low antigenicity.

25.5 MMP INHIBITORS AS TUMOUR STROMA FORMING AGENTS

In our laboratory we have established a series of ovarian carcinoma xenografts which grow as mucinous ascites in the peritoneal cavity of the nude mouse [19]. Following treatment of two of these xenografts with TNF, ascitic disease is resolved and the surface of the peritoneum becomes covered in multiple solid nudules of tumour in a manner reminiscent of the human disease [20]. We set out to determine if this phenomenon could be modified by matrix metalloproteinase inhibitors. In doing so we determined that matrix metalloproteinase inhibitors had the effect of resolving ascites. Late stage ovarian cancer is frequently complicated by the accumulation of ascites for which there is no adequate treatment. We have recently reported that treatment of ascites bearing nude mice with a broad spectrum synthetic matrix metalloproteinase, BB-94, converts ascites to solid tumour and decreases tumour burden and increases survival [18].

25.5.1 BB-94: A SYNTHETIC MMP INHIBITOR

BB-94, [4-(N-hydroxyamino)-2R-isobutyl-3S-(thiophen-2-ylthiomethyl)-succinyl]-L-phenylalanine-N-methylamide, was provided by British Biotechnology Ltd, Cowley, Oxford, UK. BB-94 has a molecular weight of 478, contains a peptide backbone which binds the molecule to matrix metalloproteinases and a hydroxamic acid group which binds to the catalytically active zinc atom. The concentrations (nM) of BB-94 required for half maximal inhibition of MMPs are as follows: interstitial collagenase, 3; stromelysin, 20; 72 kd type IV collagenase, 4; 92 kd type IV collagenase, 1–10. BB-94 is a fine white powder and was sonicated into suspension at 2.5 mg/ml in PBS pH 7.2 + Tween-20 (0.01%). BB-94 was administered intraperitoneally to ascites bearing mice.

The HU and LA xenografts grew as thick mucinous ascites in the peritoneal cavity of the nude mouse. Seven days after introduction of the HU xenograft, the peritoneal cavity of the host contained 1–2 ml of mucinous ascites. By 14 days this had increased to 3–4 ml and by 21 days to 5–6 ml. Treatment of mice with BB-94 daily intraperitoneally from three days after tumour transplantation prevented formation of ascites. A small volume of solid tumour of bright white appearance was visible in these mice and the burden of tumour was not appreciably greater on day 21 than on day 7. Fourteen days after introduction of the HU xenograft, the volume of accumulated ascites in the untreated animals was sufficient to cause the abdomen to become visibly swollen. However, when the animals were treated with BB-94, their abdomens did not swell and they appeared healthy. Figure 25.3 shows the appearance of the peritoneal cavity of mice bearing the HU xenograft at 14 days after treatment with vehicle alone (25.3a) or with BB-94 (25.3b). The position of solid tumour is indicated by the large arrow. In the animals treated with vehicle alone, mucinous ascites covered all of the peritoneal organs. In BB-94 treated animals the tumour burden was low; typically each animal had one large tumour of maximum dimension approximately 8 mm which was free floating in the peritoneal cavity or attached to fat. Such tumours were often located at the rectum end of the colon or at the base of the spleen. They were only loosely attached to the fat and were of bright white appearance because they were avascular.

A similar pattern was observed with the LA xenograft. Mice treated with diluent alone became swollen by 14 days due to an accumulation of mucinous ascites whereas those treated with BB-94 appeared normal. Post mortem examination revealed solid white tumours loosely attached to peritoneal organs, typically at the colon and base of the spleen. Accumulations of drug were also visible in BB-94 treated animals. These appeared as small white deposits (small arrows in Figure 25.3b) attached to fat, peritoneal organs and the omentum. These deposits were observed in a non-tumour bearing mouse treated with drug. Histological examination of these deposits demonstrated that they were not tumour and had no inflammatory infiltrate.

The observed antitumour effects of BB-94 were unlikely to be caused by any direct cytotoxic effect towards the tumour cells themselves. BB-94 had no effect on the growth of various cell lines tested including SKOV (human ovarian carcinoma), CHO cells, human foreskin fibroblasts, mouse BALB-C2Y fibroblasts and Shionagi mouse breast carcinoma cells as determined by enumeration of cells and incorporation of ^{3}H-thymidine.

BB-94 caused a dramatic decrease in tumour burden. Tumour weight in mice treated with vehicle alone was 156 ± 103 mg (mean $\pm$ SD 8 separate determinations) seven days after introduction of the tumour and this had more than doubled to 542 ± 307 mg (n=8) by 14 days. Limited survival in mice treated with vehicle alone beyond 14 days prevented reliable quantitation. However, in BB-94 treated animals the tumour burden was low at seven days (46.4 ± 16.3 mg, n=8) compared to animals treated with vehicle only ($p<0.001$) and did not increase significantly during the first 28 days after introduction of the

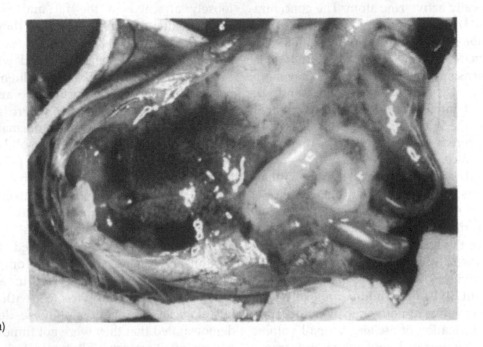

(a)

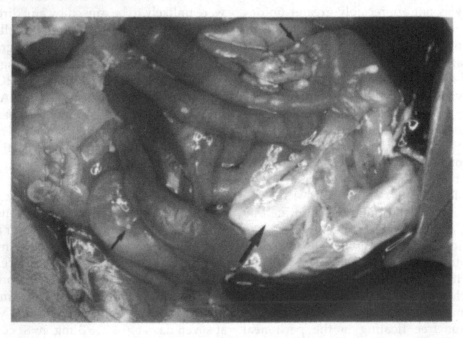

(b)

Figure 25.3 Internal appearance of peritoneal cavity of mice bearing the HU xenograft following treatment with vehicle alone (a) or BB-94 40 mg kg^{-1} day^{-1} (b). Mice were treated from day 3 after the introduction of xenograft until sacrifice at day 14. Solid tumour indicated by large arrow. Small arrow indicates white deposit, representing an accumulation of drug.

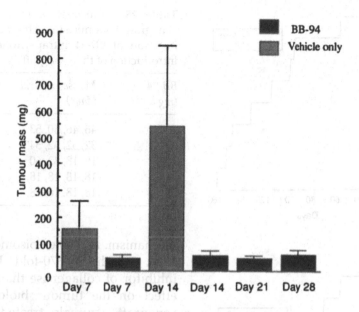

Figure 25.4 Tumour burden of mice bearing the HU xenograft. Solid tumour was dissected from the peritoneal cavity of BB-94 treated mice and weighed. The tumour burden of mice bearing ascites was determined by washing the peritoneal cavity with PBS and weighing the resulting pellet after centrifugation. Mice were treated with BB-94 40 mg kg^{-1} day^{-1} or vehicle only as indicated from day 3 after introduction of the xenograft until sacrifice. Each value shown is the mean value of eight separate determinations and the error bars are the standard deviation of the measurements.

xenograft (61.8±19.0 mg, n=8 at 28 days) (Figure 25.4)

This decreased tumour burden was associated with a dramatic increase in survival. When BB-94 was given daily on days 3–21 after introduction of the xenograft, the median survival was increased from 19 days (vehicle only treated) to 129 days (BB-94 treated) (Figure 25.5a) ($p<0.001$). When BB-94 was given on days 7–21, survival was still greatly increased (median survival of vehicle only treated group 18 days, median survival of BB-94 treated group 105 days) ($p<0.001$) (Figure 25.5b). BB-94 treated mice eventually died from abdominal swelling caused by an accumulation of solid tumour and ascites.

In most experiments mice were dosed daily with BB-94 but the drug was also effective if given less regularly than this. Ascites was resolved in mice injected once on day 3 with 40 mg kg^{-1}. The effect of a single injection of

BB-94 on increasing survival was dose dependent. When 40 mg kg^{-1} was given on day 3 after introduction of HU xenograft, 4/4 mice were still alive at day 45; when treated with 30 mg kg^{-1}, 3/4 mice were alive at 45 days whilst in the group treated with 10 mg kg^{-1}, 3/4 mice were dead by day 22. All four mice treated with diluent control died on day 18 (Table 25.2).

The HU and LA xenografts consisted of small clumps of tumour cells floating in mucin (Figure 25.6a,c). In both xenografts the transition from ascites to solid tumour was associated with encapsulation of the clumps of tumour cells by host cells and in the case of the HU xenograft, the solid tumour which resulted from treatment with BB-94 had a relatively high proportion of stroma to tumour cells (Figure 25.6b). Isolated clumps of tumour cells were visible in the stroma and some of these appeared to be necrotic (Figure 25.6b).A

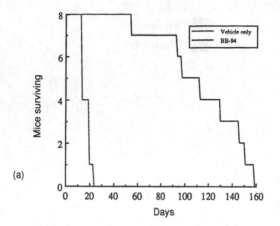

(a)

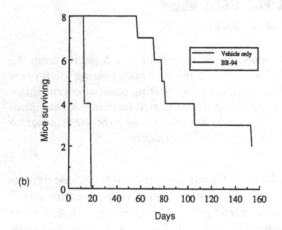

(b)

Figure 25.5 Survival of mice bearing the HU xenograft following treatment with BB-94 40 mg kg^{-1} day^{-1} or vehicle control as indicated. Mice were treated either from day 3 (a) or day 7 (b) after the introduction of xenograft until day 21 or death, whichever was first.

Table 25.2 Survival of mice bearing the HU xenograft. Four mice in each group were given one injection of BB-94 intraperitoneally day 3 after introduction of the xenograft

BB-94 (mg kg^{-1})	Mouse survival (days)	Mean survival (days)
40	46, 46, 50, 53	48.8
30	32, 32, 32, 54	37.5
10	18, 18, 32, 60	32.0
1	18, 18, 18, 18,	18.0
0	18, 18, 18, 18,	18.0

mechanism. A diastereoisomer of BB-94, BB-1268, which is 670-fold less potent an inhibitor of collagenase than BB-94, had no effect on the tumour biology of the HU xenograft. Animals treated with BB-1268 developed ascites in an identical manner to those treated with vehicle alone.

25.6 MMP INHIBITORS MAY RESOLVE ASCITIC DISEASE

Thus, inhibition of MMP activity in the peritoneal cavity of the host caused a transition from ascites to solid tumour, probably by shifting the balance from matrix breakdown to matrix synthesis. We examined the MMP activity in HU bearing mice treated with BB-94 or vehicle alone by zymography. Inactive proforms of the 92 kd and 72 kd enzymes were detected in ascites from mice treated with vehicle alone but no activated forms of these enzymes could be detected. It was not possible to determine interstitial collagenase or stromelysin expression by this technique due to lack of sensitivity. Ascites from xenograft bearing mice is extremely thick and mucinous and this limits the amount of material which can be loaded onto polyacrylamide gels. After treatment with BB-94, ascites resolves and the large amounts of mucin are no longer present, enabling larger amounts of material to be loaded onto gels. When 80 mg

similar transition occurred when mice bearing the LA xenograft were treated with BB-94 (Figure 25.6d). The proportion of tumour cells to stroma was much higher in LA solid tumours than in HU tumours but some necrosis was visible towards the centre of the tumour (Figure 25.6d).

The observed antitumour effects of BB-94 were dependent upon its MMP inhibiting properties and not to some other non-specific

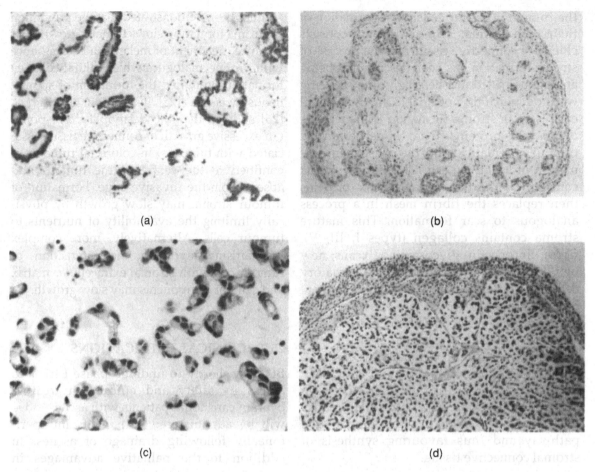

Figure 25.6 Histology of HU and LA xenografts. HU xenograft (a,b), LA xenograft (c,d). Mice were treated with vehicle only control (a,c) or BB-94 40 mg kg^{-1} day^{-1} (b,d) from day 3 after introduction of the xenograft until sacrifice on day 14. See text for explanation.

of solid tumour from a BB-94-treated, HU bearing mouse was analysed by gel substrate analysis, activated 92 kd enzyme was detected in addition to the inactive forms of the 92 and 72 kd enzymes (Figure 25.7). As stated above, the active and inactive forms of the human 92 kd collagenase cannot be resolved by zymography, but we have found resolution of the murine enzymes in several experiments. This suggests that the proteases in the xenografts are murine enzymes induced by signals from the human tumours.

We propose that activity of MMP in HU bearing mice keeps the tumour in the ascitic phase and prevents laying down of extracellular matrix proteins and formation of solid tumour. Consequently when these enzymes are inhibited by BB-94, stroma formation is favoured.

In addition to their role in blocking metastasis, synthetic inhibitors such as BB-94 may have additional beneficial effects by inhibiting angiogensis [21] and promoting the formation of stroma, causing encapsulation of

253

the tumour. Tumour cells cause formation of their own stroma. Tumour stroma consists chiefly of connective tissue and the process of stroma formation has been described as being analogous to wound healing, tumours being wounds which do not heal [22]. An essential early step in stroma formation is the leakage of plasma proteins from hyperpermeable tumour vasculature and the consequent formation of a fibrin mesh [23]. Mature stroma consisting of extracellular matrix proteins then replaces the fibrin mesh in a process analogous to scar formation. This mature stroma contains collagen (types I, III, V), fibrin, fibronectin, glycosaminoglycans, new blood vessels, fibroblasts and inflammatory cells [24]. Tumours and associated stromal cells also express MMPs (see above) capable of degrading extracellular matrix proteins. Tumour associated stroma is clearly a dynamic structure continually undergoing remodelling. Treatment of tumour with MMP inhibitors may disrupt the balance between synthesis and lysis of extracellular matrix components by blocking the degradative pathway and thus favouring synthesis of stromal connective tissue.

It has been demonstrated that the promotion of stroma formation slows tumour growth. For instance, treatment of melanoma bearing mice with proline analogues which inhibit collagen formation promoted the formation of spontaneous metastasis [25]. In addition, Hewitt *et al.* [26] showed that the desmoplastic response (an excessive growth of connective tissue associated with tumours) in colorectal tumours is confined to the centre of the tumour and absent from the invasive edge. Formation of tumour stroma may slow growth by physically limiting the availability of nutrients to tumour cells. Alternatively, more complex mechanisms involving the interaction of tumour cells with stromal extracellular matrix and cellular components may slow growth.

25.7 CLINICAL IMPLICATIONS

BB-94 is shortly to undergo phase I trials to assess its safety and efficacy in treating ovarian carcinoma patients with ascites. BB94 will be administered to patients intraperitoneally following drainage of ascites. In addition to the palliative advantages in

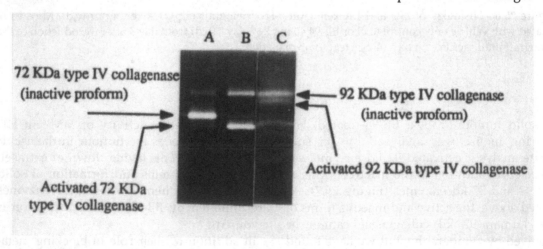

Figure 25.7 Zymography of tumour from mouse bearing HU xenograft. Lane A, conditioned media from PMA-stimulated HT-1080 cells; lane B, RPMI 7951 conditioned medium; lane C, 80 µg of solid tumour from HU bearing mouse. Tumour was taken from mouse 21 days after introduction of HU xenograft. Mouse was treated with BB-94, 40 mg kg^{-1} day^{-1}, days 3–20.

removal of ascites, it is hoped that the tumour stroma forming properties of BB-94 will cause a slowing or termination of tumour growth as was observed in the xenograft models.

In addition to this, MMP inhibitors such as BB-94 may be of therapeutic benefit to ovarian cancer patients with less advanced disease. Ovarian tumour biopsies contained significant levels of type IV collagenases (regardless of their histological grade) which may explain why this type of tumour is particularly prone to cause extensive local invasion in the peritoneum.

REFERENCES

1. Siegal, G.P., Barsky, S.H., Terranova, V.P. and Liotta, L.A. (1981) Stages of neoplastic transformation of human breast tissue as monitored by dissolution of the basement membrane components. *Invasion Metastasis*, **1**, 54–65.

2. Liotta, L.A. and Stetler-Stevenson, W.G. (1991) Tumour invasion and metastasis: an imbalance of positive and negative regulation. *Cancer Res.*, **51**, 5054s–9s.

3. Chin, J.R., Murphy, G. and Werb, Z. (1985) Stromelysin, a connective tissue-degrading metalloendopeptidase secreted by stimulated rabbit synovial fibroblast in parallel with collagenase. *J. Biol. Chem.*, **260**, 12367–76.

4. Wilhelm, S.M., Collier, I.E., Kronberger, A. *et al.* (1987) Human skin fibroblast stromelysin: structure, glycosylation, substrate specificity, and differential expression in normal and tumorigenic cells. *Proc. Natl. Acad. Sci. USA*, **84**, 6725–9.

5. Templeton, N.S., Brown, P.D., Levy, A.T. *et al.* (1990) Cloning and characterisation of human tumour cell interstitial collagenase. *Cancer Res.*, **50**, 5431–7.

6. Collier, I.E., Wilhelm, S.M., Eisen, A.Z. *et al.* (1988) H-ras oncogene-transformed human bronchial epithelial cells (TBE-1) secrete a single metalloproteinase capable of degrading basement membrane collagen. *J. Biol. Chem.*, **263**, 6579–87.

7. Hibbs, M.S., Hoidal, J.R. and Kang, A.H. (1987) Expression of a metalloproteinase that degrades native type V collagen and denatured collagens by cultured human alveolar macrophages. *J. Clin. Invest.*, **80**, 1644–50.

8. Ward, R.V., Atkinson, S.J., Slocombe, P.M. *et al.* (1991) Tissue inhibitor of metalloproteinase-2 inhibits the activation of 72 kd progelatinase by fibroblast membranes. *Biochim. Biophys. Acta*, **1079**, 242–6.

9. Ogata, Y., Enghild, J.J. and Nagase, H. (1992) Matrix metalloproteinase 3 (Stromelysin) activates the precursor for the human matrix metalloproteinase 9. *J. Biol. Chem.*, **267**, 3581–4.

10. Brown, P.D., Levy, A.T., Margulies, I.M.K. *et al.* (1990) Independent expression and cellular processing of Mr 72,000 type IV collagenase and interstitial collagenase in human tumourigenic cell lines. *Cancer Res.*, **50**, 6184–91.

11. Davies, B., Miles, D.W., Happerfield, L.C. *et al.* (1993) Activity of type IV collagenases in benign and malignant breast disease. *Br. J. Cancer*, **67**, 1126–31.

12. Pyke, C., Ralfkiaer, E., Tryggvason, K. and Dano, K. (1993) Messenger RNA for two type IV collagenases is located in stromal cells in human colon cancer. *Am. J. Pathol.*, **142**, 359–65.

13. Pyke, C., Ralfkiaer, E. Huhtala, P. *et al.* (1992) Localisation of messenger RNA for Mr 72,000 and 92,000 type IV collagenases in human skin cancers by *in situ* hybridization. *Cancer Res.*, **52**, 1336–41.

14. Emonard, H.P., Remacle, A.G., Noel, A.C. *et al.* (1992) Tumour cell-surface-associated binding site for the Mr 72,000 Type IV collagenase. *Cancer Res.*, **52**, 5845–8.

15. Seltzer, J.L., Adams, S.A., Grant, G.A., and Eisen, Z.A. (1981) Purification and properties of a gelatin-specific neutral protease from human skin. *J. Biol. Chem.*, **256**, 4662–8.

16. Goldberg, G.I., Wilhelm, S.M., Kronberger, A. *et al.* (1986). Human fibroblast collagenase. Complete structure and homology to an oncogene transformation-induced rat protein. *J. Biol. Chem.*, **261**, 6600–5.

17. Welgus, H.G., Campbell, E.J., Cury, J.D. *et al* (1990). Neutral metalloproteinases produced by human mononuclear phagocytes. *J. Clin. Invest.*, **86**, 1496–502.

18. Davies, B., Brown, P.D., East, N. *et al.* (1993) A synthetic matrix metalloproteinase inhibitor decreases tumour burden and prolongs survival of mice bearing human ovarian carcinoma xenografts. *Cancer Res*, **53**, 2087–91.

19. Ward, B.G., Wallace, K., Shephard, J.H. and Balkwill, F.R. (1987) Intraperitoneal xenografts of human epithelial ovarian cancer in nude mice. *Cancer Res.*, **47**, 2662–7.

20. Malik, S.T.A., Griffin, D.B., Fiers, W. and Balkwill, F.R. (1989) Paradoxical effects of tumour necrosis factor in experimental ovarian cancer. *Int. J. Cancer*, **44**, 918–25.

21. Moses, M.A., Sudhalter, J. and Langer, R. (1990) Identification of an inhibitor of neovascularization from cartilage. *Science*, **248**, 1408–10.

22. Dvorak, H.F. (1986) Tumours: wounds that do not heal. *N. Engl. J. Med.*, **315**, 1650–9.

23. Nagy, J.A., Brown, L.F., Senger, D.R. *et al.* (1988) Pathogenesis of tumour stroma generation: a critical role for leaky blood vessels and fibrin deposition. *Biochim. Biophys. Acta*, **94**, 305–26.

24. Barsky, S.H., Rao, C.N., Grotendorst, G.R. and Liotta, L.A. (1982) Increased content of type V collagen in desmoplasia of human breast carcinoma. *Am. J. Pathol.*, *108*, 276–83.

25. Barsky, S.H. and Gopalakrishna, R. (1987) Increased invasion and spontaneous metastasis of BL6 melanoma with inhibition of the desmoplastic response in C57 BL/6 mice. *Cancer Res.*, **47**, 1663–7.

26. Hewitt, R.E., Powe, D.G., Carter, G.I. and Turner, D.R. (1993) Desmoplasia and its relevance to colorectal tumour invasion. *Int. J. Cancer*, **53**, 62–9.

Chapter 26

Signal transduction therapy: a new paradigm

E.C. KOHN

26.1 INTRODUCTION

The advent of molecular medicine has brought new approaches to the treatment, diagnosis and evaluation of malignant disease. The molecular medicine of cancer has gone from cytotoxic chemotherapy to immunotherapy and now has entered into gene therapy interventions. Through recent scientific advances, immunotherapy has been brought from the laboratory bench to the clinic in the form of biological response modification, treatment with directed antibodies and combinations of cytokines and activated lymphocytes primed against the tumor. The optimal use and outcome of these forms of immunotherapy for ovarian cancer are still under investigation. The explosion in knowledge of how specific genes are involved in the process of cancer growth and metastasis has led to the areas of transgenic animal experimentation and human gene therapy. The concept of gene therapy for general cancer treatment is in the early stages of investigation and specific applications to ovarian cancer have not yet been introduced clinically. The last new target to be identified is that of signal transduction.

Signal transduction is the process whereby information is transferred across the cell membrane from the external environment or from cell to cell. The result of this transmembrane signal transduction can be stimulation or inhibition of effector functions at the membrane, within the cytoplasm and cytoskeleton and at the nucleus. There are three major categories of transmembrane signal transduction: activation of ion channels, transfer of information through guanine nucleotide binding (G) protein intermediates causing the generation of second messengers, and phosphorylation or dephosphorylation events [1–5]. These signaling events may be directly receptor activated or be immediate downstream events related to ligand–receptor interactions. In all cases, the signal(s) causes secondary or tertiary biochemical events to occur within the cell, ultimately resulting in stimulation or inhibition of cellular behavior.

The three broad categories defined above may be narrowed by the identification of common denominators underlying their regulation. Candidates for common signal regulators include cell cycle, specific cellular behavior or activity or selected signals themselves. Review of the literature has suggested that intracellular calcium may be a common underlying regulator which can modulate and also result from signals transduced through ion channels, G protein related pathways and phosphorylation–dephosphorylation events. These observations are not related

257

only to malignancy but may be seen broadly in normal and diseased states.

Calcium homeostasis is a balance between stimulation of calcium influx, efflux and intracellular release and storage. Two types of calcium influx channels have been described. Voltage gated calcium channels (VOCC) have been cloned and sequenced [6] and may be inhibited by one of three classes of inhibitors: phenylalkylamines, benzothiazepines and dihydropyridines [7]. They may be stimulated by receptor activation or by voltage changes across the cellular membrane. In contrast, receptor operated calcium channels are not inhibited by the organic inhibitors of VOCCs but may be inhibited by inorganic ions such as manganese, magnesium, cadmium and lanthanum which compete for transport. These channels are regulated by ligand–receptor interactions [2]. For example, calcium is an important regulator of muscarinic acetylcholine receptor stimulated potassium channels in the heart through its regulation of arachidonic acid release by phospholipase A2 [8–10]. Calcium can be mobilized in response to certain subtype muscarinic receptors (m1, m3, m5), those which do not stimulate the potassium channels and therefore may function as modulators. Researchers have shown that calcium is a necessary cofactor for formyl peptide, fMLP, stimulation of monocyte second messenger release and subsequent monocyte migration and biochemical activities [11,12]. Recent evidence has shown that calcium regulates receptor stimulated tyrosine phosphorylation of downstream effector enzymes such as phospholipase C-γ (PLC-γ) effecting normal and malignant processes [13–15].

Calcium is also important in cellular functions where the specific cellular signal events have not yet been elucidated fully. A key example of this is the process of pseudopodial protrusion. It is known that pseudopodia form in response to chemoattractants which stimulate normal cell and tumor cell motility. These attractants may be tumor derived motility factors, growth factors or extracellular matrix proteins [16–18]. The process of pseudopod formation requires actin polymerization and cytoskeletal restructuring, membrane flow and environmental sensing [19]. Calcium has long been known to be important in the process of cellular adhesion in general and may regulate many of the steps in pseudopodial protrusion and locomotion. Other events that may be at least in part regulated by calcium include protein secretion, proteinase activity and apoptosis as suggested in Figure 26.1 [20–23].

26.2 SIGNAL TRANSDUCTION THERAPY: HYPOTHESIS

We focused our attention on how calcium mediated signal transduction may be important in tumor invasion and screened for agents which might affect components of invasion in *in vitro* experiments. Our hypothesis was that intervention at the regulatory level might be more specifically directed at invasion and metastasis and yet still be effective in inhibition of proliferation. We reasoned that the plasticity of normal cell regulation might afford protection and that the altered signaling pathways in malignant cells, as a result of oncogenic deletion, overexpression and amplification, may make the malignant cells more vulnerable to biochemical interventions.

There were three important obstacles to overcome in the proposition of signal transduction therapy as a new paradigm for cancer treatment. The first was the question of selectivity. Most, if not all of these signaling pathways are found in every cell, normal and malignant. Without selectivity of action and therefore specificity, agents which alter calcium homeostasis might be uniformly toxic or demonstrate selective toxicity of key organs, thus preventing their safe utilization. The second obstacle, toxicity and the definition of a safe therapeutic window, was therefore partly dependent upon demonstration of

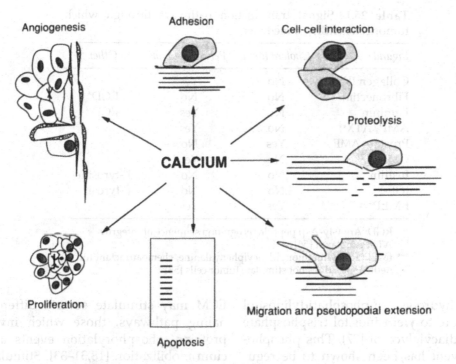

Figure 26.1 Calcium mediates components of tumorigenesis.

selectivity. Lastly, if the agent was shown to be specific and selectively toxic, demonstration of efficacy was the last hurdle prior to initiation of clinical studies.

The remainder of this discussion will focus on the biochemical role of calcium in signal transduction and the biological effects of modulation of calcium concentrations on proliferation and metastatic potential. It will close with a discussion of CAI, a novel anticancer agent which inhibits stimulated calcium influx. How CAI overcomes the aforementioned obstacles will be described.

26.3 IMPORTANCE OF SIGNAL TRANSDUCTION PATHWAYS IN CANCER

26.3.1 GROWTH FACTORS AND ONCOGENES

Several approaches have been used to elucidate the role of signal transduction pathways in the process of malignant proliferation and invasion with subsequent metastatic spread. The first uses specific ligands for which the malignant cell has known receptors and functions and simply determines if any common signal pathways are triggered by cellular interaction with these ligands and investigates the effector functions. This approach has identified categories of growth factors and motility factors. These are analysed by the primary pathway of signal transmission shown in Table 26.1. Many oncogenic growth factors are ligands for transmembrane receptors which have tyrosine kinase activity. Ligand–receptor interaction results in receptor autophosphorylation or phosphorylation of important related proteins, such as other effector enzymes [24]. These other effector enzymes may be enzymes which produce second messengers, such as the activation of PLC-γ by receptor tyrosine kinase mediated tyrosine phosphorylation [14,15,25,26]. Activation of PLC-γ by phosphorylation

Table 26.1 Signal transduction pathways through which tumor cell motility is mediated

Ligand	Cholera toxin	Pertussis toxin	Other
Collagen IV	No	Yes	
Fibronectin	No	No	RGD*
Laminin	No	Yes	RGD
AMP/ATX**	No	Yes	
Prostate AMF	Yes	No	
GM-CSF	No	Yes	
Insulin	No	No	P-tyrosine
IGF-I	No	No	P-tyrosine
f-MLP***	Yes	Yes	

* RGD: Arg-Gly-Asp peptide recognition sequence of integrins
** ATX: Autotaxin [56]
*** fMLP: formylmethionyl-leucylphenyalanine, chemoattractant for
   neutrophils, does not stimulate tumor cells [53]

stimulates hydrolysis of phosphatidylinositol bisphosphate to yield inositol trisphosphate (IP3) and diacylglycerol [27]. This phosphorylation event has been shown to be regulated by calcium in many settings and ultimately causes the internal release of calcium by IP3. Receptor activation with subsequent phosphorylation of PLC-γ or other effector proteins may be linked to malignancy. Epidermal growth factor (EGF) which causes receptor autophosphorylation upon binding is mitogenic for a wide variety of cancers including ovarian cancer [28] and has been shown to stimulate motility of human adenocarcinoma cell lines *in vitro* [29]. Cells which overexpress the EGFR secondary to amplification of *c-erb* B, such as ovarian cancers [30], may have increased sensitivity to EGF and therefore increased activity of these pathways, especially when compared to normal cells.

26.3.2 EXTRACELLULAR MATRIX PROTEINS

Another class of ligands which mediate their effects through calcium requiring activities is the extracellular matrix (ECM) proteins.

ECM may stimulate several different signaling pathways, those which involve G proteins, phosphorylation events and calcium mobilization [18,31–33]. Stimulation of melanoma cell migration in *in vitro* motility assays by type IV collagen has been shown to require mobilization of intracellular calcium [33]. The migration response to type IV collagen is inhibited by cellular treatment with pertussis toxin [18] and chelation of intracellular calcium by BAPTA [33]. Pertussis toxin, from *Bortadella pertussis*, irreversibly ADP-ribosylates selected alpha subunits of G proteins. This ADP-ribosylation uncouples the heterotrimeric inactive G protein from the effector enzyme [1]. Similar calcium dependent results were not seen when cells were stimulated with fibronectin [18,33]. Fibronectin, however, does stimulate tumor cell migration through activation of integrin receptors [18,34]. Integrins are heterodimeric transmembrane receptors which signal cell migration, shape change, adhesion, proliferation and activation through several pathways, including tyrosine phosphorylation and intracellular alkalinization [32]. The role of calcium as a regulator of integrin function has not yet been defined. However, activation of selected integrins in neutrophils has been shown to induce calcium transients in the cytoplasm, thus demonstrating a secondary effector function of calcium in that setting [35]. Thus, the evaluation of growth and migration stimulatory factors has defined the role of many signal transduction events.

26.3.3 ONCOGENIC TRANSMEMBRANE RECEPTORS

Another approach is the ectopic placement of transmembrane receptors or signal proteins of known signal activity and the subsequent ligand specific stimulation or inhibition of malignant behavior by the activation of these receptor or signal proteins. Several examples in the literature all point to calcium mediated events underlying the stimulation or reversal of the malignant phenotype. Julius and colleagues transfected the serotonin 5HT1C receptor into recipient NIH-3T3 fibroblasts and investigated the response of ligand stimulation [36]. They found that receptor activation with serotonin led to focus formation *in vitro* and colony formation in soft agar, as long as the serotonin ligand was present. Mesulergine, a specific antagonist of the 5HT1C receptor, reversed these behaviors. Cells bearing the transfected receptor were tumorigenic after inoculation into nude mice. The investigators linked the increase of intracellular calcium caused by serotonin stimulation of the transfected 5HT1C receptors to the phenotypic tumorigenic changes.

Similar results were seen by Allen and coworkers with transfection of the adrenergic α-1B receptor into NIH-3T3 and RAT1 fibroblasts [37]. In their studies, catecholamine ligands stimulated proliferation of the stably transfected cells and a reversible morphological change which could be inhibited by receptor specific antagonists. Ligand binding of the α-1B adrenergic receptor resulted in production of inositol phosphates. A genetically engineered mutant receptor which constitutively stimulated inositol phosphate production without requirement for catecholamine ligands also increased cell proliferation, focus formation and tumorigenicity in nude mice. The ability of the mutant receptor to produce the same second messenger, thereby implicating the same signaling pathway, without requirement for ligand confirms the importance of this signal pathway in tumorigenesis. Production of inositol phosphates by the seven transmembrane α-1B adrenergic receptor is stimulated through G protein intermediates. The generation of the inositol phosphates through phospholipase C-β action secondarily causes release of calcium from intracellular stores and stimulates calcium influx.

The muscarinic receptor family of acetylcholine receptors has been used for similar studies. The family consists of five receptor subtypes of which the odd-numbered and even-numbered have similar but independent signaling footprints [38,39]. Upon stimulation, the odd-numbered muscarinic receptors (m1, m3, m5) result in the production of cAMP, generation of inositol phosphates, release of arachidonic acid, tyrosine phosphorylation and mobilization of calcium from extracellular and intracellular stores [9,10,39]. Placement of the odd-numbered muscarinic receptors into NIH-3T3 cells and subsequent stimulation with a stable acetylcholine analog, carbachol, resulted in focus formation in culture [40]. Functional receptor stimulation of phospholipase C-β (PLC-β) with resultant formation of IP3 and stimulation of increase in intracellular calcium was demonstrated, as was release of arachidonic acid. The release of arachidonic acid has been shown previously to require influx of extracellular calcium [10]. All of these transfection experiments have in common the activation of calcium stimulating or calcium mediated signaling pathways.

26.3.4 RECEPTOR MEDIATED INHIBITION OF TUMORIGENESIS

In contrast, when a similar approach was taken using a different cell substrate, opposite effects were demonstrated. We have studied the behavior of the odd-numbered muscarinic receptors after stable transfection into Chinese hamster ovary cells. The parental cell line as well as the transfected cells are very pleomorphic in culture with a rapid growth rate and an epithelioid morphology [39]. These cells readily form tumors at the site of subcutaneous inoculation in nude mice. When the m5 receptor was activated by carbachol, the morphology of the cell monolayer changed dramatically. Agonist stimulation resulted in a morphological change from pleomorphic and disordered to fibroblastoid with smaller nuclei and orderly organization. In addition, cells demonstrated a density dependent growth pattern and had poor colony forming capacity in soft agar [39]. Application of carbachol to CHOm5 cell inoculation site of nude mice prevented tumor formation, demonstrating that the morphological differentiation observed *in vitro* translated into a non-tumorigenic phenotype *in vivo*. Though carbachol stimulation of the muscarinic receptor results in activation of many effector systems including ion channel activation [10], G protein mediated events (IP3) and phosphorylation [13], the differentiation behavior correlated with receptor stimulated calcium influx directly [39]. CAI, an inhibitor of receptor operated calcium influx to be discussed in more detail below, confirmed the role of calcium by reversing the fibroblastoid morphology caused by carbachol as it inhibited carbachol stimulated calcium influx [39].

26.4 SIGNALING IN INVASION AND METASTASIS

The process of invasion and metastasis is a complex one which can be broken down into component parts, including angiogenesis, adhesion, proteolysis and migration (Figure 26.1) [41]. Angiogenesis, the process of new blood vessel formation, occurs physiologically during pregnancy, menstruation, development and growth and wound healing [42]. It is a crucial component of cancer progression and metastasis. The process of tumor cell adhesion is important in several ways. First, cell–cell interactions are involved in maintenance of tissue organization and integrity. Secondly, tumor cells must adhere to endothelial cell basement membrane during intravasation and to endothelial cells and their underlying basement membrane during extravasation at secondary sites [41]. The process of entrance and exit from the vascular conduits is an active one in which local basement membrane degradation occurs. Several classes of proteinases have been shown to be important in the process of invasion. These include the neutral metalloproteinases, such as the type IV collagenase (MMP-2) [43], cysteine proteinases (cathepsin D and L) [44] and serine proteinases (urokinase and tissue plasminogen activator) [45]. The final component is the ability of tumor cells to migrate from the primary sites and into the secondary sites where proliferation ensues to produce the metastatic focus. Tumor cells migrate in response to growth factors and extracellular matrix proteins and ECM protein fragments. Recent investigations have probed the signal regulation of these components of invasion and metastasis.

Many classes of adhesion molecules have been described. The integrin transmembrane receptors can mediate adhesion of normal and malignant cells [32]. Extracellular matrix protein receptors, such as the family of laminin receptors, provide anchoring between cells and basement membrane. Cell adhesion molecules, CAMs, are a broad family of related molecules including L-CAM (liver), N-cadherin (neural), P-cadherin (placental) and E-cadherin (epithelial, formerly called uvomorulin) [46]. These adhesion molecules have been conserved in nature and have roles in normal growth and development. They are calcium dependent for their normal action of cell sorting, cell polarity and tissue morphology [46]. CAMS are very specific in their activity and have only homophilic interactions [46]. They are associated with the cell cytoskeleton through associated proteins and calcium. The signaling mediated by CAMs has not yet been fully characterized; other than the requirement for calcium, only tyrosine phosphorylation has been demonstrated.

E-cadherin is critical in the process of invasion and metastasis, where it has been shown to play a suppressor role [47,48]. A highly metastatic ovarian cancer cell line had very low amounts of E-cadherin expression when compared with the less metastatic control cell line [46]. In breast cancer tissues, a significant correlation was found between decreased E-cadherin expression and aggressive behavior [48]. The importance of calcium in the metastasis suppressor function of the E-cadherin complex was demonstrated by Shimoyama and coworkers [49]. They demonstrated that normal E-cadherin was present in a lung cancer cell line; however, the expression of α-catenin, the calcium binding link between E-cadherin and the cytoskeleton, was reduced. This resulted in decreased cell–cell adhesiveness.

Proteolysis is the next step in tumor cell invasion. It is also required for wound healing, tissue remodeling, angiogenesis and normal growth and development. The neutral metalloproteinases are zinc metal ion requiring enzymes [50]. Laboratory assays use calcium for renaturation and activation of enzyme activity [20]. Transforming growth factor-β has been shown to upregulate transcription of MMP-2 type IV collagenase in tumor cells as well as increase the amount of activated MMP-2 [20]. Thrombin and urokinase plasminogen activator also have been shown to regulate activation of the MMP-2 [51]. The thrombin receptor is a seven trans-

membrane domain receptor of the G protein family. Signal events mediated through the thrombin receptor include calcium mobilization, tyrosine phosphorylation and production of inositol phosphates [15]. Which of these signal pathways of thrombin mediates activation of MMP-2 has not yet been elucidated.

Migration is the final requirement for invasion and metastasis of tumor cells [52]. Laboratory studies have shown that different tumor cell lines may still respond to the same chemoattractants [17]. Several signal transduction pathways have been linked to tumor cell migration due to these different families of attractants. Lester and colleagues investigated the prevalence of G protein α subunits in highly and minimally metastatic B16 melanoma sublines [53]. They demonstrated increased pertussis toxin substrate in the highly invasive cell line and identified that substrate as the Giα2 or Gα2i subunit. They correlated this observation with pertussis toxin mediated decrease in chemoinvasion using the Matrigel assay and decrease in chemotaxis to fibronectin, laminin and type IV collagen. The specific second messenger transduced through the Giα2 or Gα2i subunit in this model system has not been elucidated.

The A2058 human melanoma cell line secretes novel motility stimulating factors, autocrine motility factor (AMF) [54] and autotaxin [55]. Migration to both is inhibited by cellular treatment with pertussis toxin, indicating the involvement of a G protein signal pathway [55,56]. AMF was shown to stimulate inositol trisphosphate production [57] and calcium mobilization (Kohn, unpublished results). Tumor cell migration to AMF is inhibited by cell treatment with CAI (see below) and voltage gated calcium channel blockers such as verapamil and diltiazem (Kohn, unpublished results). These results indicate the importance of calcium in the process of tumor cell migration to AMF. In contrast, Evans and coworkers [58] identified an AMF-like attractant activity in the conditioned media of rat prostate adenocarcinoma cells. This chemoattractant was inhibited by cholera toxin, which inhibits GTP-ase activity of the G protein α subunit and creates a constitutively 'on' effector. Cholera toxin has been linked primarily with stimulation of cAMP production. Evans *et al.* showed that forskolin, which stimulates cAMP production directly, also inhibited migration in response to the prostate AMF [58]. These results demonstrate the variability in signaling pathways which mediate the same end function.

Pertussis toxin treatment of the A2058 cells also inhibited migration to laminin and type IV collagen but not to fibronectin [18]. Further studies showed that type IV collagen stimulated intracellular release of calcium in a pertussis toxin independent fashion. Blockade of this intracellular release of calcium inhibited tumor cell migration [33], further strengthening the link between calcium and migration. Pertussis toxin treatment of these cells did not inhibit migration to the insulin polypeptide growth factor family [17]. This expected difference demonstrates that tumor cell migration is a multifactorial process which is mediated through multiple chemoattractants and multiple signal transduction pathways.

The complex process of invasion and metastasis is a coordinated effort of many different cell functions including those of the malignant cells, endothelial cells and stromal cells. While these functions are disparate, the requirement for calcium is a common intermediate for many and as more is understood about these processes, its importance may become more widespread.

26.5 IDENTIFICATION AND INVESTIGATION OF CAI

The understanding that both extracellular and intracellular calcium play important roles in the process of invasion and metastasis led us to search for novel agents which would affect invasion and metastasis through modulation of cellular calcium. This approach was two-pronged, using biological assays of tumor cell adhesion to plastic and extracellular matrix substrata, stimulated motility and proliferation assays *in vitro*, in combination with evaluation of the effects of calcium on these biological parameters and direct analysis of cellular calcium fluxes. In the initial screening using biological assays, over 25 different compounds were evaluated. These compounds included known agents such as indomethacin and isoniazid and novel compounds which had been submitted for our evaluation. Of these many compounds, CAI was distinguished as the most potent in all of the parameters tested [59]. CAI is a small molecular weight, hydrophobic compound with limitations of aqueous solubility. It has a steep dose–response curve in its inhibition of adhesion, migration and proliferation.

As discussed above, three important criteria must be met in the evaluation of CAI for clinical use. These three, efficacy, toxicity, and selectivity, are especially important in the signal transduction therapy category. This is because of the ubiquitous presence of the same signaling pathways in normal cells and malignant cells.

26.5.1 EFFICACY

Initial screening for activity consisted of tumor cell migration assays. The chemoattractant ligands used were autocrine motility factor [17,54], type IV collagen (Kohn, unpublished results) and insulin like growth factor-I (IGF-I) [17,60]. Adhesion to tissue culture plastic [60] and extracellular matrix components such as type IV collagen and laminin were also tested. The A2058 human melanoma cell line and OVCAR3 human ovarian cancer cell lines were used most commonly. In these experiments, CAI was effective in the inhibition of motility and adhesion in the concentration range of 1–10 μM. A notable exception was the lack of inhibition of motility stimulated by IGF-I; this was expected as IGF-I transduces its signals through tyrosine phosphorylation [24]. Inhibition was demonstrated with as little as one hour of pretreatment with CAI, but appeared optimal with longer exposures. The results with the OVCAR3 line confirmed the observations with the A2058 cell line with inhibition of migration to laminin and autocrine motility factor of up to 80% and 50% respectively, given concentrations of CAI of 2 μM. OVCAR3 adhesion to tissue culture plastic was similarly inhibited over 75% in the same concentration range (Kohn, unpublished results).

The ability of CAI to inhibit proliferation *in vitro* was studied using an array of human cancer cell lines (Table 26.2). Growth inhibition was demonstrated using two techniques, nuclear staining as a measure of total cell number and measurement of DNA synthesis with tritiated thymidine incorporation. In the concentration range 1–10 μM, CAI inhibited proliferation over 80% of control growth for all human tumor cell lines tested. Similar striking results were seen when colony forming assays in soft agar were done. CAI inhibited colony formation in soft agar of A2058, OVCAR3 and CHOm5 cells by 75% to greater than 95% at 20 μM. The inhibitory concentration at 50% (IC50) for inhibition of proliferation for all cell lines was in the range of 1 μM [61]. These data indicated efficacy of CAI in *in vitro* models of invasion, metastasis and proliferation.

Experiments to demonstrate efficacy *in vivo* and for preliminary determination of toxicity were done using human xenograft models of melanoma and ovarian cancer with the A2058 cell line and OVCAR3 cell lines respectively [61]. CAI was administered orally by gavage in solution in PEG-400 vehicle. The results indicated that oral administration of CAI inhibited the growth and metastatic capacity of OVCAR3 xenografts in nude mice with

Table 26.2 Human cell lines growth inhibited by CAI treatment [61,62]

Cell line	Tumor type/site
MCF-7	Breast
MDA-231	Breast
HT-29	Colon
WIDR	Colon
OVCAR3	Ovary
OVCAR4	Ovary
PC-3	Prostate
PANC-1	Pancreas
T24	Bladder
RD	Rhabdomyosarcoma
HuT78	Mycosis fungoides
RPMI 8226	Plasmacytoma
UMSSC38	Squamous cell carcinoma of head and neck
H4	Neuroglioma
A172	Glioblastoma

decrease in tumor size, ascites volume and metastatic dissemination [61]. It arrested growth and inhibited tumor development of subcutaneously inoculated A2058 cells. Oral administration of CAI resulted in measurable plasma levels of CAI in mice in the range of 1–10 μM. These plasma levels were in the potentially therapeutic range identified by the studies of proliferation and invasion and metastasis. Observation of the mice over 30–40 days of oral CAI administration and at both gross and histological examination of necropsy revealed no overt toxicity of CAI.

26.5.2 TOXICITY

Preclinical evaluation was done in collaboration with the Developmental Therapeutics Program of the National Cancer Institute. The formulation, pharmacokinetics and toxicity of CAI were studied in three species of laboratory animals. Intravenous formulation of CAI in cremophor/ethanol, as is used for taxol, was feasible for bioavailability testing. However, it was not felt to be usable for clinical trial. An oral formulation of CAI in PEG-400 was necessary due to its considerable hydrophobicity. A long primary half life was found after oral administration of CAI in PEG-400 to mice, rats and dogs, suggesting that administration could be attempted daily, every other day and weekly. In toxicity experiments using twice daily, every day and weekly schedules, minor weight loss and emesis was seen in vehicle treated and CAI treated dogs. No other gross or histological evidence of toxicity was seen. In several dogs receiving twice daily dosing, especially at high dose, wobbly gait was seen and one dog had convulsions. No CAI was demonstrable in the cerebrospinal fluid, nor were gross or histological changes seen in the neuraxis. However, because of this toxicity, it is recommended that CAI be administered no more often than daily.

26.5.3 SELECTIVITY AND SPECIFICITY

Concomitant to preclinical toxicity and efficacy studies, the question of selectivity of signal transduction pathways was investigated. For these experiments, the well-characterized muscarinic receptor system was chosen and used in stably transfected CHO cell systems [39]. Stimulation of these receptors with the agonist carbachol in odd-numbered receptor bearing cells resulted in calcium influx, calcium requiring release of arachidonic acid and tyrosine phosphorylation and subsequent production of IP3 from both calcium sensitive and calcium insensitive PLC isozymes [39]. Simultaneous addition of CAI with carbachol inhibited calcium influx, arachidonic acid release and tyrosine phosphorylation with activation of phospholipase C-γ, without inhibition of generation of IP3 from calcium insensitive PLC-β or production of cAMP [62]. As a control, the even-numbered muscarinic receptors were studied. These receptors upon stimulation inhibit production of cAMP, but no calcium mobilization, arachidonic acid release or generation of IP3 [10]. CAI did not affect the even-numbered receptor effects on cAMP [62]. These results strongly suggest that there is selectivity of CAI for the signal transduction pathway target of calcium influx. Further experiments with molecular analogs of CAI have confirmed the selectivity of the effects of CAI [63].

26.5.4 PHASE I CLINICAL TRIAL OF CAI

A new drug investigation application for CAI was approved in January 1992 and the phase I clinical trial opened to accrual in March of that year. To date we have completed three dose escalation levels and have treated 16 patients. The only reproducible toxicity demonstrated to date is grade 1 mild nausea and rare vomiting. Both symptoms were readily treated with standard antiemetics. CAI plasma levels have been measurable in all patients as early as one hour after the first dose. An accurate and sensitive HPLC assay was developed for quantitation of CAI in patient plasma. Patient blood levels have routinely been in the range targeted by the laboratory and preclinical studies of 1–10 μM.

26.6 CONCLUSION

A new concept, signal transduction therapy, has been proposed and confirmed using modulation of calcium homeostasis as the target. Three obstacles to this approach were identified as efficacy, toxicity, and specificity and were overcome. This new paradigm for cancer treatment uses a novel biochemical target aimed to produce a cytostatic effect and biomodulation. This modulation of key signaling pathways upon which cancer cells may be more heavily dependent offers a method by which cancer proliferation and metastasis may be interrupted at early stages and potentially, with minimal toxicity.

REFERENCES

1. Spiegel, A. (1988) G proteins in clinical medicine. *Hosp. Pract.*, **June**, 93–111.
2. Rink, T.J. (1990) Receptor-mediated calcium entry. *FEBS Lett.*, **268**, 381–5.
3. Bean, B.P. (1989) Classes of calcium channels in vertebrate cells. *Ann. Rev. Physiol.*, **51**, 367–84.
4. Simon, M.I., Strathmann, M.P., and Gautam, N. (1991) Diversity of G proteins in signal transduction. *Science*, **252**, 802–8.
5. Aaronson, S.A. (1991) Growth factors and cancer. *Science*, **254**, 1146–53.
6. Tanaabe, T., Tadeshima, H., Mikami, A. *et al.* (1987) Primary structure of the receptor for calcium-channel blockers from skeletal muscle. *Nature*, **328**, 313–18.
7. Zernig, G. (1990) Widening potiential for Ca^{2+} antagonists: non-L-type Ca^{2+} channel interaction. *TiPS*, **11**, 38–44.
8. Kim, D., Lewis, D.L., Graziafei, L. *et al.* (1989) G-protein $\beta\gamma$-subunits activate the cardiac muscarinic K^+-channel via phospholipase A2. *Nature*, **337**, 557–60.
9. Brooks, R.C., McCarthy, K.D., Lapetina, E.G. and Morell, P. (1989) Receptor-stimulated phospholipase A2 activation is coupled to influx of external calcium and not to mobilization of intracellular calcium in C62B glioma cells. *J. Biol. Chem.*, **264**, 20147–53.
10. Felder, C.C., Dieter, P., Kinsella, J. *et al.* (1990) A transfected m5 muscarinic acetylcholine receptor stimulates phospholipse A2 by inducing both calcium influx and activation of protein kinase C. *J. Pharm. Exp. Ther.*, **255**, 1140–7.
11. Marks, P.W., and Maxfield, F.R. (1990) Transient increases in cytosolic free calcium appear to be required for the migration of adherent human neutrophils. *J. Cell. Biol.*, **110**, 43–52.
12. Hamachi, T., Hirata, M. and Koga, T. (1986) Origin of intracellular calcium and quantitation of mobilizable calcium in neutrophils stimulated with chemotactic peptide. *Biochem. Biophys. Acta*, **889**, 136–48.
13. Gusovsky, F., Leuders, J.E., Kohn, E.C. and Felder, C.C. (1993) Muscarinic receptor-mediated tyrosine phosphorylation of phospholipase C-gamma: alternative mechanism for cholinergic receptor-induced phosphoinositide breakdown. *J. Biol. Chem.*, **268**, 7768–72.
14. Bianchini, L., Todderud, G. and Grinstein, S. (1993) Cytosolic [Ca2+] homeostasis and tyrosine phosphorylation of phospholipase Cgamma2 in HL60 granulocytes. *J. Biol. Chem.*, **268**, 3357–63.
15. Tanaguchi, T., Kitagawea, H., Yasue, S. *et al.* (1993) Protein-tyrosine kinase p72^{syk} is activated by thrombin and is negatively regulated through Ca2+ regulation in platelets. *J. Biol. Chem.*, **268**, 2277–9.
16. Guirguis, R., Margulies, I., Taraboletti, G. *et al.* (1987) Cytokine-induced pseudopodial protrusion is coupled to tumor cell migration. *Nature*, **329**, 261–3.
17. Kohn, E.C., Francis, E.A., Liotta, L.A. and Schiffmann, E. (1990) Heterogeneity of the motility responses in malignant tumor cells: a biological basis for the diversity and homing of metastatic cells. *Int. J. Cancer*, **46**, 287–92.
18. Aznavoorian, S.A., Stracke, M.L., Krutzsch, H. *et al.* (1990) Signal transduction for chemotaxis and haptotaxis by matrix molecules in tumor cells. *J. Cell. Biol.*, **110**, 1427–38.
19. Bar-Sagi, D. and Feramisco, J.R. (1986) Induction of membrane ruffling and fluid-phase pinocytosis in quiescent fibroblasts by ras proteins. *Science*, **233**, 1061–8.
20. Brown, P.D., Levy, A.T., Margulies, I.M.K. *et al.* (1990) Independent expression and cellular processing of Mr 72,000 type IV collagenase and interstitial collagenase in human tumorigenic cell lines. *Cancer Res.*, **50**, 6184–91.
21. Ojcius, D.M., Zychlinsky, A., Zheng, L.M. and Young, J.D.E. (1991) Ionophore-induced apoptosis: role of DNA fragmentation and calcium fluxes. *Exp. Cell. Res.*, **197**, 43–9.
22. Klee, C.B. (1988) Ca2+-dependent phospholipid- (and membrane-) binding proteins. *Biochemistry*, **27**, 6645–53.
23. Kojima, I., Matsunaga, H., Kurokawa, K. *et al.* (1988) Calcium influx: an intracellular message of the mitogenic action of insulin-like growth factor-I. *J. Biol. Chem.*, **263**, 16561–7.
24. Kadowski, T., Koyasu, S., Nishida, E. *et al.* (1987) Tyrosine phosphorylation of common

and specific sets of cellular proteins rapidly induced by insulin, insulin-like growth factor I, and epidermal growth factor in an intact cell. *J. Biol. Chem.*, **262**, 7342–50.

25. Nishibe, S., Wahl, M.I., Hernández-Sotomayor, S.M.T. *et al.* (1990) Increase of the catalytic activity of phospholipase C-γ1 by tyrosine phosphorylation. *Science*, **250**, 1253–6.

26. Kim, H.K., Kim, J.W., Zilberstein, A. *et al.* (1991) PDGF stimulation of inositol phospholipid hydrolysis requires PLC-gamma1 phosphorylation on tyrosine residues 783 and 1254. *Cell*, **65**, 435–41.

27. Wahl, M.I., Nishibe, S., Suh, P.G. *et al.* (1989) Epidermal growth factor stimulates tyrosine phosphorylation of phospholipase C-II independently of receptor internalization and extracellular calcium. *Proc. Natl Acad. Sci. USA*, **86**, 1568–72.

28. Kurachi, H., Morishige, K., Amemiya, K. *et al.* (1991) Importance of transforming growth factor alpha/epidermal growth factor receptor autocrine growth mechanism in an ovarian cancer cell line *in vivo*. *Cancer Res.*, **51**, 5956–9.

29. Blay, J. and Brown, K.D. (1985) Epidermal growth factor promotes chemotactic migration of cultured rat intestinal epithelial cells. *J. Cell. Physiol.*, **124**, 107–12.

30. Berchuck, A., Kamel, A., Whitaker, R. *et al.* (1990) Overexpression of HER-2/neu is associated with poor survival in advanced epithelial ovarian cancer. *Cancer Res.*, **50**, 4087–91.

31. Kornberg, L.J., Earp, H.S., Turner, C.E. *et al.* (1991) Signal transduction by integrins: increased protein tyrosine phosphorylation caused by clustering of β1 integrins. *Proc. Natl Acad. Sci. USA*, **88**, 8392–6.

32. Hynes, R.O. (1992) Integrins: versatility, modulation, and signaling in cell adhesion. *Cell*, **69**, 11–25.

33. Savarese, D.M.F., Russel, J.T., Fatatis, A. and Liotta, L.A. (1992) Type IV collagen stimulates an increase in intracellular calcium: potential role in tumor cell motility. *J. Biol. Chem.*, **267**, 21928–35.

34. McCarthy, J.B., Hagen, S.T. and Furcht, L.T. (1986) Human fibronectin contains distinct adhesion and motility-promoting domains for metastatic melanoma cells. *J. Cell. Biol.*, **102**, 179–88.

35. Jaconi, M.E.E., Theler, J.M., Schlegel, W. *et al.* (1991) Multiple elevations in cytosolic-free Ca2+ in human neutrophils: initiation by adherence receptors of the integrin family. *J. Cell. Biol.*, **112**, 1249–57.

36. Julius, D., Livelli, T.J., Jessell, T.M. and Axel, R. (1989) Ectopic expression of the serotonin 1c receptor and the triggering of malignant transformation. *Science*, **244**, 1057–62.

37. Allen, L.F., Lefkowitz, R.J., Caron, M.G. and Cotecchia, S. (1991) G-protein-coupled receptor genes as protooncogenes: constitutively activating mutation of the alpha1B-adrenergic receptor enhances mitogenesis and tumorigenicity. *Proc. Natl Acad. Sci. USA*, **88**, 11354–8.

38. Bonner, T.I. (1989) The molecular basis of muscarinic receptor diversity. *TINS*, **12**, 148–51.

39. Felder, C.C., MacArthur, L., Ma A.L. *et al.* (1993) Tumor-suppressor function of muscarinic acetylcholine receptors is associated with activation of receptor-operated calcium influx. *Proc. Natl Acad. Sci. USA*, **90**, 1706–10.

40. Gutkind, J.S., Novotny, E.A., Brann, M.R., and Robbins, K.C. (1991) Muscarinic acetylcholine receptor subtypes as agonist-dependent oncogenes. *Proc. Natl Acad. Sci. USA*, **88**, 4703–7.

41. Liotta, L.A. (1986) Tumor invasion and metastases – role of the extracellular matrix. *Cancer Res.*, **46**, 1–7.

42. Furcht, L.T. (1986) Critical factors controlling angiogenesis: cell products, cell matrix, and growth factors. *Lab. Invest.*, **55**, 505–9.

43. Liotta, L.A., Steeg, P.S. and Stetler-Stevenson, W.G. (1991) Cancer metastasis and angiogenesis; an imbalance of positive and negative regulation. *Cell*, **64**, 327–36.

44. Tandon, A.K., Clark, G.M., Chamness, G.C. *et al.* (1990) Cathepsin-D and prognosis in breast cancer. *N. Engl. J. Med.*, **322**, 297–302.

45. Hollas, W., Blasi, F. and Boyd, D. (1991) Role of urokinase receptor in facilitating extracellular matrix invasion by cultured colon cancer. *Cancer Res.*, **51**, 3690–5.

46. Takeichi, M. (1991) Cadherin cell adhesion receptors as a morphogenetic regulator. *Science*, **251**, 1451–5.

47. Vleminck, K., Vakaet, L., Mareel, M. *et al.* (1991) Genetic manipulation of E-cadherin expression by epithelial tumor cells reveals an invasion suppressor role. *Cell*, **66**, 107–19.

48. Oka, H., Shiozaki, H., Kobayashi, K. *et al.* (1993) Expression of E-cadherin cell adhesion molecules in human breast cancer tissues and its relationship to metastasis. *Cancer Res.*, **53**, 1696–701.

49. Shimoyama, Y., Nagafuchi, A., Fujita, S. *et al.* (1992) Cadherin dysfunction in a human cancer cell line: possible involvement of loss of alpha-catenin expression in reduced cell–cell adhesiveness. *Cancer Res.*, **52**, 5770–4.

50. Stetler-Stevenson, W., Krutzsch, H.C., Wacher, M.P. *et al.* (1989) The activation of human type IV collagenase proenzyme. *J. Biol. Chem.*, **264**, 1353–6.

51. Keski-Oja, J., Lohi, J., Tuuttila, A. *et al.* (1992) Proteolytic processing of the 72,000 Da type IV collagenase by urokinase plasminogen activator. *Exp. Cell. Res.*, **202**, 471–6.

52. Stossel, T.P. (1989) From signal to pseudopod. *J. Biol. Chem.*, **264**, 18261–4.

53. Lester, B.R., McCarthy, J.B., Sun, Z. *et al.* (1989) G-protein involvement in matrix-mediated motility and invasion of high and low experimental metastatic B16 melanoma clones. *Cancer Res.*, **49**, 5940–8.

54. Liotta, L.A., Mandler, R., Murano, G. *et al.* (1986) Tumor cell autocrine motility factor. *Proc. Natl Acad. Sci. USA*, **83**, 3302–6.

55. Stracke, M.L., Krutzsch, H.C., Unsworth, E.J. *et al.* (1992) Identification, purification, and partial sequence analysis of autotaxin, a novel motility-stimulating protein. *J. Biol. Chem.*, **267**, 2524–9.

56. Stracke, M.L., Guirguis, R., Liotta, L.A. and Schiffmann, E. (1987) Pertussis toxin inhibits stimulated motility independently of the adenylate cyclase pathway in human melanoma cells. *Biochem. Biophys. Res. Commun.*, **146**, 339–45.

57. Kohn, E.C., Liotta, L.A. and Schiffmann, E. (1990) Autocrine motility factor stimulates a three-fold increase in inositol trisphosphate in human melanoma cells. *Biochem. Biophys. Res. Commun.*, **166**, 757–64.

58. Evans, C.P., Walsh, D.S., and Kohn, E.C. (1991) An autocrine motility factor secreted by the Dunning R-3327 rat prostatic adenocarcinoma cell subtype AT2.1. *Int. J. Cancer*, **49**, 109–13.

59. Bochis, R., Chabala, J.C. and Fisher, M.H. 5-amino or substituted amino 1,2,3-triazoles. US Patent 4,590,201, May 1986.

60. Kohn, E.C. and Liotta, L.A. (1990) L651582, a novel antiproliferative and antimetastasis agent. *J. Natl Cancer Inst.*, **82**, 54–60.

61. Kohn, E.C., Sandeen, M.A. and Liotta, L.A. (1992) *In vivo* efficacy of a novel inhibitor of selected signal transduction pathways including calcium, arachidonate, and inositol phosphates. *Cancer Res.*, **52**, 3208–12.

62. Felder, C.C., Ma A.L., Liotta, L.A. and Kohn, E.C. (1991) The antiproliferative and antimetastatic compound L6511582 inhibits muscarinic acetylcholine receptor-stimulated calcium influx and arachidonic acid release. *J. Pharm. Exp. Ther.*, **257**, 967–71.

63. Kohn, E.C., Felder, C.C., Jacobs, W. *et al.* (1994) Structure–function analysis of signal and growth inhibition by carboxyamido-triazole, CAI. *Cancer Res.*, **54**, 935–42.

Chapter 27

Radiotherapy as salvage or consolidation therapy in advanced epithelial ovarian cancer

G.M. THOMAS

27.1 INTRODUCTION

Survival results after treatment of advanced epithelial ovarian cancer are disappointing. While cisplatin alone or in combination produces response rates of approximately 60–80% in advanced disease, the initial optimism that overall cure rates in ovarian cancer would be substantially improved has not been fulfilled. The duration of relapse-free time has been increased over that achieved with single agent alkylating agents, but only 5–10% more patients are long term disease-free survivors [1]. Overall cure rates in advanced disease remain about 20–30% [2–4]. One strategy that has been generally pursued in improving treatment outcomes in solid tumours has been to attempt to combine effective therapies sequentially or concurrently, particularly if their toxicities are non-overlapping.

Whole abdominal and pelvic radiotherapy has been shown to be curative in certain subsets of patients with optimal disease (Figure 27.1) [5]. As a consequence of the recognition of the relative effectiveness of surgery, chemotherapy and radiation in reducing tumour burden, it is reasonable to investigate the possible advantage of combinations of therapy in advanced disease. Fuks

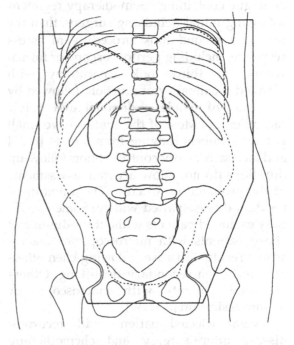

Figure 27.1 Line drawing from a simulator radiograph showing the treatment volume for abdominopelvic radiotherapy. A generous margin is allowed between the treatment field edges and the peritoneum, indicated by a dotted line. Note that the field extends outside the iliac crests. The kidney shielding is from the posterior to keep the renal dose between 1800 and 2000 cGy. The pelvic boost field is not shown. This is the posterior (prone) projection.

271

and coworkers have reviewed the rationale for sequential chemotherapy, secondary explorative and cytoreductive surgery and radiotherapy in advanced ovarian cancer in the platinum chemotherapy era [6].

27.2 OVERVIEW OF STUDIES IN THE LITERATURE

Sequential multimodality therapy has been used by many. Twenty-eight studies have currently been identified in the literature [6–33]. Twenty-four are single arm studies [11–33]. The common features of these studies are the use of mainly platinum or platinum analogue containing chemotherapy regimens following initial debulking surgery, then the use of a second look procedure to assess response, including peritoneoscopy or formal second or third look laparotomy with planned maximal cytoreduction, followed by a course of whole abdominal and pelvic radiotherapy. Most of the studies have small patient numbers ranging from 8 to 44 [6–33] and lack satisfactory controls. Short follow-up durations do not allow accurate assessments of the probabilities of cure. The amounts of residual disease varied widely. Some specifically excluded patients without residuum and chose patients with microscopic or macroscopic residual disease following chemotherapy and even secondary debulking. Others excluded patients with macroscopic or >5 mm residuum [8,11,30].

Several selected patients with recurrent disease after surgery and chemotherapy [12,14,15,19,22–24,33]. The chemotherapy regimens employed were probably the standard regimens employed at the various institutes over the years of reporting. Many patients received prolonged chemotherapy initially, one series reporting treatment with up to 28 courses of cyclophosphamide and platinum [32] and most series reporting 6–12 courses of therapy with some using second line chemo-

therapy after first line failure [13]. Some patients were known to be resistant to their induction chemotherapy. It is unclear in many of these studies whether salvage radiotherapy had been a part of the initial therapeutic plan.

The most common radiation technique employed is open field irradiation of the whole abdomen and pelvis, although some were treated with the moving strip technique [29] and others were treated with split-field techniques where the abdomen was radiated sequentially in sections rather than with an open beam [14,20,25]. Generally, the planned whole abdominal radiation dose varied between 20 Gy [27] and 30 Gy [14,24,25,32]. The majority of studies used a routine boost to the pelvis to bring the pelvic dose to 45 or 50 Gy regardless of the site of residuum. The use of the pelvic boost is presumably a direct extrapolation from its standard use where radiotherapy is the sole postoperative treatment. Several also employed a boost to the para-aortic nodes [6,17,18].

The results of these studies have been interpreted by the various investigators as positive (Table 27.1), negative or equivocal for a survival benefit. The volume of residual disease, prior to initial chemotherapy, is unclear in many of the reviewed series. While data are incomplete on the extent of disease prior to radiation therapy, many series did allow categorization of patients into three broad groups: zero residuum, microscopic or <5 mm and macroscopic or >5 mm (Table 27.1). From these data it is possible to broadly examine the outcome by the amount of disease residuum prior to radiation therapy. Table 27.2 shows a summary of the 28 available literature series, both randomized and non-randomized, for 713 patients. For those with no residuum, the disease-free survival, at variable times after treatment, was 76% (86 of 113), for those with microscopic or <5 mm residuum 49% (77 out of 158) and for greater than microscopic residuum 17% (34 of 202).

Table 27.1 Survival results reporting benefit for sequential therapy in patients with zero or microscopic residual disease prior to radiation therapy

Author	Number surviving/ number at risk	
	Zero residuum	Microscopic or <5 mm
Chiara *et al.* [12]	6/9	5/11
Greiner *et al.* [15]	14/15	5/9*
Reddy *et al.* [19]	–	4/5
Kuten *et al.* [20]	5/5	12/18
Solomon *et al.* [22]	–	4/12
Kong *et al.* [23]	–	3/5
Rosen *et al.* [24]	4/4	3/4
Haie *et al.* [26]	14/23	–
Kersh *et al.* [28]	1/4	10/15
Goldhirsch *et al.* [29]	19/24	–
Menczer *et al.* [31]	9/10**	–
Morgan *et al.* [32]	–	8/8*

* <1 cm residuum
** Result interpreted as negative by authors

Table 27.2 Survival following sequential surgery, chemotherapy and whole abdominopelvic radiation therapy appears dependent on tumour residuum prior to radiation. Data extracted from 28 literature series containing 713 patients, of which 473 had sufficient information to estimate residum

No residuum	Microscopic or <5 mm	Macroscopic
76% (86/113)	49% (77/158)	17% (34/202)

Most studies provided some data on the observed toxicity of combined therapy, specifically addressing the questions of bone marrow toxicity and resultant delays or incompletion of the planned radiation therapy. Some report negligible toxicities, with no significant delays or failures to complete radiation therapy [22,26,29,31–33]. Others report significant therapy delays and inability to complete radiation therapy in up to 60% of patients [11,13–15,18,24]. Throm-

bocytopenia was the predominant reason for failure to complete therapy, but leukopenia was also a problem in some series. The incidence of bowel obstruction was variable. In 13 series, bowel obstruction occurred in less than 10% of patients [7,8,12,16,20,22,24,26,28, 29–33,39] whereas in a small number of series, obstruction occurred in 30–75% of patients [11,14,18,21].

Four randomized studies have been performed [7–10]; two have appeared only as abstracts with relatively short follow-up times. Each was designed to examine the role of consolidative radiotherapy versus continued chemotherapy with the same or different agents to those used for induction. The consolidative chemotherapy regimens in each study were respectively chlorambucil [10], carboplatin [8], platinum and epirubicin [9] and platinum, cyclophosphamide with or without adriamycin, or carboplatin, adriamycin, cyclosphosphamide [7]. Each of the studies selected patients with residual disease after chemotherapy and none appeared to intentionally include those with no residuum after chemotherapy. One study described disease as being of minimum residuum but in fact included patients with >2 cm residual disease [9]. The study of Lawton *et al.* included only patients who had residual disease after chemotherapy but in some complete secondary surgical debulking was accomplished prior to the consolidative therapy [10]. The numbers of evaluable patients on the randomized portion of these studies were small (from 25 to 58 patients). Two studies suggest that radiation is inferior to continued chemotherapy when persistent disease is found at second look surgery [7,9] and the two larger studies suggest that abdominopelvic irradiation and chemotherapy, using either carboplatin [8] or chlorambucil [10], were equivalent. Since none of these studies had a 'no treatment' arm, it is impossible to determine whether the addition of either consolidative radiotherapy or chemotherapy provided additional benefit over that achieved with standard surgery and induction chemotherapy alone.

27.3 DISCUSSION

It is disappointing that, although a large number of patients (713 in 28 literature series) have been treated with multimodality therapy including salvage consolidation therapy, it is impossible to reach a definitive conclusion about the value of such a strategy. Overall, the balance of evidence is against a significant curative benefit for radiotherapy as salvage or consolidation therapy, at least in the situations where it has been used. Because of the diversity of criteria for patient selection and the variability in the chemotherapy, surgery and radiation employed, sweeping generalizations about the results of these trials should be interpreted with caution. However, it is important to consider the possible causes of treatment failure in order to guide the design of future studies which may examine the role of salvage radiotherapy in epithelial ovarian cancer.

27.3.1 PATIENT SELECTION

The first is inappropriate patient selection based on large volume residuum. Many studies are flawed because patients had macroscopic residual abdominal disease [10,13,14,18,19,24,28,32]. The 17% survival (Table 27.1) of those with greater than microscopic disease is probably no different to that achieved with primary surgery and chemotherapy. It suggests that salvage radiotherapy is inappropriate for most patients with disease residuum which is in excess of microscopic after chemotherapy.

However, the overall disease-free survival of 76% and 49% for those without residual disease and with microscopic disease respectively could be interpreted as suggestive of some possible benefit in these patient groups

and helps guide the future selection of those in whom such therapy should be explored in a controlled fashion. Some authors have claimed therapeutic advantage for patients with no macroscopic residuum [23,29] or residuum that is <5 mm [11,18] (Table 27.1). The observed outcomes, however, are compatible with the variability of already known prognostic factors in ovarian cancer such as age, grade and previous response to chemotherapy, and therefore do not establish a treatment effect for radiotherapy. Patients with a pathological complete response to chemotherapy after surgery and induction chemotherapy without consolidative therapy have reported survivals ranging between 30% and 60% depending on the patient age, grade and tumour residuum present [34]. While most series had insufficient patients to do meaningful analyses of possible prognostic factors determining the observed outcome, the data of Schray *et al.* are valuable because of the method of analysis and presentation [18]. They performed a multivariate analysis of factors significant for disease-free survival and established significance for the grade of tumour: 1, 2 versus 3,4, 70% versus 10% survival, the initial residuum, prior to chemotherapy: <2 cm versus >2 cm, 50% versus 14% survival, and patient age: less than or greater than 50 years, 54% versus 20% survival. They also looked at the amount of residual disease at the time of radiation therapy. Where disease was microscopic, three out of five remained disease-free following radiotherapy, whereas if disease was macroscopic and debulked to microscopic prior to consolidative radiation therapy, only five of 21 remained disease-free. Figure 27.2 shows the results of their analysis and, although the patient numbers are small, the presented information may be useful in guiding future directions. Of importance was their analysis of outcome versus the number of favourable factors present, i.e. the prechemotherapy residuum, the preradio-

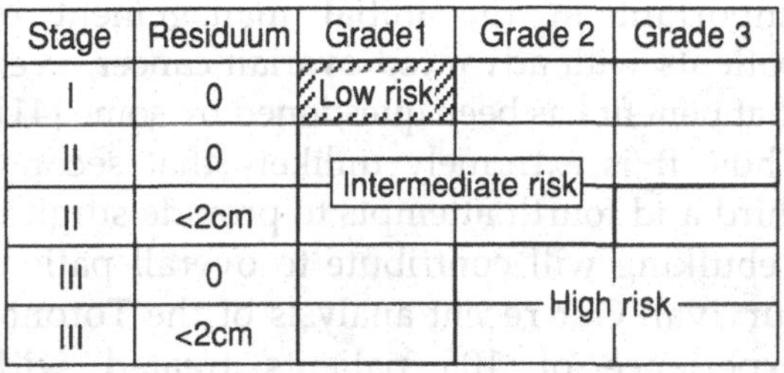

Stage	Residuum	Grade1	Grade 2	Grade 3
I	0	Low risk		
II	0	Intermediate risk		
II	<2cm			
III	0		High risk	
III	<2cm			

Figure 27.2 Prognostic subgroupings according to stage, residuum and grade in patients with stages I–III, small or no tumor residuum. Abdominopelvic radiotherapy is recommended as the sole postoperative treatment in the intermediate risk patient group.

therapy residuum and the grade of the tumour. If no favourable factors were present, 0% (0 of 17) remained disease-free; one factor present, 29% (four of 14); two factors present, 53% (eight of 15) and three factors present, 67% (four of six). Rosen *et al.* [24], in a small series, suggest that tumour grade may be another factor correlating with survival: four of five with grade 1 or 2 tumours versus three of 11 with grade 3 survived.

Appropriate selection of patients for studies of salvage radiotherapy should be guided by this type of information and by extrapolation from the pertinent situations where radiation used as the sole postoperative therapy has been shown to be of curative benefit. Abdominopelvic radiotherapy encompasses only the peritoneal cavity and retroperitoneum, so its use as primary treatment is restricted to stages I, II and III. A multifactorial classification of patients has been developed and refined with validation studies on sequential patient cohorts in Toronto in 1982 [35,36], 1985 [5] and 1991 [37]. This classification system has identified that radiation therapy is only appropriate as the sole postoperative therapy for patients with no macroscopic disease in the upper abdomen and small or no macroscopic residual disease in the pelvis. This classification

system allows identification of the 'intermediate' risk group of patients who receive the most significant benefit from postoperative radiation therapy and in whom this therapy appears to be curative. The five year survival rate is over 75% for these patients [5,37,38]. On the other hand, within the patient groups with no residual or small volume pelvic residual disease, there is a group of patients shown as high risk (Figure 27.2). They have a poor outcome, equivalent to 20% 10 year failure-free rate when treated with abdominopelvic radiotherapy alone [5]. If radiation is not beneficial as initial therapy, it is probable that it would be even less beneficial in similar patients who have already received extensive surgery including secondary debulking and chemotherapy to which resistance may have already developed. These biological factors, which may be operative in this setting, will be discussed subsequently.

We have recently reported on the use of 'consolidation' abdominopelvic radiotherapy following six cycles of cisplatin based combination chemotherapy in the high risk, optimally cytoreduced patients [39]. Forty-four out of 51 eligible patients seen between 1981 and 1985 with optimally cytoreduced stage II or III disease were entered into the non-randomized study. Their survival was compared to that of 48 eligible control patients matched for age, stage and residual disease, treated with radiation alone between 1978 and 1981. The median follow up on study was 6.6 years. The combined therapy led to an extension of the median survival from 2.4 to 5.7 years and 42.6% of patients receiving combined therapy were free of relapse at five years compared to 21.6% ($p = 0.03$) in the historical control group treated with abdominopelvic irradiation alone. Since the control group received radiation therapy alone, we cannot be certain that the entire benefit observed was attributable to the combined sequential therapy, i.e. whether the 'consolidation' radiation therapy provided improvement over that

275

achievable in a comparable group treated with chemotherapy alone. There is evidence, however, that the radiotherapy did appear to be additive [39]. Thus, the summary of the literature results (Table 27.1), the detailed analysis of Schray *et al.* [18] and our own data [39] all support the concept that, if patients are to be selected for salvage radiotherapy, they have microscopic or no residual disease.

27.3.2 THERAPY RELATED TOXICITY

In addition to inappropriate patient selection, a second possible explanation for the observed treatment failure in the published series is the high degree of toxicity which was encountered, resulting in delayed or incomplete radiotherapy. The literature series do not allow any statistically meaningful analysis of factors leading to bone marrow toxicity but several investigators comment on an increased incidence in patients who received increasing courses of chemotherapy. Rosen *et al.* report ability to complete therapy in 10 of 11 patients treated with less than eight courses of cyclophosphamide, adriamycin and platinum, whereas only two of five completed therapy if they received greater than eight courses [24]. There is now general agreement that extending chemotherapy past six cycles is unlikely to provide additional benefit. Others reported apparent decreases in toxicity when the radiation doses were modified downward from the planned maximums [18,20].

In general, reports of abdominopelvic radiotherapy after chemotherapy have suggested higher bowel complication rates than when radiotherapy is used alone. Surgical detail is lacking, but many patients appear to have undergone three or four laparotomies, often with maximal attempts at cytoreduction prior to radiotherapy [14]. In one series [22], six of 18 patients had undergone pelvic exenteration as part of their sequential therapy. While primary cytoreductive surgery may be

important in the initial management of patients with advanced ovarian cancer, even that benefit has been questioned by some [41]. Thus, it is extremely unlikely that second, third and fourth attempts to provide surgical debulking will contribute to overall patient survival. Our recent analysis of the Toronto experience of 105 patients treated with sequential chemotherapy and radiation suggests that increased complications are associated with the combined presence of two factors: higher radiation doses, pelvic dose above 45 Gy, or abdominal dose above 22.5–25 Gy with multiple previous abdominal explorations or second look laparotomy [40]. The use of whole abdominal radiation doses in excess of 22.5–25 Gy may result in unacceptable long term morbidity for surviving patients. The routine use of a pelvic boost in salvage radiation therapy plans should be questioned. It may be appropriate to use such a boost in patients where the site of residuum prior to chemotherapy was in the pelvis, but it is unlikely to benefit patients whose residuum was in other places in the abdomen. Inability to complete the planned sequential therapy in a timely fashion in a significant proportion of patients may be a contributing factor to the lack of overall benefit.

Thus, if sequential multimodality therapy is to be tested, it is important to keep the risk of complications to a minimum, and the probability of completing radiotherapy to a maximum by restricting the radiation dose in patients who have had second look surgery and by limiting the chemotherapy to six courses of the best available agents.

27.3.3 TUMOUR BIOLOGY

In addition to inappropriate patient selection and therapy toxicity, unfavourable biological phenomena may be operative to limit any significant curative benefit from sequential radiotherapy used for salvage or consolidation. While it is hoped that subsequent radiotherapy may provide independent cytotoxicity from that of cisplatin chemotherapy, tumour cellular cross resistance may exist between the two. This has been demonstrated for human ovarian cancer cell lines *in vitro* [42]. The data suggest that tumour persisting after cisplatin chemotherapy may also be relatively radio-resistant. Prolonged cytoreductive therapy (with radiation or chemotherapy) may be associated with accelerated proliferation of clonogenic tumour cells. Withers and coworkers [43] and others have shown that protraction of planned radiotherapy courses results in diminishing local control rates. The data suggest that proliferation rates of the clonogenic compartment, i.e. tumour stem cells, appear to accelerate after the first four weeks of a fractionated course of radiotherapy. The magnitude of the extra radiation dose required to overcome this accelerated population was estimated to be approximately 60 cGy per day. Thus, a prolonged course of cytoreductive therapy, either radiotherapy or chemotherapy, may cause accelerated tumour proliferation and contribute to treatment failure. This may be particularly relevant for the radiotherapy required in epithelial ovarian cancer where the large radiation volume and tolerance of the bowel impose limitations on the radiation dose. Thus, the model of sequential chemotherapy–radiotherapy in ovarian cancer may be invalid in some situations because of these two possible causes of relative radioresistance.

27.4 STRATEGIES FOR INVESTIGATING THE ROLE OF CONSOLIDATION RADIOTHERAPY

It is probable that treatment strategies employing sequential multimodality therapy, including whole abdominopelvic radiotherapy, will be beneficial in a small, select group of patients. Patient selection should be based on identification of those who fail following

chemotherapy and those most likely to benefit from salvage radiotherapy. It would be appropriate to apply such therapy to patients who have a negative second look laparotomy after chemotherapy but who are at high risk of relapse. Approximately 50% of patients with negative second look laparotomy do relapse and some of the factors predicting relapse are known: that is, patients who had large residual stage III presentations prechemotherapy, who are over 50 years of age or have grade 3 tumours [34]. The other patients are those with microscopic positive second look laparotomies where the tumour is well differentiated.

The constituent modalities of sequential therapy must be chosen to minimize complications and give a high likelihood of completion.

Lastly, in order to be meaningful, a model of sequential surgery, chemotherapy and radiotherapy must be examined in the context of a randomized trial, preferably in comparison to standard induction chemotherapy alone. The design and conduct of such a trial is not trivial since large numbers of patients would be required to receive 'induction' chemotherapy to result in sufficient patients with zero or microscopic residuum to enter the subsequent randomized phase of the trial. Such a study could only be performed in a large, cooperative group. The literature reports over 700 patients already treated with sequential multimodality therapy but possible benefits of this treatment strategy are unassessable.

REFERENCES

1. Neijt, J.P., ten Bokkel Huinink, W.W., van den Burg, M.E.L. *et al.* (1991) Long term results of chemotherapy in advanced (FIGO Stages III or IV) ovarian cancer. *Int. Gynecol. Cancer Soc.*, (abstract), 36.
2. Neijt, J.P., ten Bokkel Huinink, W.W., van den Burg, M.E.L. *et al.* (1987) Randomized trial

comparing two combination chemotherapy regimens (CHAP-5 vs CP) in advanced ovarian carcinoma. *J. Clin. Oncol.*, **5**, 1157–68.

3. Vogl, S.E., Pagano, M., Kaplan, B.H. *et al.* (1983) Cisplatin based combination chemotherapy for advanced ovarian cancer: high overall response rate with curative potential only in women with small tumour burdens. *Cancer*, **51**, 2024–30.

4. Omura, G.A., Blessing, J.A., Ehrlich, C.E. *et al.* (1986) A randomized trial of cyclophosphamide and doxorubicin with or without cisplatin in advanced ovarian carcinoma: a Gynecologic Oncology Group study. *Cancer*, **57**, 1725–30.

5. Dembo, A.J. (1984) Abdominopelvic radiotherapy in ovarian cancer: a 10-year experience. *Cancer*, **55**, 2285–90.

6. Fuks, Z., Rizel, S. and Biran, S. (1988) Chemotherapeutic and surgical induction of pathological complete remission and whole abdominal irradiation for consolidation does not enhance the cure of Stage III ovarian carcinoma. *J. Clin. Oncol.*, **6**, 509–16.

7. Bruzzone, M., Repetto, L., Chiara, S. *et al.* (1990) Chemotherapy versus radiotherapy in the management of ovarian cancer patients with pathological complete response or minimal residual disease at second look. *Gynecol. Oncol.*, **38**, 392–5.

8. Lambert, H.E., Rustin, G.J.S., Gregory, W.M. and Nelstrop, A.E. (1993) A randomised trial comparing single agent carboplatin with carboplatin followed by radiotherapy for advanced ovarian cancer. A North Thames Ovary Group Study. *J. Clin. Oncol.*, **11**, 440–8.

9. Mangioni, C., Epis, A., Vassena, L. *et al.* (1987) Radiotherapy (RT) versus chemotherapy (CH) as second line treatment of minimal residual disease (MRD) in advanced epithelial ovarian cancer (EOC) *Proceedings of the International Gynecological Cancer Society*, October, Amsterdam.

10. Lawton, F., Luesley, D., Blackledge, G. *et al.* (1990) A randomized trial comparing whole abdominal radiotherapy with chemotherapy following cisplatinum cytoreduction in epithelial ovarian cancer. West Midlands Ovarian Cancer Group Trial II. *Clin. Oncol.*, **2**, 4–9.

11. Hacker, N.F., Berek, J.S., Burnison, C.M. *et al.* (1985) Whole abdominal radiation as salvage therapy for epithelial ovarian cancer. *Obstet. Gynecol.*, **65**, 60–6.

12. Chiara, S., Orsatti, M., Franzone, P. *et al.* (1991) Abdominopelvic radiotherapy following surgery and chemotherapy in advanced ovarian cancer. *Clin. Oncol.*, **3**, 340–4.

13. Peters III W.A., Blasko, J.C., Bagley Jr, C.M. *et al.* (1986) Salvage therapy with whole-abdominal irradiation in patients with advanced carcinoma of the ovary previously treated by combination chemotherapy. *Cancer*, **58**, 880–2.

14. Hoskins, W.J., Lichter, A.S., Whittington, R. *et al.* (1985) Whole abdominal and pelvic irradiation in patients with minimal disease at second-look surgical reassessment for ovarian carcinoma. *Gynecol. Oncol.*, **20**, 271–80.

15. Greiner, R., Goldhirsch, A., Davis, B.W. *et al.* (1984) Whole-abdomen radiation in patients with advanced ovarian carcinoma after surgery, chemotherapy and second-look laparotomy. *J. Cancer Res. Clin. Oncol.*, **107**, 94–8.

16. Piver, M.S., Barlow, J.J., Lee, F.T. and Vongtama, V. (1975) Sequential therapy for advanced ovarian adenocarcinoma: operation, chemotherapy, second-look laparotomy and radiation therapy. *Am. J. Obstet, Gynecol.*, **122**, 355–7.

17. Hainsworth, J.D., Malcolm, A., Johnson, D.H. *et al.* (1983) Advanced minimal residual ovarian carcinoma: abdominopelvic irradiation following combination chemotherapy. *Obstet. Gynecol.*, **61**, 619–23.

18. Schray, M.F., Martinez, A., Howes, A.E. *et al.* (1988) Advanced epithelial ovarian cancer: salvage whole abdominal irradiation for patients with recurrent or persistent disease after combination chemotherapy. *J. Clin. Oncol.*, **6**, 1433–9.

19. Reddy, S., Hartsell, W., Graham, J. *et al.* (1989) Whole-abdomen radiation therapy in ovarian carcinoma: its role as a salvage therapeutic modality. *Gynecol. Oncol.*, **35**, 307–13.

20. Kuten, A., Stein, M., Steiner, M. *et al.* (1988) Whole abdominal irradiation following chemotherapy in advanced ovarian carcinoma. *Int. J. Radiat. Oncol. Biol. Phys.* **14**, 273–9.

21. Linstadt, D.E., Stern, J.L., Quivey, J.M. *et al.* (1990) Salvage whole-abdominal irradiation following chemotherapy failure in epithelial ovarian carcinoma. *Gynecol. Oncol.* **36**, 327–30.

22. Solomon, H.J., Atkinson, K.H., Coppleson, J.V.M. *et al.* (1988) Ovarian carcinoma: abdominopelvic irradiation following reexploration. *Gynecol. Oncol.*, **31**, 396–401.

23. Kong, J.S., Peters, L.J., Wharton, J.T. *et al.* (1988) Hyperfractionated split-course whole abdominal radiotherapy for ovarian carcinoma: tolerance and toxicity. *Int. J. Radiat. Oncol. Biol. Phys.*, **14**, 737–43.

24. Rosen, E.M., Goldberg, I.D., Rose, C. *et al.* (1986) Sequential multi-agent chemotherapy and whole abdominal irradiation for stage III ovarian carcinoma. *Radiother. Oncol.*, **7**, 223–32.

25. Rothenberg, M.L., Ozols, R.F., Glatstein, E. *et al.* (1992) Dose-intensive induction therapy with cyclophosphamide, cisplatin, and consolidative abdominal radiation in advanced-stage epithelial ovarian cancer. *J. Clin. Oncol.*, **10**, 727–34.

26. Haie, C., Pejovic-Lenfant, M.H., George, M. *et al.* (1989) Whole abdominal irradiation following chemotherapy in patients with minimal residual disease after second look surgery in ovarian carcinoma. *Int. J. Radiat. Oncol. Biol. Phys.*, **17**, 15–19.

27. Cain, J.M., Russell, A.H., Greer, B.E. *et al.* (1988) Whole abdomen radiation for minimal residual epithelial ovarian carcinoma after surgical resection and maximal first-line chemotherapy. *Gynecol. Oncol.*, **29**, 168–75.

28. Kersh, C.R., Randall, M.E., Constable, W.C. *et al.* (1988) Whole abdominal radiotherapy following cytoreductive surgery and chemotherapy in ovarian carcinoma. *Gynecol. Oncol.*, **31**, 113–20.

29. Goldhirsch, A., Greiner, R., Dreher, E. *et al.* (1988) Treatment of advanced ovarian cancer with surgery, chemotherapy, and consolidation of response by whole-abdominal radiotherapy. *Cancer*, **62**, 40–7.

30. Rustin, G.J.S., Minton, M., Southcott, B. *et al.* (1987) Surgery, chemotherapy and whole abdominal radiotherapy in the management of advanced ovarian carcinoma. *Clin. Radiol.*, **38**, 269–72.

31. Menczer, J., Modan, M., Brenner, J. *et al.* (1986) Abdominopelvic irradiation for Stage II–IV ovarian carcinoma patients with limited or no residual disease at second-look laparotomy after completion of cisplatinum-based combination chemotherapy. *Gynecol. Oncol.*, **24**, 149–54.

32. Morgan, L., Chafe, W., Mendenhall, W. and Marcus, R. (1988) Hyperfractionation of whole-abdomen radiation therapy: salvage treatment of persistent ovarian carcinoma following chemotherapy. *Gynecol. Oncol.*, **31**, 122–34.

33. Coltart, R.S., Nethersell, A.B.W. and Brown C.H. (1986) A pilot study of high dose abdominopelvic radiotherapy following surgery and chemotherapy for Stage III epithelial carcinoma of the ovary. *Gynecol. Oncol.*, **23**, 105–10.

34. Shelly, W.E., Carmichael, J.C., Brown, L.B. *et al.* (1988) Adriamycin and cisplatin in the treatment of Stage III and IV epithelial ovarian carcinoma. *Gynecol. Oncol.*, **29**, 208–21.

35. Dembo, A.J. and Bush, R.S. (1982) Choice of postoperative therapy based on prognostic factors. *Int. J. Radiat. Oncol. Biol. Phys.*, **8**, 893–7.

36. Dembo, A.J., Bush, R.S. and Brown, T.C. (1982) Clinicopathological correlates in ovarian cancer. *Bulletin du Cancer (Paris)*, **69**, 292–8.

37. Carey, M., Dembo, A.J., Fyles, A.W. and Simm, J. (1993) Testing the validity of a prognostic classification in patients with surgically optimal ovarian carcinoma: a 15-year review. *Int. J. Gynecol. Cancer*, **3**, 24–35.

38. Lindner, H., Willich, H. and Atzinger, A. (1990) Primary adjuvant whole abdominal irradiation in ovarian carcinoma. *Int. J. Radiat. Oncol. Biol. Phys.*, **19**, 1203–6.

39. Ledermann, J.A., Dembo, A.J., Sturgeon, J.F.G. *et al.* (1991) Outcome of patients with unfavourable optimally cytoreduced ovarian cancer treated with chemotherapy and whole abdominal radiation. *Gynecol. Oncol.*, **41**, 30–5.

40. Whelan, T.J., Dembo, A.J., Bush, R.S. *et al.* (1992) Complications of whole abdominal and

pelvic radiotherapy following chemotherapy for advanced ovarian cancer. *Int. J. Radiat. Oncol. Biol. Phys.*, **22**, 853–8.

41. Hoskins, W.J., Rubin, S.C. (1991) Surgery in the treatment of patients with advanced ovarian cancer. *Semin. Oncol.* **18**, 213–21.

42. Louie, K.G., Behrens, B.C., Kinsella, T.J. *et al.* (1985) Radiation survival parameters of anti-neoplastic drug-sensitive and resistant human ovarian cancer cell lines and their modification by buthionine sulfoximine. *Cancer Res.*, **45**, 2110–15.

43. Withers, H.R., Taylor, J.M.G. and Maciejewski, B. (1988) The hazard of accelerated tumour clonogen repopulation during radiotherapy. *Acta Oncol.*, **27**, 131–46.

Chapter 28

Ethical decision making in the care of seriously ill and dying patients. Theory and practice

E.J. LATIMER

28.1 INTRODUCTION

In the care of patients with ovarian cancer, the physician and health care team will need to make many decisions about how best to treat the patient. This is particularly true of those patients who are seriously ill and dying.

The physician needs to have a working knowledge of the theory of biomedical ethics and an approach to the process of decision making, as it is important to understand the nature and impact of decisions which are made and the basis upon which they can be seen as ethical and sound. It is also important to understand how patient care practices like effective symptom control and non-initiation and cessation of treatment differ from euthanasia (acting with the intention to take life) [1–6].

Physicians, other health professionals and lay people alike, all of whom share a great desire to relieve patient suffering, may be confused about the ethical, moral and legal dimensions of interventions that might be considered in various clinical situations. Utilizing case examples, this paper will provide an overview of theory and present an aid to decision making.

There are three theoretical perspectives upon which the physician may draw when considering the ethical dimensions of a particular patient problem and/or the relation-

ship between physician and patient. These are the cardinal principles of biomedical ethics, the notion of an ethic of caring and the notion of the particular virtues of the physician as a ethical agent.

The principles of biomedical ethics [6–9] provide the science whereby one might apply analysis to a problem. They is similar to rules and they provide a means of overt, dispassionate analysis of a problem.

Four cardinal principles form the basis for an ethical consideration of treatment practices. These are autonomy, beneficence, non-maleficence and justice. There is also a number of rules and obligations that relate to the principles and influence their implementation in clinical work. These include the obligation to tell the truth and to act in a trustworthy way in professional relationships with patients. The reader is directed to references for further considerations of the cardinal principles [6–11].

28.2 AUTONOMY

Respect for autonomy recognizes an individual's right or ability to decide for herself, according to beliefs, values and a life plan. Respect for autonomy in medical practice recognizes that patients' decisions are uniquely their own and that these decisions may be opposite to the course that is advised or deemed wise in a given situation. Autonomy exists when patients act intentionally, with understanding and without controlling influences. Respect for autonomy is the opposite of paternalism, which says 'I know what is best for you'. Respect for autonomy relies upon truth telling, the conveying of accurate information and the determination that a patient understands the facts of the situation and the implications of decisions. It recognizes that the patient may value certain components of the situation differently from the physician or health care team.

The patient is assumed to have the capacity to understand and make decisions unless there is real evidence to the contrary. Patients who are incompetent in one aspect of their lives, for example in managing financial affairs, may still have the capacity to understand clinical issues and to make decisions about their care.

Although very important, respect for autonomy is not the only principle to be considered in medical decision making. For example, the exercise of autonomy does not necessarily imply an obligation upon others to act [13]. However, it is very compelling because it is based in moral thought, cultural practice and legal precedent.

Respect for autonomy is central to the care of dying patients. Gentle truth telling and exchange of accurate information about status, options, planned care and future expectations is essential.

28.3 NON-MALEFICENCE

This principle is embodied in the concept 'one ought not to inflict evil or harm'. Causing unnecessary physical or psychological pain to patients while performing tests or procedures or during history taking, physical examination or the conveying of information is a violation of the principle of non-maleficence.

Insensitive truth telling (the 'assault of truth') is a violation, as is any denigration of the individual person in the process of caring for him or her.

Patients must not be over- or undertreated. Continued aggressive life prolonging or cure oriented treatment that is not suited to their needs or wishes may be a violation of non-maleficence. Unnecessary and unwanted oversedation or premature, unrequested or uniformed withdrawal of treatment may be another.

28.4 BENEFICENCE

This concept states that 'one ought to prevent or remove evil or harm, and do or promote good' [6]. Beneficence implies positive acts and includes all of the strategies that health care professionals employ to support patients and families and reduce suffering. This includes the effective treatment of pain and other symptoms, sensitive interpersonal support and the acknowledgement of the patient as a unique human being to be respected and valued.

Various proposed treatments can be evaluated in terms of their potential to prevent or remove distressing symptoms or suffering and thereby promote good. Cessation of treatment can, in an appropriate clinical context, be viewed as an act of beneficence where continued life is viewed by the patient as an 'evil or harm'. Treatment plans that are in line with the goals of care that a patient sees for him or herself (Figure 28.1) would convey beneficence.

28.5 JUSTICE

Justice deals with the concept of fairness or what is deserved by people. It describes what individuals are legitimately entitled to and what they can claim. For the individual, it may serve to limit autonomy; what the individual wishes, chooses or feels entitled to may not be allowable in the context of the greater good. This may be regrettable but necessary to maintain the particular values upon which society is based.

Decisions and actions that may seem morally compelling and appropriate for a particular person may not be allowable because of the wider risk they present to other members of society. Euthanasia may be one such action [1,5]. Seriously ill or dying people should not automatically be deprived of certain therapies if they wish to attempt them and have full knowledge of what is entailed. The issue of what constitutes 'futile treatment' is fraught with complexities [14–16]. Cardiopulmonary resuscitation of the patient with far advanced cancer in the event of sudden cardiac arrest prior to the dying phase of illness may be an example of this [16].

Justice also demands that dying patients have access to care equal to others. Sadly, this has not always been the case in that the dying patient may be viewed as less of a priority with regard to health care resources.

The principle of double effect is not one of the cardinal ethical principles but is utilized in helping to decide whether some evil effects can be accepted in an action. It applies to situations in which there is a difference between the intended effects and the non-intended, albeit foreseen effects of an action. To invoke this principle, intentions and motives must be evident and the practitioner must clearly intend a desirable outcome while recognizing the possibility of other undesirable and unavoidable outcomes. The undesirable secondary effect must in no way be wished or planned. The most common clinical application of this principle arises in situations of intractable symptoms like pain or suffocation, where there is a compelling need to act in using opioid analgesics and sedative medications to realize the moral goal of patient relief. The physician may recognize the possibility that a secondary effect, for example respiratory depression, may shorten life but does not primarily intend this effect.

28.6 VIRTUES AND THE ETHIC OF CARING

When an ethical dilemma, with its opposing tensions, presents itself it can be considered from the viewpoint of each principle. For example, the physician might ask what respect for autonomy dictates in a particular situation. Does justice guide thinking? What of beneficence and non-maleficence? A consideration of the impact of the four cardinal ethical principles provides the basis of analytical ethics or ethics as a discipline or exercise. Double effect is a way of considering situations where necessary actions may result in undesired outcomes.

The ethic of caring [17,18] is one which might be seen as very germane to the relationship between physician and patient, particularly in situations of life and death care and decision making. This way of considering an ethical dilemma also utilizes the biomedical principles but is much more likely to be influenced by the uniqueness of the individuals involved, the relationships they have and the context in which the problem occurs. This ethic relies as heavily on beneficence as on autonomy and emphasizes social relationships and connection in addition to individual rights.

The notion of virtue ethics [19–20] describes the qualities of the professional, in this case the health professional. Virtues are related to character and describe the dimension of the physician's role as a moral agent or one who is ethical. The traditional virtues include those of honesty, privacy, temperance, justice, courage, prudence and charity. Pellegrino underlines the tremendous potential of the professions as moral communities with the ability to influence society for good [19].

The relationship of physicians with patients has been described as a covenant [20], the key ingredients of which are the essence of a promise and the fidelity to that promise which the physician brings. This relationship holds aspects of descriptive truth (the facts) and performance truth (the faithfulness to that promise) [19]. The physician becomes committed to the well-being of the patient and effaces self-interest to this well-being in the context of his on her professional calling. The physician goes a 'step beyond' what is 'contracted' or 'required' for a patient.

28.7 AN APPROACH TO DECISION MAKING IN CLINICAL PRACTICE

28.7.1 INCLUDING THE PATIENT AND FAMILY IN THE PROCESS [21,31]

The inclusion of seriously ill and dying patients and their families in decisions about their care is a difficult clinical challenge for physicians and other health care professionals for several reasons. These patients are often very frail and sad and it may seem to their physicians that they are vulnerable. It can seem unkind to burden them with more stress and the issues themselves necessitate speaking of death, something which professionals may find more distressing than patients themselves. Interpersonal communication itself may be difficult due to sedation, ventilation or sensorium changes.

Nevertheless, their participation in decision making is vital to the maintenance of integrity for patients themselves and for the health professions. Patients must be gently informed that death will occur, so that they can maintain control, deal with their relationships and leave life in a manner consistent with the way they would choose.

For professionals, the patient's participation is also vital. Although they have information and experience and may advise patients, professionals are philosophically in no position to unilaterally decide such personal issues as the manner, conduct and timing of another person's dying. They must, wherever possible, allow patients to participate in this by providing information, options and facilitating choices with available resources within the confines of professional codes of ethics and law.

Certain patterns of practice will enhance patient autonomy and participation in decision making. The physician and team are encouraged to consider the following approach.

• Try to gain a 'capsule' of the patient as a person, in terms of their way of being, values, hopes and dreams. Remain curious about people. This information comes ideally from patients themselves but can often be reflected by those closest to them. It is invaluable in formulating treatment and care plans that match the person.

• Be accessible to patients. Practice sitting at the bedside to exchange information, rather than standing. It opens an entirely different path to dialogue and establishes the patient as partner. Ask patients what they understand their situation to be and what information they would like about their illness, treatment plans and overall status.

• Ask patients what they would like to see happen and what you can do to help them. What goals does the patient have? Inquire directly about their thoughts for the future. What are their wishes, hopes and fears? What is important to them?

• Be knowledgeable about the patient's illness and status, potential options, likely outcomes. What are you and the patient dealing with, what is the reality? What are the possibilities and limitations?

• Be sure that the patient has the type of information that he or she wants and needs. Learn gentle but accurate ways of conveying this. Be prepared to deal with the emotional accompaniment to these types of conversations.

• Help patients to think through their options, giving guidance not only about what is possible but also what you as a professional, with knowledge and experience, might recommend. Try to avoid personal bias but do not present choices as being equal if they are not so.

• Do not try to predict certain outcomes where certainty does not exist. Do not try to foretell the future beyond what is generally known to be likely to happen and try not to burden patients with unnecessary worry about events that only might occur. In other words, give patients and families the information that they need to have but do not feel compelled to outline every conceivable eventuality.

• Always balance reality and truth with hope. Emphasize what is possible rather than what is not. Use creative imagination in helping patients to set goals that are reachable and that enhance their sense of themselves.

• Utilize a similar approach when speaking with families. It may be wise to meet with them apart from the patient on occasion, but with her permission and knowledge.

• Discuss ethical conundrums openly with colleagues of all disciplines. Create a forum where this can occur. These issues can be very complex and ethical, humane practice is more likely to occur when a variety of viewpoints can be heard.

28.7.2 A SCHEMA FOR DECISION MAKING

Figure 28.1 illustrates an approach to decision making for the dying patient [7].

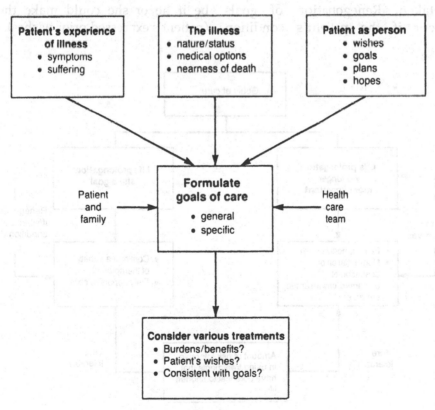

Figure 28.1 Medical decision making with dying patients.

285

Consideration is given to the illness and to the patient's experience, goals and plans. Goals of care are established jointly by patient and family together with the health care team. The process of decision making undertaken by the physician and health team and an examination of the way in which they have considered the competing moral principles involved are as important as the decision reached [7–11].

In this approach, various treatment options are considered in relation to their ability to enhance established goals. Once it has been decided whether prolongation of life is viewed as a paramount goal or not, two broad paths of care become evident (Figure 28.2) [7]. Full supportive care is necessary in both paths but they vary in the types of treatments that are appropriate and the degree of risk that is acceptable as supportive therapies are undertaken. Renegotiation of goals should occur if the patient's condition changes significantly, either towards improvement or deterioration.

28.7.3 NON-INITIATION OR CESSATION OF TREATMENT

Certain treatments or therapies should not be undertaken if they are unwanted or unwarranted. The competent patient is assumed to have the capacity for voluntary participation in decision making through the process of informed consent. Such a patient may decline to start a course of management on the basis of the information provided and previously held views, beliefs and values (the exercise of autonomy). Where the patient is found to lack the capacity to act autonomously, proxy consent is sought. Usually this will be from family, who are seen to be in a position to know best what the patient's wishes would be if he or she could make them known (patient's expressed prior wishes).

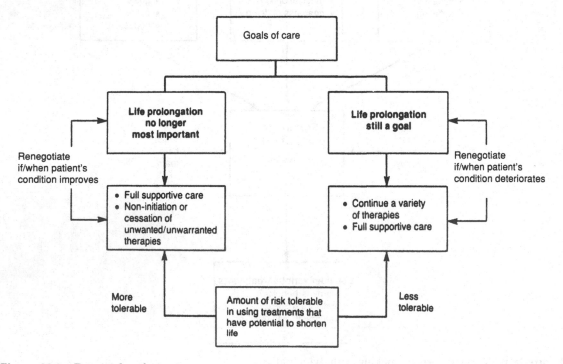

Figure 28.2 Potential paths to care.

If discussion with family is not sufficiently revealing of the patient's wishes, the concept of a 'reasonable person' might be invoked. In this situation, the benefits and burdens of the proposed therapy or treatment are described and clinicians, families, ethics committees and sometimes courts attempt to determine what a reasonable person would choose to do. It is apparent that decision making on behalf of the incompetent patient will remain one of the most challenging and controversial areas in ethical decision making since the concepts of benefit and burden may be assessed differently by the various participants and this can give rise to vastly disparate views of what a 'reasonable person' might choose.

There is also still considerable controversy over what constitutes treatment and what is simply supportive care to which everyone is entitled. This is particularly evidenced by the issues of withholding or not starting artificial feeding or hydration and the definition, in this context, of 'artificial' itself [8–9].

Cessation of treatment, as opposed to non-initiation, must also be considered in each of two general contexts described above: that of the competent patient who requests that treatment be stopped and the non-competent patient who is unable to do so. Cessation of treatment, although sometimes psychologically and emotionally more problematic for professionals, patients and families, is no different, ethically, than never having started it in the first place [6–12]. In fact, treatment once started may at times be stopped with somewhat more confidence, because all parties have had an opportunity to assess more accurately the actual experienced benefits and burdens of therapy.

As with non-initiation of therapy, cessation of treatment is most problematic when it is considered for non-competent patients, not only because it can be difficult to know what the patient might have wanted but also because the onus of acting on behalf of another is a burden shared by society as a whole, particularly when life and death decisions are being made. In this situation, motives and outcomes must be carefully and honestly considered.

28.7.4 CONTINUED TREATMENT

Treatment is continued when it is consistent with the goals of care for the patient. Such goals are based on the status of the illness, the range of possible treatments and the patient's wishes about them and the benefits and burdens involved. Open negotiation before commencing a trial of therapy can allow for its cessation by mutual agreement if outcomes are not as expected. A course of therapy, once embarked upon, should not be considered irrevocable.

The ethical soundness of a particular decision can only be judged in the clinical context. For example, it would be ethically wrong to withhold potentially beneficial treatment from an incompetent patient if its benefits clearly outweighed its burdens and it was clear that this patient or a reasonable person would choose to have it. On the other hand, even the patient's expressed refusal of treatment may sometimes be overruled, particularly if there is very sound reason to believe that the decision is not well informed or that the patient is not acting in a manner consistent with her own prior values, wishes and life-plan or that she lacks the capacity to decide [13].

Decisions made for or with one patient may not necessarily apply to another. Such decisions cannot be made categorically, on the basis of policies, protocols or impersonal generalizations about age or diagnosis. Rather, they must be based on thoughtful analysis of the issues in a particular patient's situation and a clear exchange of information among patient, family and health professional team. Such an open examination of issues and the viewpoints of all will give a firmer ethical foundation upon which to decide and to act.

28.7.5 NECESSARY ACTIONS THAT INCREASE THE RISK OF DEATH

Treatments in this group have the potential for shortening life. They may be necessary either in the setting of continued treatment or the setting in which treatments are stopped or not begun. In essence, such decisions may be morally and ethically defensible if there is a compelling need to act. In patients with advanced diseases, such need may exist in the treatment of such symptom crises as intractable pain, suffocation or choking, in which the compelling moral obligation is the relief of distress in accordance with the principle of beneficence. The physician acts with the knowledge of potential shortening of life (in actual practice, the risk may be quite low) but does not primarily act to bring about death. Most important, the physician does not fail to act when the need exists, because the moral need to relieve suffering is recognized as being paramount.

Physicians should provide more reassurance to patient and family that definitive and effective treatment will be provided should these sorts of symptom crises occur. This gentle but open dialogue and action when necessary would do much to relieve suffering and the anticipated fear of it. Such actions can be clearly distinguished from the primary intention to take life (euthanasia).

28.7.6 SOUND TREATMENT DECISIONS VERSUS EUTHANASIA

It is important to recognize that well-taken decisions to cease or not start treatments in the care of seriously ill and dying patients can be distinguished from euthanasia. The distinction lies in the motivation or intention of the physician, which is to relieve the patient of treatments which he or she does not want or which are not of benefit. Death may occur if it is inevitable, from the disease process, because obstacles are removed or not placed in its way. Direct control over life and death is not taken, as it would be in euthanasia,

where the goal of the physician's actions is not only to remove burdensome treatment but to go one step further and to take actions to ensure that the death of the patient occurs.

To avoid confusion with carefully considered ethical decision making and acceptable patterns of practice in that regard, it would be best if the word *euthanasia* were limited to describe that pattern of practice which acts specifically with the intention and goal to end life. Euthanasia is not part of medical practice and represents a topic of considerable controversy [1–6,22–30,32].

28.8 CASE EXAMPLES

Case 1

A 38 year old woman is known to be dying of ovarian cancer. She has been comfortable on low doses of opioid analgesia for pain. She develops a sudden severe chest pain and becomes severely hypotensive. The clinical diagnosis is pulmonary embolus and the patient is assessed to be in shock. Her pain is severe and she is restless and moaning. She requires several intravenous bolus doses of morphine to restore comfort. Her clinical condition continues to deteriorate and she dies within the hour.

Case 2

A 42 year old woman with advanced ovarian cancer presents with ascites and subsequently develops a pleural effusion and dyspnea. She has been placed on a ventilator to support her during chemotherapy but the chemotherapy does not produce the expected positive response. She continues to deteriorate. Two weeks into treatment, she asks to have the ventilator removed so she can die. She feels that her present existence is intolerable.

Case 3

A 71 year old woman with endstage ovarian cancer is very frail and mostly bedridden. She is physically comfortable but, in her own experience, feels she is 'lingering too long'. She feels she is suffering because of her incapacity and asks that she be given something to help her die.

28.8.1 DISCUSSION OF CASE EXAMPLES

The foregoing discussion can be applied in the consideration of the three clinical cases.

Case 1 illustrates a potential application for the principle of double effect. However, this can only be true if the physician's actions are motivated by the intention to relieve pain and not to end the life of the patient and provided that the doses of morphine used are appropriate to the clinical situation.

The patient did die, in all probability due to the pulmonary embolus and the shock it induced. How can the action of giving her bolus doses of morphine be viewed? Although the possibility of shortening her life may have been foreseen, her death is not desired or intended. The possibility that the patient's life may have been at all shortened as a result of giving the morphine can be seen as a regrettable and unwished consequence of required intervention for a morally compelling reason to relieve severe intractable pain. Indeed, were it not for the need to relieve the pain, the physician would not have acted. Were the physician to have wished or intended the death of the patient by his or her actions, or were there no clear and compelling need to act, the action could not be justified on the basis of the principle of double effect.

Perhaps most important of all is the fact that the physician did take necessary action to relieve the patient's pain. The physician did not hesitate to do what was necessary for fear of 'killing the patient'. Beneficence required action for pain relief.

Continued treatment against the wishes of the autonomous patient in case 2 can be seen as a violation of the principles of respect for autonomy and non-maleficence if continued ventilation is viewed as doing harm and a violation of beneficence if removal from the ventilator were seen as a good. Alternatively, one could define death as the greater harm and conclude that her continued ventilation was most beneficent and least harmful to her, although this would be difficult to defend because the necessity to preserve life at all costs is no longer seen as paramount.

The principle of respect for autonomy would be very compelling in case 2. The continued treatment of a competent patient against her consistently expressed wishes to the contrary, which is occurring in the absence of modifiable factors like a clinical depression, is not ethically sound [6–8,10–12]. The ventilator may be seen as an impediment to her natural death. The intention in removing the ventilator is to allow death, if it is inevitable, by cessation of unwanted treatment.

Although the decision to remove a ventilator may be ethically sound, it cannot be taken lightly or in haste. In clinical practice, the management of such a request as this patient's may be extremely complicated [12]. Patients must be provided with ample opportunities to explore all options open to them. Adequate staff resources in the spheres of counselling and psychosocial and spiritual care are necessary for them to do this.

The woman in case 3 is asking the physician to take her life. Her physical and psychological situation is compelling. She is not asking for cessation of treatment because, in essence, there is nothing to be stopped. Pain relief is not an issue for her but relief of her suffering is and she sees this relief as coming via her death. She is asking for euthanasia, where the intention of any action by a physician or other person would be to take her life. Is this a morally permissible act by the physician or, indeed, by anyone? Viewpoints vary, but the weight of thought would say no.

What, then, are appropriate professional obligations to her? She requires care based upon a palliative or hospice approach. The first need is to explore her request fully, to come to know its origins, her thoughts, feelings, hopes and despairs in order to seek avenues for intervention [31–34]. She should be reassured that while euthanasia is not possible, nothing will be done to prolong her life. She should be involved in open conversations about her options to decline resuscitation, artificial feeding, hydration and antibiotics. A trial of antidepressants may lift her mood. She should be reassured that any symptoms will be vigorously controlled with appropriate therapeutics. She should receive ongoing support of a tender, personal and caring type using a palliative care or hospice care type of philosophy. This will require the use of an interdisciplinary team and special volunteers. Every effort should be made to treat her as the unique person that she is and to involve her in life as much as she wishes to participate. She should be provided with opportunities to tell her story and to express her thoughts about her life, illness, present and future.

This approach to her care will present a great challenge to the health care team, but it can be mutually enhancing for patient and caregivers alike.

28.9 CONCLUSIONS

Ethical decision making in the care of seriously ill and dying patients is a dynamic process requiring ongoing reflection, questioning and discussion. Physicians and members of the health care team must be knowledgeable about the fundamental principles of ethical thought that may guide analysis of complex decisions. They must engage in a process of decision making that primarily involves the patient as the unique person for whom they care, but also extends to include the people who share the patient's life.

Open dialogue with patients, families and other health professionals encourages the expression of diverse perspectives on these very complex issues.

When all is said and done, it can sometimes be difficult to know that the 'right' decision has been made. This is the particular crux of a classic moral dilemma. However, it is important for health professionals, as moral beings, to have struggled with the issues and, after careful consideration, to have arrived at the best decision possible given the circumstances. The maintenance of society's values and the ethics of the professions themselves depend on it.

REFERENCES

1. Grisez, G. and Boyle, J.M. Jr. (1979) *Life and Death with Liberty and Justice. A Contribution to the Euthanasia Debate*, University of Notre Dame Press, Notre Dame, Indiana.
2. Gula, R.M. (1986) *What are They Saying about Euthanasia?* Paulist Press, New York.
3. Ramsey, P. (1978) *Ethics at the Edges of Life*, Yale University Press, Newhaven.
4. Horan, D.J. and Mall, D. (1977) *Death, Dying and Euthanasia*, University Publications of America, Inc, Washington DC.
5. Latimer, E.J. (1991) Euthanasia: a physician's reflections. *J. Pain Symptom Man.*, **6**, 487–91.
6. Beauchamp, T.L. and Childress, J.F. (1989) *Principles of Biomedical Ethics*, Oxford University Press, New York.
7. Latimer, E.J. (1991) Ethical decision-making in the care of the dying and its applications to clinical practice. *J. Pain Symptom Man.*, **6**, 329–36.
8. *Guidelines on the Termination of Life-sustaining Treatment and the Care of the Dying.* A report of the Hasting's Centre, Briarcliff Manor, New York, 1987.
9. Lynn, J. (1986) *By No Extraordinary Means. The Choice to Forego Life-sustaining Food and Water*, Indiana University Press, Indianapolis.
10. Gostin, L. (ed.) (1989) Life and death choices. *Law, Med. Health Care*, **17**, 205–82.

11. Dickens, B. (1990) Terminal care and related decisions. A review of legal developments. *Modern Med. Canada*, **45**, 296–306.

12. Thomas, J.E. and Latimer, E.J. (1989) When families cannot 'let go': ethical decision-making at the bedside. *CMAJ*, **141**, 389–91.

13. Jackson, D.L. and Younger, S. (1979) Patient autonomy and 'death with dignity'. *N. Engl. J. Med.*, **301**, 404–8.

14. Callaghan, D. (1991) Medical futility, medical necessity. The problem-without-a-name. *Hastings Centre Report*, July–August, 30–5.

15. Schneiderman, L.J., Jecker, N.S. and Jonsen, A.R. (1990) Medical futility: its meaning and ethical implications. *Ann. Intern. Med.*, **112**, 949–54.

16. Tomlinson, T. and Brody, H. (1990) Futility and the ethics of resuscitation. *JAMA*, **264**, 1277.

17. Gilligan, C. (1982) *In a Different Voice. Psychological Theory and Women's Development*, Harvard University Press, Cambridge, Mass.

18. Levine, R.J. Medical ethics and personal doctors; conflicts between what we teach and what we want. *Am. J. Law Med.*, **13**, 351–64.

19. Pellegrino, E. and Carrol, J. (1989) Character, virtue, and self-interest in the ethics of the professions. *Loma Linda University Centre for Christian Bioethics*, **5**, 1–6.

20. May, W.F. (1975) Code, covenant, contract or philanthropy. A basis for professional ethics. *Hastings Centre Report*, **5**, 29–38.

21. Latimer, E.J. (1991) Making decisions with dying patients – the ethics and art. Pain *Man. Newsletter*, **4**, 8–9.

22. Maguire, D.C. (1984) *Death by Choice*, Image Books (Doubleday), New York.

23. Lifton, R.J. (1986) *The Nazi Doctors. Medical Killing and the Psychology of Genocide*, Basic Books Inc, New York.

24. Rachels, J. (1986) *The End of Life. Euthanasia and Morality*, Oxford University Press, Oxford.

25. Gostin, L. (ed.) (1987/88) Euthanasia. *Law Med. Health Care*, **15**, 4.

26. Kass, L.R. (1989) Neither for love nor money: why doctors must not kill. *Public Interest*, **94**, 25–46.

27. Campbell, C. and Crigger, B.J. (eds) (1989) Mercy, murder and morality: perspectives on euthanasia. *Hastings Centre Report* (special supplement), Jan/Feb, 2–32.

28. De Wachter, M.A.M. (1989) Active euthanasia in the Netherlands. *JAMA*, **262**, 3316–19.

29. Righter, H., Borst-Eilers, E. and Leenan, H.J.J. (1988) Euthanasia across the North Sea. *BMJ*, **297**, 1593–5.

30. Lynn, J. (1988) The health care professional's role when active euthanasia is sought. *J. Pall. Care*, **4**, 100–2.

31. Latimer, E.J. (1990) The pain of cancer: helping patients and families. I & II. *Humane Med.*, 6(2) & 6(3), 96–100.

32. Scott, J.F. (1988) Lies and lamentation – A solid no to euthanasia. *J. Pall. Care*, **4**, 119–21.

33. Hauerwas, S. (1986) *Suffering Presence. Theological Reflection on Medicine, the Mentally Handicapped and the Church*. University of Notre Dame Press, Notre Dame, Indiana.

34. Hauerwas, S. (1981) *Vision and Virtue. Essays in Christian Ethical Reflection*. University of Notre Dame Press, Notre Dame, Indiana.

Part Five
Immunotherapy and Gene Therapy

Chapter 29

Overcoming drug resistance of ovarian carcinoma cell lines by treatment with combination of TNF-α/anti-Fas antibody and chemotherapeutic drugs or toxins

B. BONAVIDA, J.T. SAFRIT, H. MORIMOTO, Y. MIZUTANI, S. YONEHARA and J.S. BEREK

29.1 INTRODUCTION

Current conventional therapies in the treatment of neoplastic diseases consist of surgery, chemotherapy, radiotherapy and combination therapy. While these forms of treatment have resulted in cures and prolonged survival, recurrent tumors and metastases continue to be very common. Treatment of these recurrent tumors has posed a major challenge to oncologists since these tumors become refractory to chemotherapeutic drugs and metastases are not amenable to surgery or radiotherapy. Thus, the development of tumor cell resistance to cytotoxic drugs has provoked the search for new means to overcome resistance. During the last few years, a surge of new approaches in cancer therapy has emerged that include biological response modifiers to boost the immune response, the use of activated cytotoxic cells such as LAK and TIL and the preparation of 'magic bullets' consisting of targeted antibody-drug/toxin conjugates, the use of recombinant cytokines (e.g. TNF-α, IFN-γ, IL-2 etc.) and more recently, genetic engineering techniques to modify tumor cells or lymphocytes. Furthermore, new agents to reverse the multidrug resistance phenotype have been considered.

While most of these approaches have been tested in experimental systems and a few in humans, they all share a common premise that tumor cells resistant to chemotherapy or radiation will remain sensitive to immunocytotoxic effector systems. Alternatively, there exists the possibility that the development of resistance to chemotherapeutic drugs could also result in resistance to cytotoxic effector cells, cytokines, toxins and vice versa. We designed a study to determine whether there existed any correlation between the sensitivity and resistance of tumor cells to chemotherapeutic drugs, immune effector cells or factors and toxins.

We compared the sensitivity of tumor cells to cytotoxicity mediated by recombinant tumor necrosis factor (rTNF), cytotoxic effector cells (natural killer cells, moncytes, LAK cells), chemotherapeutic drugs (CDDP, ADR) and microbial toxins (DTX, PEA). Human tumor cell lines sensitive and resistant to rTNF or drugs were used. Cell lines tested consisted of several histological types such as that of the brain, lung, colon and ovarian tumors. Cell lines made resistant to rTNF by

295

coculture with TNF were also relatively resistant to unactivated monocytes and their supernatants. However, these lines were sensitive to all other methods tested including activated monocytes, natural killer and LAK cells, drugs and toxins. The tumor lines naturally resistant to rTNF were found to have various degrees of sensitivity and resistance to these other systems. Upon the analysis of our data, a pattern suggested a hierarchy of sensitivity and resistance of the tumor cells to the cytotoxic mechanisms explored. From a majority of cell lines resistant to rTNF to a minority of lines resistant to LAK, we found an interesting gradation of sensitivity and/or resistance to the other cytotoxic modalities employed [1].

These findings suggested that there exist common pathways of sensitivity and resistance to different cytotoxic agents. Therefore, we propose that the resistance pattern of the tumor cells in question should be evaluated prior to application of other cytotoxic modalities. Furthermore, the phenomenon of cross resistance to therapies other than chemotherapeutic drugs must not be overlooked.

We hypothesized that if common pathways exist in tumor cell sensitivity and resistance to various cytotoxic modalities, then it was probable that resistance to one or two agents can be overcome by combination treatment with the two agents. This hypothesis was tested in many *in vitro* experimental systems. We initially focused on studying the biologically active molecule TNF-α in combination with drugs (ADR, CDDP, tamoxifen) and/or toxins (DTX, PEA, ricin) in reversing tumor cell resistance. TNF was first discovered as a macrophage derived factor that mediates tumor necrosis in endotoxin treated mice [2]. It has since been shown to have significant antitumor activity against many tumor types but has had limited clinical success, partly due to its high *in vivo* toxicity [3].

We describe below our recent findings in reversing tumor cell resistance by combination treatments with TNF-α and other agents as well as our investigations on the possible underlying mechanisms involved.

29.2 COMBINATION TREATMENT WITH TNF-α AND ADRIAMYCIN

Tumor necrosis factor has been shown to be cytotoxic against some ovarian cell lines [4]. We examined the cytotoxic effect of a combined modality using a variety of concentrations of recombinant tumor necrosis factor (rTNF) (a cytotoxic cytokine) with adriamycin (ADR) on human ovarian carcinoma cell lines. Five cell lines were used: PA-1, 222, OVCAR-3, SKOV-3 and OVCAR-8. Concentrations of rTNF that were minimally cytotoxic resulted in significant cytotoxicity and synergy when used with optimal and suboptimal concentrations of ADR. Interestingly, the rTNF and drug resistant SKOV-3 cell line was sensitive to the synergistic effect of adriamycin and rTNF. The synergistic effect was specific to rTNF. These studies clearly demonstrate that significant synergistic antitumor cytotoxic activity can be achieved against human ovarian carcinoma cell lines with combination rTNF and ADR at low concentrations [5].

One mechanism of drug resistance is the development of multiple drug cross resistance (MDR) to vinca alkaloids and anthracyclines. MDR has been associated with the presence of a 170 kd membrane glycoprotein (GP-170) on the surface of these cells [6]. GP-170 is thought to function as a unidirectional transport channel that actively pumps drugs and toxins out of the cell [7].

The mechanism of enhancement by TNF-α of doxorubicin (DOXO) topoisomerase targeted drug cytotoxicity is not known. Both TNF-α [8] and DOXO cause DNA fragmentation and apoptosis and thus may complement each other in the synergy. TNF-α could be acting by its suggested ability to cause DNA damage that combines with that caused by DOXO to kill the cell. Alternatively, TNF-α could act by increasing the sensitivity of the cell to DOXO induced damage, perhaps by affecting the uptake or efflux of the drug.

To understand the possible mechanisms involved in overcoming resistance by the combined effect of TNF-α and DOXO, we examined whether the drug influx/efflux is affected by the cytotoxic combination and whether TNF-α or TNF-α and DOXO has any effect on MDR function or on the regulation of MDR mRNA expression.

We have examined four human ovarian tumor lines (A2780, AD10, OVC-8 and SKOV-3) selected for their sensitivity and/or resistance to the recombinant human tumor necrosis factor alpha (TNF-α) and the chemotherapeutic drug DOXO. The tumor lines were either sensitive to both agents, resistant to one or the other, or resistant to both. Of the four lines examined, only the DOXO resistant line AD10 exhibited the multidrug resistance (MDR) phenotype. Enhanced cytotoxicity was seen with the combination of TNF-α and DOXO in each line regardless of their sensitivity or patterns and thus demonstrates that drug resistance due to the expression of the MDR phenotype or its absence can be overcome by TNF-α and DOXO. We then examined whether TNF-α or TNF-α and DOXO modulated the MDR phenotype in AD10 as a possible mechanism of overcoming drug resistance. TNF-α had no effect on either DOXO intake or efflux as measured by flow cytometry. Further, TNF-α treatment showed no effect on the level of MDR-1 mRNA. These results suggest that the enhanced cytotoxicity seen with the combination of TNF-α and DOXO is not the result of any modulation of drug influx or efflux by TNF-α. Overall, these findings suggest that combination treatment with TNF-α and DOXO can overcome resistance inflicted by different mechanisms [9].

In a recent study, we further examined the mechanism of overriding resistance by TNF-α and ADR using renal carcinoma cell lines (RCC) but the findings are also applicable to ovarian lines. Specifically, the study addressed four questions concerning the renal lines' sensitivity or resistance to drugs and TNF:

1. Is there a correlation between the sensitivity and/or resistance of the lines to TNF and adriamycin (ADR)?
2. Is there a correlation between the sensitivity and/or resistance to TNF and the TNF mRNA and TNF protein levels in these lines?
3. Is there a correlation between the sensitivity and/or resistance to TNF and the expression of the MDR phenotype?
4. Can combination treatment of the renal lines with TNF + ADR alter the TNF or MDR mRNA expression by these lines?

These questions were investigated with six human RCC lines of different sensitivities to TNF and ADR.

Induction of TNF mRNA and protein have been suggested as mechanisms of resistance to TNF in certain tumors [10]. Resistant and sensitive lines were capable of upregulating TNF mRNA after treatment with TNF or PMA and ionophore for periods as short as one hour, but only the resistant lines were able to secrete detectable levels of TNF protein. Therefore, a positive correlation existed between resistance to TNF and production and secretion of TNF by the cell lines. In the presence of the protein synthesis inhibitor cycloheximide (CHX), the TNF mRNA level in the TNF resistant lines was increased while the sensitive lines required an additional signal such as exogenous TNF to upregulate the mRNA. Due to the enhanced cytotoxicity seen with the combination of TNF and ADR, we determined the effect of this combination on the levels of TNF mRNA. As examined in a constitutively TNF expressing line, ADR alone reduced the constitutive mRNA level and, in combination with TNF, reduced the level of induction produced by TNF. We suggest that the downregulation of TNF mRNA by ADR may play a role in the enhanced cytotoxicity seen with combined TNF and ADR treatment [11].

Future directions will examine the specificity of TNF mRNA downregulation by ADR and the role of ADR in regulating other inducible resistant genes like MnSOD [12].

29.3 COMBINATION TREATMENT WITH TNF-α AND CIS-DIAMMINEDICHLOROPLATINUM (II) (CDDP)

Since the initial report of the antitumor efficacy of CDDP, this drug has played a major role in the treatment of several human cancers including ovarian cancer. The overall response rate of patients with ovarian cancer has significantly improved because of the aggressive use of regimens containing CDDP. We along with others have reported that combination of TNF-α and CDDP results in synergistic effects. In a further study, we investigated the cytotoxic effect of CDDP and TNF-α used in combination on CDDP resistant human ovarian tumor cell lines.

Treatment of the CDDP resistant C30 cells with CDDP and TNF-α overcomes the resistance of C30 cells to CDDP or TNF-α. In addition, the combination of CDDP and TNF-α resulted in a synergistic effect on the C30 resistant line, the CDDP sensitive parental cell line, A2780 and on two freshly derived ovarian carcinoma cell cultures. Treatment of C30 cells with CDDP followed by TNF-α showed a synergistic effect, while treatment with TNF-α followed by CDDP demonstrated a less cytotoxic effect. A possible mechanism of resistance to TNF-α in tumor cells is the induction of TNF-α mRNA and protein. C30 cells do not constitutively produce mRNA for TNF-α; however, treatment of C30 cells with TNF-α induces the expression of TNF-α mRNA. When CDDP was used in combination with TNF-α, the level of TNF-α mRNA induced by TNF-α was markedly reduced [13].

This study demonstrates that the combination of CDDP and TNF-α can overcome the CDDP resistance of tumor cells and that downregulation of TNF-α mRNA by CDDP may play a role in the enhanced cytotoxicity seen with the combination of CDDP and TNF-α. The synergistic effect obtained with established ovarian tumor cell lines and in short term cultures of freshly isolated ovarian tumors suggests that combination treatment with TNF-α and CDDP may have clinical applications in the therapy of drug resistant tumors.

In a recent study, we explored the effect of antioxidants like glutathione (GSH) on the sensitivity of lines resistant to TNF-α, CDDP or combination. GSH is a tripeptide thiol and is the most abundant non-protein sulfhydrylic compound in mammalian cells [14]. GSH plays an important role in the detoxification of various hazardous agents such as free radicals and xenobiotic compounds, either by itself or in reactions catalysed by GSH peroxidase and GSH S-transferase. It has further been associated with the development of drug resistance. Tumor cells which acquire resistance to certain cytotoxic agents are found to contain a much greater concentration of GSH [15,16]. When cellular GSH content is depleted, an increased sensitivity to these cytotoxic challenges has been demonstrated. We have investigated whether the resistance of C30 human ovarian cell lines to TNF-α or CDDP can be overcome by treatment with BSO in combination with TNF-α and/or CDDP.

Combination treatment of C30 cells with BSO and CDDP can overcome the resistance to CDDP. The combination of BSO and TNF-α resulted in a synergistic cytotoxic effect.

Furthermore, combination treatment with BSO, CDDP and TNF-α also showed a synergistic cytotoxic activity against C30 cells. This study demonstrates that treatment with BSO in combination with TNF-α or CDDP can overcome the TNF-α or CDDP resistance of tumor cells and that depletion of intracellular GSH and downregulation of TNF-α mRNA by BSO may play a role in the enhanced cytotoxicity observed with the combination of BSO and TNFα [unpublished].

29.4 COMBINATION TREATMENT WITH TNF-α AND TOXINS (DTX, PEA)

Diphtheria toxin (DTX) is a toxin secreted by *Corynebacterium diphtheriae* and is best characterized by its ability to inhibit protein synthesis. We have shown that DTX also has a cytotoxic activity. DTX mediated lysis results in early DNA fragmentation [17] with the same hallmarks as programmed cell death or apoptosis.

We hypothesized that DTX and TNF-α, used in combination, may result in either additive or synergistic cytotoxic activity. This was examined on three human ovarian carcinoma cell lines chosen for their differing sensitivities to TNF-α and DTX: 222, sensitive to both TNF-α and DTX; 222TR, a TNF-α resistant DTX sensitive variant of 222; and SKOV-3 resistant to both DTX and TNF-α. The simultaneous use of DTX and TNF-α at suboptimal concentrations resulted in synergistic cytotoxic activity against all three lines tested thus overcoming the TNF-α resistance of 222TR and the double resistance of SKOV-3. DNA fragmentation was observed in all three lines treated with DTX and TNF-α and occurred as early as 4 hours following treatment. Cycloheximide, actinomycin-D or emetine at concentrations causing >90% protein synthesis inhibition did not result in cytotoxicity alone or synergy with TNF-α, suggesting that synergy with DTX was not due

to its ability to inhibit protein synthesis. The use of energy poisons and pH conditions that inhibit DTX mediated cytotoxicity resulted in the abrogation of synergy. These findings show that the two cytotoxic agents TNF-α and DTX, when used at suboptimal concentrations, synergize in their cytotoxic activity against sensitive and resistant cell lines. Since the SKOV-3 cell line used here is also resistant to chemotherapeutic drugs, combination treatment with DTX and TNF-α may be beneficial in overcoming drug resistance [18].

A recent study was undertaken to further elucidate the pathway of DTX and *Pseudomonas* exotoxin A (PEA) mediated lysis and its role in the synergy obtained between DTX and TNF-α. Specifically, we investigated the role of DTX mediated catalytic reaction of ADP-ribosylation of EF-2 in both the cytolytic reaction and synergy with TNF-α. Using a DTX sensitive tumor cell line, we first examined the activity of the mutant CRM 197 which does not catalyse the ADP-ribosylation of elongation factor-2 (EF-2). CRM 197 was not cytolytic for target cells and did not mediate intranucleosomal DNA fragmentation of viable cells. The failure of CRM 197 to mediate target cell lysis suggested that the catalytic activity of DTX is a prerequisite for target cell lysis. This was corroborated by demonstrating that MeSAdo, which blocks the biosynthesis of dipthamide, inhibited DTX mediated protein synthesis inhibition and also blocked target cell lysis. Moreover, the addition of nicotinamide, which competes with NAD+ on DTX action site of EF-2, also blocked DTX mediated lysis. These findings suggest that ADP-ribosylation of EF-2 may be a necessary step in the pathway leading to target cell lysis. In contrast to the sensitive line, the SKOV-2 tumor cell line is sensitive to protein synthesis inhibition by DTX but is not susceptible to cytolysis and apoptosis by DTX. Thus, protein synthesis inhibition by DTX is not sufficient to mediate target cell lysis. Like the direct lysis by DTX, synergy was significantly reduced by MeSAdo and by nicotinamide. Further, synergy was not observed with the combination of CRM 197 and TNF-α. These results demonstrate that, in synergy, DTX or PEA may utilize the same pathway required for its cytolytic activity. *Pseudomonas* exotoxin A (PEA) shared all the properties shown for DTX. Altogether, these findings demonstrate that DTX mediated apoptosis is initiated at a step beyond the ADP-ribosylation of EF-2 [19].

29.5 COMBINATION WITH ANTI-FAS ANTIBODY AND TNF-α (DRUGS/TOXINS)

An ideal approach to overcoming drug resistance is to find cytotoxic agents that are highly selective to the tumor cells and minimally or non-toxic to the host. Thus, an agent that can mimic TNF in its cytotoxic and synergistic activity but that is devoid of other undesired activities may be a superior and selective agent in immunotherapy. With this objective, we investigated the cytotoxic effect of anti-Fas antibody in combination with drugs or toxins. Monoclonal mouse anti-Fas antibody is directed against Fas antigen, a 36 kd encoded polypeptide that belongs to the family of cell surface proteins which includes nerve growth factor receptor, TNF receptors, B cell antigen CD40 and T cell antigen OX40. Anti-Fas antibody mimics TNF-α in its cytolytic activity but not in other TNF-α mediated activities [20]. Thus, we examined whether anti-Fas antibody synergizes in cytotoxicity with toxins and drugs.

Anti-Fas antibody in combination with DTX, ADM or CDDP results in enhanced cytotoxicity and synergy and also overrides resistance to TNF, drugs or toxins when tested against a battery of human tumor cell lines. Synergy between anti-Fas and DTX indicates that DTX is enzymatically active since inhibitors of DTX mediated protein synthesis

inhibition resulted in loss of synergy. When the plant toxin ricin was used, there was no synergy with the anti-Fas antibody but there was an additive effect. The synergy was not obtained in a TNF-receptor negative line but was achieved with other anti-Fas resistant lines. Cell lines resistant either to ADM or CDDP were rendered sensitive by a combination of drug and anti-Fas antibody. Further, combination treatment of anti-Fas ovarian lines and ADM overcame resistance of gp 170 by expressing multidrug resistance (MDR). In all cases, cytotoxicity was augmented by pretreatment of target cells with IFN-γ which upregulates Fas antigen expression. These results show that anti-Fas antibody can synergize in cytotoxicity with toxins and chemotherapeutic drugs and combination treatment can reverse resistance to TNF, toxins and/or drugs [18].

29.6 CONCLUSION

It is well documented that resistance of cancerous cells to chemotherapy poses a threat to the patient. It is clear that new approaches to overcome resistance are urgently needed and in this vein, several potential avenues have been explored in experimental systems and in the clinics. The application of biological molecules in cancer therapy was first heralded by the use of IL-2 alone or in combination with LAK or TIL. Another molecule which was considered of therapeutic potential is TNF-α. However, TNF-α alone has proved ineffective in phase I and phase II clinical trials due to its toxicity *in vivo*.

In ovarian cancer, trials of intraperitoneal administration of TNF have been reported. In one study, prolonged exposure to high concentrations of TNF was achieved with minimal systemic toxicity; however, there was no objective response [21]. In a second trial, 17 of 32 patients had complete resolution of ascites by ultrasound [22].

Combinations of TNF and other agents in ovarian cancer therapy are at a preliminary stage and phase I data are available. The combination of IFN-γ with TNF reduced the maximum tolerated dose of TNF. Antitumor activity was observed in biliary cancer, pancreatic cancer and sarcoma [23,24]. IL-2 was also used in combination with TNF since IL-2 and TNF showed synergistic activation of LAK cells [25]. Investigators at the M.D. Anderson Cancer Center treated 16 patients with advanced non-small cell carcinoma of the lung with IL-2 and TNF and observed four regressions [26]. Studies with combinations of TNF and cytotoxic drugs are scarce. In a study reported *in vitro*, topoisomerase II inhibitors (e.g. etoposide) synergized with TNF for cytotoxicity [27]. One etoposide and TNF trial showed increased toxicity but marked myelosuppression limited the administration of TNF [28].

The studies reported in this chapter exemplify the potential use of combination treatment with TNF and various drugs/toxins in overcoming drug resistance and exerting a significant synergistic cytotoxicity. The synergy with small doses of TNF-α and drugs should minimize the toxicity induced by these drugs when used alone. Further, the findings showing that resistance of different types (MDR+, MDR−) can be overcome suggest that combination treatment is a viable approach for *in vivo* clinical trials.

The findings reported here have also opened new therapeutic avenues for exploration. For instance, *in vivo* stimulation of TNF-α secretion can be used instead of exogenous administration or the introduction of cells transfected with the TNF gene. Further, understanding the molecular mechanisms of the synergistic activity and intracellular pathways resulting in toxicity may well provide means to directly intervene into the cell to potentiate the cytotoxic effect.

ACKNOWLEDGEMENTS

The authors acknowledge the research support provided by the Boiron Research Foundation, France, and Institut Henri Beufour, France. The authors acknowledge the secretarial assistance of Ms Katty Kim and Samantha Nguyen.

REFERENCES

1. Safrit, J., Tsuchitani, T., Zighelboim, J. and Bonavida, B. (1992) Hierarchy of sensitivity and resistance of tumor cells to cytotoxic effector cells, cytokines, drugs and toxins. *Cancer Immunol. Immunother.*, **34**, 321–8.
2. Carswell, E.A., Old L.J., Kassel, R.L. *et al.* (1975) An endotoxin-induced serum factor that causes necrosis in tumors. *Proc. Natl. Acad. Sci. USA*, **72**, 3666–70.
3. Sherman, M.L., Spriggs, D.R., Arthur, K.A. *et al.* (1988) Recombinant human tumor necrosis factor administered as a five days infusion in cancer patients: phase I toxicity and effects on lipid metabolism. *J. Clin. Oncol.*, **6**, 344–50.
4. Balkwill, D.E., Ward, B.G., Woodie, E. *et al.* (1987) Therapeutic potential of tumor necrosis factor α and γ interferon in experimental human ovarian cancer. *Cancer Res.*, **47**, 4755–8.
5. Bonavida, B., Tsuchitani, T., Zighelboim, J., *et al.* (1990) Synergy is documented *in vitro* with low dose recombinant tumor necrosis factor, cisplatin, and doxorubicin in ovarian cancer cells. *Gynecol. Oncol.*, **38**, 333–9.
6. Riordan, J.R. and Ling, V. (1985) Genetic and biochemical characterization of multidrug resistance. *Pharmacol. Ther.*, **28**, 51–75.
7. Horio, M., Gottesman, N.M. *et al.* (1988) ATP-dependent transport of vinblastine vesicles from human multidrug-resistant cells. *Proc. Natl. Acad. Sci. USA*, **85**, 3580–4.
8. Schmid, D.S., Honung, R., McGrath, K.M. *et al.* (1987) Target cell DNA fragmentation is mediated by lymphotoxin and TNF-α. *Lymphokine Res.*, **6**, 195–202.
9. Safrit, J.T., Berek, J.S. and Bonavida, B. (1992) Sensitivity of drug resistant human ovarian

tumor cell lines to combined effects of tumor necrosis factor (TNF-α) and doxorubicin. Failure of the combination to modulate the MDR phenotype. *Gynecol. Oncol.,* **48**, 214–20.

10. Spriggs, D., Imanura, K., Rodriguez, D. *et al.* (1987) Induction of tumor necrosis factor expression and resistance in a human breast tumor cell line. *Proc. Natl. Acad. Sci. USA,* **84**, 6563.

11. Safrit, J.T., Belldegrun, A. and Bonavida, B. (1993) Sensitivity of human renal cell carcinoma lines to TNF, adriamycin and combination: role of TNF-mRNA induction in overcoming resistance. *J. Urol.,* **149**, 1202–8.

12. Wong, G.H.W., Elwell, J.H., Oberly, L.W. *et al.* (1989) Manganous superoxide dismutase is essential for cellular resistance to cytotoxicity of tumor necrosis factor. *Cell,* **58**, 923.

13. Mizutani, Y. and Bonavida, B. (1993) Overcoming CDDP resistance of human ovarian tumor cells by combination treatment with CDDP and TNF-α. *Cancer,* **72**, 809–18.

14. Coleman, C.N., Glove, D.J. and Turrisi, A.T. (1990) Radiation and chemotherapy sensitizers and protectors. In *Cancer Chemotherapy,* (eds B.A. Chabner and J.M. Collins), J.B. Lippincott, Philadelphia, pp. 424–48.

15. McGown, A.T. and Gox, B.W. (1986) A proposed mechanism of resistance to cyclophosphamide and phosphoramide mustard in a Yoshida cell line *in vitro. Cancer Chemother. Pharmacol.,* **17**, 223–9.

16. Mans, D.R.A., Schuurhuis, G.J., Treskes, M. *et al.* (1992) Modulation by D,L-buthionine-S, R-sulphoximine of etoposide cytotoxicity on human non-small cell lung, ovarian and breast carcinoma cell lines. *Eur. J. Cancer,* **28**, 1447–52.

17. Chang, M.P., Bramhall, J., Graves, S. *et al.* (1989) Internucleaosomal DNA cleavage preceded diphtheria toxin-induced cytolysis. Evidence that cell lysis is not a simple consequence of translation inhibition. *J. Biol. Chem.,* **264**, 15261.

18. Morimoto, H., Safrit, J.T. and Bonavida, B. (1991) Synergistic effect of tumor necrosis factor-alpha- and diphtheria toxin-mediated cytotoxicity in sensitive and resistant human ovarian tumor cell lines. *J. Immunol.,* **147**, 2609.

19. Morimoto, H. and Bonavida, B. (1992) Diphtheria-toxin and *Pseudomonas,* a toxin-mediated apoptosis: ADP-ribosylation of EF-2 is required for DNA fragmentation and cell lysis and synergy with tumor necrosis factor-α. *J. Immunol.,* **149**, 2089–94.

20. Yonehara, S., Ishii, A. and Yonehara, M. (1991) A cell-killing monoclonal antibody (anti-Fas) to a cell surface antigen co-downregulated with the receptor of tumor necrosis factor. *J. Exp. Med.,* **169**, 1747–56.

21. Reichman, B., Markman, M., Inotti, N. *et al.* (1989) Phase I trial of intraperitoneal recombinant tumor necrosis factor. *Proc. Am. Soc. Clin. Oncol.,* **8**, 64.

22. Raeth, U., Schmid, H., Karck, U. *et al.* (1991) Phase II trial of recombinant human tumor necrosis factor in patients with malignant ascites from ovarian carcinomas and non-ovarian tumors with intraperitoneal spread. *Proc. Am. Soc. Clin. Oncol.,* **10**, 187.

23. Abbruzzese, J.L., Levin, B., Ajani, J.A. *et al.* (1989) Phase I trial of recombinant human gamma-interferon and recombinant human tumor necrosis factor in patients with advanced gastrointestinal cancer. *Cancer Res.,* **49**, 4057–61.

24. Schiller, J.H., Alberti, D.B., Arzoomanian, R.Z. *et al.* (1990) Phase I trial of combination of recombinant gamma interferon and recombinant tumor necrosis factor alpha. *Proc. Am. Assoc. Cancer Res.,* **31**, 183.

25. McIntosh, J.K., Mule, J.J., Krosnick, J.A. *et al.* (1989) Combination cytokine immuno-therapy with tumor necrosis factor alpha, interleukin 2, and alpha-interferon and its synergistic antitumor effects in mice. *Cancer Res.,* **49**, 1408–14.

26. Yang, S.C., Owen, S.L., Mendiguren, R.A. *et al.* (1990) Combination immunotherapy for non-small cell lung cancer. Results with interleukin-2 and tumor necrosis factor-alpha. *J. Thorac. Cardiovasc. Surg.,* **99**, 8–12.

27. Alexander, R.B., Nelson, W.G. and Coffey, D.S. (1987) Synergistic enhancement by tumor necrosis factor of *in vitro* cytotoxicity from chemotherapeutic drugs targeted at DNA topoisomerase II. *Cancer Res.*, **47**, 2403–6.

28. Orr, D., Oldham, R., Lewis, M. *et al.* (1989) Phase I study of the sequenced administration of etoposide and recombinant tumor necrosis factor in patients with advanced malignancy. *Proc. Am. Soc. Clin. Oncol.*, **8**, 741.

Chapter 30

Potential for immunotherapy: PEM as a target antigen

J. TAYLOR-PAPADIMITRIOU, N. PEAT, J. BURCHELL, P. BEVERLEY and M. SMITH

30.1 INTRODUCTION

In looking for novel therapies for the effective treatment of ovarian cancer, particularly as an adjuvant to surgery, immunotherapy is an option which is ready to be explored. Two reasons why this option may now be a realistic one are that potential target antigens are being identified and considerable advances have been made in understanding the underlying mechanisms involved in tumour rejection and in antigen presentation and recognition by the various components of the immune system. The possibility of extending immunotherapy to prevention (at least for prevention of recurrence of the disease) is also a real one since active specific immunotherapy (ASI) appears to be unaccompanied by obvious serious side effects.

When an ovarian cancer or any other malignant tumour is detected clinically, the cells making up the tumour have clearly not been rejected by the host immune system. The implications of this are that even if the tumour does express antigens which can potentially be recognized by some or all of the compartments of the immune system, they are either not being presented effectively or are not being recognized by effector cells. The challenge is therefore two-fold, that is, to identify relevant antigens and to find a way

to present these so that an immune response is generated which is effective in rejecting the tumour cells. In this chapter, we will focus on a specific antigen, the polymorphic epithelial mucin (PEM, the product of the MUC1 gene), explain why it may be a candidate target antigen for immunotherapy or preventative vaccination of ovarian cancer and discuss the model systems which are available to explore its efficacy as an immunogen. We will also briefly review some of the general problems associated with effective antigen presentation and with tumour cell killing and what strategies can be adopted to achieve successful tumour rejection.

30.2 TUMOUR ASSOCIATED ANTIGENS IN OVARIAN CANCER

While most information available from patients relates to PEM, there are other antigens which may be important targets. Overexpression of the c-erbB2 antigen is seen in a proportion of patients [1] and this is being largely considered as a target for therapies based on antibodies (see below). The folate binding protein, recognized by the MOv18 antibody, is overexpressed in ovarian cancer and could also represent a suitable target for immunotherapy as well as for conjugated or bispecific antibodies [2]. As in other tumours, the p53 gene is mutated in 36% of ovarian cancers [3]. Even though this is an internal antigen, antibodies to it have been detected in cancer patients [4]. Moreover, p53 peptides have been identified which can be presented by HLA class I molecules (A2) and recognized by cytotoxic T cells from ovarian cancer (K. Melief, personal communication). There is also a possibility that the MAGE antigens identified by Boon and colleagues [5] may be present on ovarian cancers, but this needs to be verified. The CA125 antigen (Chapter 19) has not yet been cloned but if it is, it could in the future also be considered a possible immunogen.

30.3 ANTIBODIES AS A TREATMENT MODALITY

The appeal of ASI is that by injecting an immunogen or immunogens, there is the prospect of mobilizing the whole spectrum of the host's cellular and humoral immune responses. In administering an unlabelled antibody directed to one epitope of a target antigen, inevitably the attack on the immune system is confined to a single component of one compartment, albeit present in high concentration. The effect of the antibody can, of course, be boosted by coupling to a toxin or radioactivity, or a bispecific antibody may be generated which, reacting in one arm with the T cell receptor, can recruit cells of the immune system. Recent studies suggest that with a single radiolabelled antibody, it is possible to affect the survival of ovarian cancer patients. Thus a study by Hird *et al.* [6] indicates that only one injection of yttrium-labelled HMFG-1 antibody (directed to PEM) given intraperitoneally can have a dramatic effect on the survival of ovarian cancer patients who have minimal disease after conventional treatment. In colon cancer, several injections of unlabelled anti-

body have also been found to have a significant effect on survival, providing the tumour burden postsurgery was not large (G. Reithmuller, personal communication). Studies with bispecific antibodies are also beginning in the clinic.

The results with the antibodies are very encouraging. They emphasize what the immunologist have predicted for some time, that the immune system or components thereof are most likely to be effective where the tumour burden is low. This is particularly important in the case of solid tumours, where it is clearly going to be easier for antibodies or leucocytes to reach tumours cells when they are single or in small clusters and not in a large solid mass. The study with the HMFG-1 antibody is now moving to a phase II trial and the relevance of mouse versus humanized monoclonal antibodies will also be investigated.

30.4 MECHANISMS OF TUMOUR REJECTION

Before discussing in detail the PEM antigen, its expression in ovarian cancer and why it may be an excellent target antigen, it may be relevant to consider the current ideas as to which components of the immune system may be relevant to tumour rejection mediated by specific antigens. Clearly antibodies could play a role but whether this is direct, that is, by recruiting macrophages through the Fc receptor, or indirect (for example, via induction of the idiotypic network) is not clear. However, a crucial role for CD8+ cytotoxic T cells supported by CD4+ helper T cells has been demonstrated in several animal models. Here, a major stimulus for activation of the T cell is the interaction of the T cell receptor with a peptide carried on the surface HLA molecule (class I in the case of CD8+ cytotoxic T cells, class II in the case of CD4+ helper T cells). For proliferation to occur, however, the secretion of IL-2 is required and this requires the interaction of costimulatory molecules on the antigen presenting cell and the T cells (Figure 30.1) (see [7] for reviews). The B7 molecule which acts as a ligand for the C28 molecule on the T cell represents such an important molecule which is expressed on antigen presenting cells. A tumour cell expressing the same antigen which activated the cytotoxic T cell (that is, peptide associated with the HLA molecule) can then be recognized and killed by it.

This view of the activation of a cytotoxic T cell requires a functional HLA and a costimulatory molecule, B7, to be present on the antigen presenting cell. These are found on

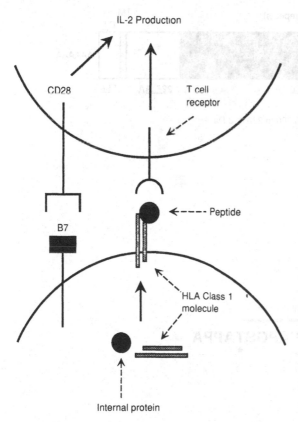

Figure 30.1 Current view of HLA restricted antigen presentation to T cells, requiring the costimulatory interaction of B7 and CD28.

professional antigen presenting cells which also express HLA class II and which can induce high IL-2 expression in helper T cells as well as activating cytotoxic T cells (Figure 30.1). It is not the case for tumour cells, which do not express B7 or, in general, HLA class II. They may also lose expression of HLA class I which means they can neither present antigen nor be targets for cytotoxic T cells. These are important concepts in the framework of immunotherapy and the importance of B7 in antigen presentation has been recently forcefully demonstrated by Linsley and colleagues who were able to convert a non-immunogenic tumour into an immunogenic tumour by transfecting and expressing B7 [8,9]. The importance of HLA class I in this classic view of antigen presentation is also to be emphasized, not only because class I expression may be lost [10] but also because only certain peptides can be presented by a particular allele. The apparent lack of requirement for HLA presentation by the PEM antigen (see below) becomes particularly important in this context.

30.5 THE POLYMORPHIC EPITHELIAL MUCIN (PEM)

Attention was focused on PEM initially because many antibodies selected for specificity of reaction with epithelial cells or carcinomas were found to react with this molecule [11]. The molecule is therefore extremely immunogenic in the mouse. The gene (MUC1) coding for the core protein of this molecule has been cloned [12–16] and the molecule has been shown to be a transmembrane protein with a cytoplasmic tail of 69 amino acids and a large extracellular domain made up largely of tandem repeats (TR) of 20 amino acids. The TR domain is rich in serine, threonine and prolines and serves as a scaffold for the addition of sugars resulting in a very extended rodlike structure

(Figure 30.2A). Since the number of tandem repeats can vary with the individual allele, the gene is highly polymorphic.

Although PEM, the MUC1 gene product, is expressed on most simple epithelial cells lining glands or ducts, it is dramatically upregulated in the mammary gland at lactation and in adenocarcinomas. The molecule is also aberrantly glycosylated in breast and other carcinomas [17,18], making it antigenically distinct from the normally processed mucin: the SM3 epitope being preferentially expressed in carcinomas (Figure 30.2B).

Although the complete structure of the core proteins of the complex gastrointestinal and lung mucins has not been elucidated, the data that are available suggest that they are probably not transmembrane molecules. Moreover, they contain cysteine rich domains which probably function to form covalently bonded aggregates. Indeed, PEM may be unique among the mucins in lacking cysteine rich

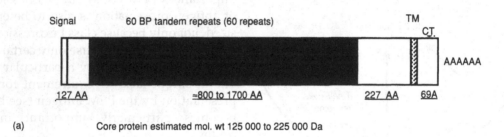

(a)   Core protein estimated mol. wt 125 000 to 225 000 Da

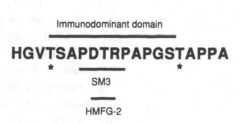

(b)   * Probable glycosylation sites

Figure 30.2 (a) Diagram of MUC1 gene. (b) Tandem repeat sequence.

308

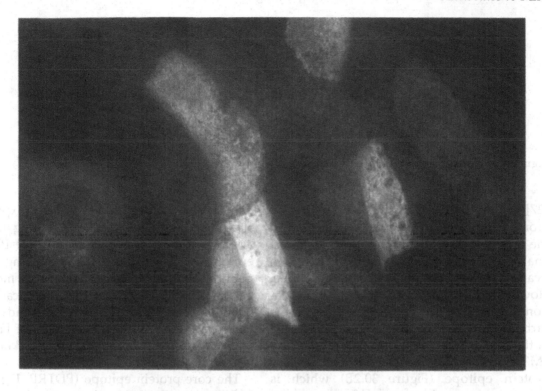

Figure 30.3 Immunohistochemical staining of ovarian cancer cell line with antibody HMFG-1.

domains and in being an intrinsic membrane glycoprotein. It is also more generally overexpressed in carcinomas. More than 90% of ovarian cancers express MUC1 and many ovarian cancer cell lines maintain expression. Figure 30.3 shows the staining of ovarian cancer cell line PEO14 [22] with the monoclonal antibody HMFG-1.

The fact that the MUC1 gene product is a transmembrane molecule which shows increased expression and aberrant glycosylation in cancer makes it an important potential target antigen for antibodies and other components of the immune system.

30.6 ANTIBODIES TO PEM

Many of the core protein epitopes detected by mouse monoclonal antibodies are found within an immunodominant domain lying between doublets of serine and threonine which are potential glycosylation sites [23,24]. Statistically it is found that only two oligosaccharide side chains are added for each tandem repeat (F.G. Hanisch, personal communication). Recent data following *in vitro* glycosylation with cell extracts suggest that the sites of attachment for these side chains are the threonines flanking the SAPDTR-PAPGS sequence (M.A. Hollingsworth, personal communication; and Figure 30.2B).

Although the sequence of the MUC1 gene coding for the core protein PEM is the same in normal and malignant cells [12,25], the length and composition of the carbohydrate side chains varies. A direct analysis of the side chains in milk mucin [26] and in the mucin derived from a breast cancer cell line

309

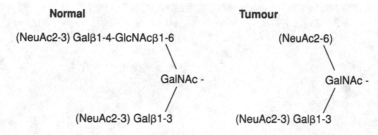

Figure 30.4 Major carbohydrate side chains on PEM.

[27] shows that the chains are larger and more complex in the normal mucin than in the breast cancer mucin (Figure 30.4). Direct analysis of the carbohydrate side chains on ovarian cancer cell lines has not been done. However, the result of the different glycosylation means that novel epitopes appear in the carbohydrate side chains and are unmasked in the core protein of the tumour mucin. The SM3 antibody [7] reacts with such a core protein epitope (Figure 30.2B) which is cryptic in the mucin expressed by the normal mammary gland and is selectively exposed in ovarian cancer [18,28]. This antibody has been effectively used to image ovarian cancers [29]. Effective imaging of ovarian cancers can also be achieved with antibodies (such as HMFG-2; Figure 30.2B) which react with epitopes which are also exposed (perhaps at low levels) on the normal mucin, suggesting that *levels* of antigen and tissue topography are important consideration, since normal PEM expressing tissues are not imaged.

30.7 EVIDENCE FOR IMMUNE RECOGNITION OF PEM IN CANCER PATIENTS

Evidence for immune recognition of the breast cancer mucin was first noted by Finn and colleagues, who isolated cytotoxic T cells which killed PEM expressing cancer cell lines [30,31]. The mechanism involved is unclear, however, since killing is not HLA restricted and indeed not dependent on HLA expression. This non-HLA restricted killing may arise from the interaction of multiple PEM epitopes with the T cell (not involving the peptide binding groove of the HLA molecule). If this is a general mechanism in cancer patients then PEM offers tremendous advantages as a target antigen, since loss of HLA will not affect the killing nor will such killing be restricted to only certain HLA alleles.

The core protein epitope (PDTRP; Figure 30.2B) recognized by the antibody SM3 [17,18] is selectively exposed in breast, ovarian and other carcinomas. Moreover, the SM3 antibody has been found to block the killing of PEM expressing breast cancer cells, suggesting that the core protein epitopes in the vicinity of the PDTRP sequence may be involved in T cell recognition. Recently it has been possible to demonstrate that ovarian cancer patients can produce antibodies to PEM, by immortalizing B cells producing such antibodies from infiltrating lymphocytes in ovarian cancers [32]. Cytotoxic T cells have also been isolated from such infiltrating lymphocytes which can recognize mucin peptides (Chapter 31).

The range of immunogens based on PEM which could be used to attempt to induce an immune response leading to tumour rejection is wide (Table 30.1). To evaluate the efficacy of the various immunogens, to optimize antigen presentation and to analyse mechanisms involved in tumour rejection, model systems are required.

Table 30.1 Possible types of immunogen based on the structure of the cancer associated polymorphic epithelial mucin

1. Cells expressing the mucin
2. Purified mucin (produced by cancer cells)
3. Recombinant core protein or different glycoforms produced by transfected cells
4. Peptides or glycopeptides based on the tandem repeat
5. Recombinant viruses (vaccines, retroviruses)
6. Recombinant BCG
7. Synthetic carbohydrates based on the short carbohydrate side chains found in the cancer associated mucin (see Figure 30.4)

30.8 RODENT MODELS FOR STUDYING TUMOUR REJECTION AND IMMUNE RESPONSES TO PEM

30.8.1 THE TA3-Ha TUMOUR FOR ANALYSIS OF CARBOHYDRATE ANTIGENS

The shorter carbohydrate side chains which are carried on the core protein of the polymorphic epithelial mucin in many carcinomas are also found on other mucin core proteins in mouse as well as in humans. The mucin expressed by an extremely aggressive mouse mammary adenocarcinoma TA3-Ha also carries these side chains and this mouse model has been used effectively to analyse the efficacy of synthetic carbohydrates as immunogens [33,34]. Antibody responses to T (Gal1-3GalNAc) coupled to KLH have been seen in immunized mice and inhibition of tumour growth was seen even when the immunogen was administered after the tumour cells were injected [33]. Ovine submaxillary mucin (carrying multiple sialylated Tn epitopes, that is, NeuAc 2-6GalNAc) and its desialylated product have also been found to be effective in both stimulating an immune response and inhibiting tumour growth in this system [34]. Although cellular responses to carbohydrates are not well studied, they

have been shown to induce delayed type hypersensitivity (DTH) responses and T cell proliferation in immunized mice [33,34]. The phase I trial in ovarian cancer patients which has begun in Canada [35] uses synthetic sialylTn coupled to KLH (keyhole limpet hemocyanin) as immunogen.

30.8.2 SYNGENEIC MODEL SYSTEM USING A MOUSE MAMMARY TUMOUR CELL LINE TRANSFECTED WITH THE HUMAN MUC1 GENE

A syngeneic model for comparing the efficacy of immunogens based on PEM was developed by introducing the MUC1 gene into the mouse mammary epithelial tumour cell line 410.4 [36]. Expression of the human PEM resulted in a reduced growth of tumours in Balb/c mice at low inoculum, but tumours did develop provided sufficient cells (10^5) were injected. A variety of immunogens can be used (see Table 30.1) and to date we have been able to show that inhibition of tumour growth can be achieved by preimmunization with transfected cells [36], peptides based on the tandem repeat sequence of PEM [37] and a recombinant vaccinia virus carrying the MUC1 gene (J. Lewis *et al.*, unpublished observations). As yet no ovarian cancer mouse model has been developed, but there is no reason to think that results from the mammary model cannot be applied to ovarian tumours.

30.8.3 TRANSGENIC MICE EXPRESSING THE HUMAN MUC1 GENE

To look at immune responses in a host where the human PEM is expressed as a self-antigen, a transgenic mouse has been developed. The MUC1 gene is compact (Figure 30.5), being closely flanked 3' by the thrombospondin 3 gene [38] and 5' by a gene giving a large transcript (13 kb) in most tissues (S.J. Gendler and T. Duhig, personal communication). Perhaps not surprisingly, therefore, we have been able to obtain accurate tissue

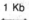

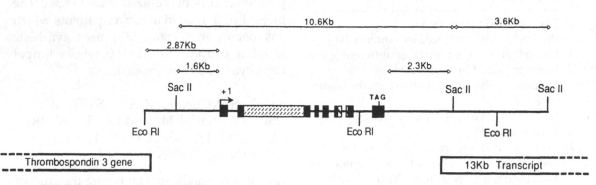

Figure 30.5 Structure of MUC1 gene.

specific expression in a transgenic mouse using a 10.6 kb fragment of genomic DNA containing only 1.5 kb of 5' sequence and 2.3 kb of 3' sequence [39]. In humans, the MUC1 gene is expressed largely by simple epithelial cells and the same distribution (as determined by staining with antibodies specific for the human PEM) is seen in the transgenic mouse. These mice therefore provide an appropriate model for toxicity testing of antibodies or antigens related to the human PEM. It is also possible to look at humoral responses to PEM based immunogens and to examine T cell proliferative responses *in vitro*. Since the mice are hybrid, it will be necessary to backcross on to a single strain in order to analyse H2 restricted cytotoxic T cell responses (cytotoxic T cell responses which are not H2 restricted can, however, be analysed). The backcrossed transgenics can then be used as recipients for PEM expressing mouse tumours, giving us a highly appropriate model for looking at tumour rejection where PEM is expressed as a self-antigen. We are also presently attempting to obtain a transgenic strain which spontaneously develops epithelial tumours by expressing an oncogene from the PEM promoter [40]. It is possible that in this way, we may develop an ovarian tumour model.

30.9   ANTIGEN PRESENTATION

Classically, antigens are administered with adjuvant, which in a general way acts to induce a more effective immune response. In this context the idea of using a recombinant BCG vaccine [41] expressing PEM is particularly attractive, since BCG has been widely administered to humans as an anti-TB vaccine and attempts to make such a construct are beginning. In classic antigen presentation through HLA class I antigen, costimulatory molecules as well as HLA class I molecules need to be present on the antigen presenting cells. As we have seen, it has been possible to obtain cytotoxic T cells from cancer patients which appear to kill PEM expressing cells in a non-HLA restricted fashion. However, it still has to be said that the tumours in these patients were not rejected, therefore these T cells were ineffective. There is still therefore a need to be concerned with antigen presentation, even with PEM. It is not yet clear whether T cell activation by PEM requires the interaction of the costimulatory B7 molecule, which is not present on tumour cells. Experiments are now underway to see whether transfection of the mouse B7 molecule into the PEM expressing mouse mammary tumour cells increases the immunogenicity of

312

PEM in this system. Hopefully similar studies can be done soon with tumours in the back-crossed transgenic mouse. It will also be important to transfect the human B7 into ovarian cancer cell lines and see if immune responses *in vitro* can be improved.

The function of the costimulatory molecules is to induce the production of IL-2 which itself can influence the production of other cytokines. One avenue which is being extensively explored in improving antigen presentation is to deliver cytokines to the tumour site or in some way to supply a specific cytokine along with the antigen for optimal recruitment of the various components of the immune system.

Mouse models have been used to examine the effect of injecting irradiated tumour cells expressing various lymphokines (e.g. interferons, interleukins, GM-CSF) on subsequent tumour development in mice challenged with tumour cells. These studies have renewed enthusiasm for the concept of cancer vaccines. In the study reported by Dranoff *et al.* [42], a variety of cytokine genes were introduced using retroviruses into B16 melanoma cells. These investigators found that irradiated cells expressing GM-CSF stimulated potent, long-lasting and specific antitumour immunity which depended on CD4+ and CD8+ T cells. The results could have important implications for the clinical use of genetically engineered tumour cells as vaccines. Retroviruses ensure that the gene may be introduced into a large number of the cells and the possibility of using irradiated cells avoids the obvious problems which may arise with the use of live tumour cells. Another possibility is to use a fusion protein which carries the antigenic determinant and the functional lymphokine. Again, a role for GM-CSF has been implicated from such studies since a GM-CSF-antigen fusion protein has been found to be an effective vaccine [43]. Such DNA based vaccines offer great advantages over cell based immunogens.

30.10 CONCLUSIONS

The identification of specific tumour associated antigens together with the improved understanding of the mechanisms underlying effective antigen presentation is bringing immunotherapy closer to implementation. The PEM antigen is expressed on most ovarian cancers, is highly immunogenic and is able to induce both cellular and humoral immunity in ovarian cancer patients. While pilot trials are beginning with PEM based antigens, studies need to be done to identify ways of presenting the antigen which will result in specific and effective tumour cell killing. These will be done in the mouse model systems and looking for immune responses *in vitro* with patient material. It is hoped that in time new immunological inroads will be made into improving the therapy of ovarian cancer.

REFERENCES

1. Hung, M.C., Zhang, X., Yen, D.H. *et al.* (1992) Aberrant expression of the c-erbB-2/neu proto-oncogene in ovarian cancer. *Cancer Lett.*, **61**, 95–103.
2. Campbell, I.G., Jones, T.A., Foulkes, W.D. *et al.* (1991) Folate-binding protein is a marker for ovarian cancer. *Cancer Res.*, **51**, 5329–38.
3. Mazars, R., Pujol, P., Maudelonde, T. *et al.* (1991) p53 mutations in ovarian cancer: a late event? *Oncogene*, **6**, 1685–90.
4. Lamb, P. and Crawford, L. (1986) Characterization of the human p53 gene. *Cancer Res.*, **6**, 1379–85.
5. Van der Bruggen, P., Traversari, C., Chomez, P. *et al.* (1991) A gene encoding an antigen recognized by cytolytic T lymphocytes on a human melanoma. *Science*, **254**, 1643–7.
6. Hird, V., Snook, D., Dhokia, B. *et al.* (1993) Adjuvant therapy of ovarian cancer with radioactive monoclonal antibody. *Br. J. Cancer*, **68**, 403–6.
7. Schwartz, R.H. (1992) Costimulation of T lymphocytes: the role of CD28, CTLA-4, and

B7/BB1 in interleukin-2 production and immunotherapy. *Cell*, **71**, 1065–8.

8. Linsley, P.S., Brady, W., Grosmaire, L. *et al.* (1992) Binding of the B cell activation antigen B7 to CD28 costimulates T cell proliferation and interleukin 2 mRNA accumulation. *J. Exp. Med.*, **173**, 721–30.

9. Chen, L., Ashe, S., Brady, W.A. *et al.* (1992) Costimulation of antitumour immunity by the B7 counterreceptor for the T lymphocyte molecules CD28 and CTLA-4. *Cell*, **71**, 1093–102.

10. Browning, M.J. and Bodmer, W.F. (1992) MHC antigens and cancer: implications for T-cell surveillance. *Curr. Opinion Immunol.* **4**, 613–18.

11. Burchell, J. and Taylor-Papadimitriou, J. (1989) Antibodies to human milk fat globule molecules. *Cancer Invest.*, **17**, 53–61.

12. Gendler, S.J., Lancaster, C.A., Taylor-Papadimitriou, J. *et al.* (1990) Molecular cloning and expression of the human tumour-associated polymorphic epithelial mucin. *J. Biol. Chem.*, **265**, 15286–93.

13. Ligtenberg, M., Vos, H., Gennissen, A. *et al.* (1990) Episialin, a carcinoma-associated mucin, is generated by a polymorphic gene encoding splice variants with alternative amino termini. *J. Biol. Chem.*, **265**, 5573–8.

14. Wreschner, D.H., Hareuveni, M., Tsarfaty, I. *et al.* (1990) Human epithelial tumor antigen cDNA sequences. *Eur. J. Biochem.*, **189**, 463–73.

15. Siddiqui, J., Abe, M., Hayes, D. *et al.* (1988) Isolation and sequencing of a cDNA coding for the human DF3 breast carcinoma-associated antigen. *Proc. Natl. Acad. Sci. USA*, **85**, 2320–3.

16. Lan, M., Batra, S., Qi, W-N. *et al.* (1990) Cloning and sequencing of a human pancreatic tumour mucin cDNA. *J. Biol. Chem.*, **265**, 15294–9.

17. Burchell, J., Gendler, S.J., Taylor-Papadimitriou, J. *et al.* (1987) Development and characterisation of breast cancer reactive monoclonal antibodies directed to the core protein of the human milk mucin. *Cancer. Res.*, **47**, 5476–82.

18. Girling, J.R., Bartkova, J., Burchell, J. *et al.*, (1989) A core protein epitope of the polymorphic epithelial mucin detected by the monoclonal antibody SM-3 is selectively exposed in a range of primary carcinomas. *Int. J. Cancer*, **43**, 1072–6.

19. Gunn, J.R., Byrd, J., Hicks, J. *et al.* (1989) Molecular cloning of human intestinal mucin cDNAs. *J. Biol. Chem.*, **264**, 6480–7.

20. Gum, J.R., Hicks, J., Swallow, D. *et al.* (1990) Molecular cloning of cDNAs derived from a novel human intestinal mucin gene. *Biochem. Biophys. Res. Commun.*, **171**, 407–15.

21. Porchet, N., van Cong, N., Dufosse, J. *et al.* (1991) Molecular cloning and chromosomal localization of a novel human tracheo-bronchial mucin cDNA containing tandemly repeated sequences of 48 base pairs. *Biochem. Biophys. Res. Commun.*, **175**, 414–22.

22. Langdon, S.P., Lawrie, S.S., Hay, F.G. *et al.* (1988) Characterization and properties of nine human ovarian adenocarcinoma cell lines. *Cancer Res.*, **48**, 6166–72.

23. Burchell, J., Taylor-Papadimitriou, J., Boshell, M. *et al.* (1989) A short sequence within the amino acid tandem repeat of a cancer associated mucin contains immunodominant epitopes. *Int. J. Cancer*, **44**, 691–6.

24. Taylor-Papadimitriou, J. (1991) Report on the First International Workshop on Carcinoma-associated Mucins. *Int. J. Cancer*, **49**, 1–5.

25. Lancaster, C., Peat, N., Duhig, T. *et al.* (1990) Structure and expression of the human polymorphic epithelial mucin gene: an expressed VNTR unit. *Biochem. Biophys. Res. Commun.*, **173**, 1019–29.

26. Hanish, F.G., Uhlenbruck, G., Peter-Katalinic, J. *et al.* (1989) Structure of neutral O-linked polylactosaminoglycans on human skim milk mucins. A novel type of linearly extended poly-N-acetyl-lactosamine backbones with Galβ(1–4) GlcNAcβ(1–6) repeating units. *J. Biol. Chem.*, **265**, 872–83.

27. Hull, S.R., Bright, A., Carraway, K.L. *et al.* (1989) Oligosaccharide differences in the DF3 sialomucin antigen from normal human milk and the BT-20 human breast carcinoma cell line. *Cancer Commun.*, **1**, 261–7.

28. Van Daam, P.A., Lowe, D.G., Watson, J.V. *et al.* (1991) Multiparameter flow cytometric quantitation of the expression of the tumor-associated antigen SM3 in normal and neoplastic ovarian tissues. *Cancer*, **68**, 169–77.

29. Granowska, M., Mather, S.J., Jobling, T. *et al.* (1990) Radiolabelled stripped mucin, SM3, monoclonal antibody for immunoscintigraphy of ovarian tumours. *Int. J. Biol. Markers*, **5**, 89–96.

30. Barnd, D.L., Lan, M.S., Metzgar, R.S. *et al.* (1989) Specific, major histocompatibilty complex-unrestricted recognition of tumor-associated mucins by human cytotoxic T cells. *Proc. Natl. Acad. Sci. USA*, **86**, 7159–64.

31. Jerome, K.R., Barnd, K.L. Bendt, K.M. *et al.* (1991) Cytotoxic T-lymphocytes derived from patients with breast adenocarcinoma recognise an epitope present on the protein core of a mucin molecule preferentially expressed by malignant cells. *Cancer Res.*, **51**, 2908–16.

32. Rughetti, A., Turchi, V., Apolonj Ghetti, C. *et al.* (1993) Human B cell immune response against the polymorphic epithelial mucin (PEM). *Cancer Res.*, **53**, 2457–90.

33. Fung, P.Y.S., Madej, M., Koganty, R. *et al.* (1990) Active specific immunotherapy of a murine mammary adenocarcinoma using a synthetic tumor-associated glycoconjugate. *Cancer Res.*, **50**, 4308.

34. Singhal, A., Fohn, M. and Hakomori, S. (1991) Induction of α-N-acetylgalactosamine-O-serine/threonine (Tn) antigen-mediated cellular immune response for active immunotherapy in mice. *Cancer Res.*, **51**, 1406–14.

35. MacLean, G.D., Bowen-Yacyshyn, M.B., Samuel, J. *et al.* (1992) Active immunization of human ovarian cancer patients against a common carcinoma (Thomsen-Friedenreich) determinant using a synthetic carbohydrate antigen. *J. Immunother.*, **11**, 292–305.

36. Lalani, E.N., Berdichevsky, F., Boshell, M. *et al.* (1991) Expression of the gene coding for a human mucin in mouse mammary tumour cells can affect their tumorigenicity. *J. Biol. Chem.*, **266**, 15420–6.

37. Ding, L., Lalani, E.N., Reddish, M. *et al.* (1993) Immunogenicity of synthetic peptides related to the core peptide sequence encoded by the human MUC1 mucin gene: effect of immunization on the growth of murine mammary adenocarcinoma cells transfected with the human MUC1 gene. *J. Cancer Immunol. Immunother.*, **36**, 9–17.

38. Vos, H.L., Devarayalu, Y., de Vries, Y. and Bornstein, P. (1992) Thrombospondin 3 (Thbs3), a new member of the thrombospondin gene family. *J. Biol. Chem.*, **267**, 12192–6.

39. Peat, N., Gendler, S.J., Lalani, E.N., (1992) Tissue-specific expression of a human polymorphic epithelial mucin (MUC1) in transgenic mice. *Cancer Res.*, **52**, 1954–60.

40. Kovarik, A., Peat, N., Wilson, D. *et al.* (1993) Analysis of the tissue specific promoter of the MUC1 gene. *J. Biol. Chem.*, **268**, 9917–26.

41. Aldovini, A. and Young, R.A. (1991) Humoral and cell-mediated immune responses to live recombinant BCG-HIV vaccines. *Nature*, **35**, 1479–82.

42. Dranoff, G., Jaffee, E., Lazenby, A. *et al.* (1993) Vaccination with irradiated tumor cells engineered to secrete murine granulocyte–macrophage colony-stimulating factor stimulates potent, specific, and long-lasting anti-tumor immunity. *Proc. Natl. Acad. Sci. USA*, **90**, 3539–43.

43. Tao, M.H. and Levy, R. (1993) A novel vaccine for B-cell lymphoma: idiotype/granulocyte-macrophage colony-stimulating factor fusion protein. *Nature*, **362**, 755–8.

Chapter 31

Ovarian tumour reactive cytotoxic T lymphocytes can recognize peptide determinants on polymorphic epithelial mucins Muc-1

C.G. IOANNIDES, B. FISK, K.R. JEROME, B. CHESAK, T. IRIMURA, J.T. WHARTON and O.J. FINN

31.1 INTRODUCTION

Tumour reactive cytotoxic T lymphocytes (CTL) have been isolated and propagated in culture from tumour infiltrating lymphocytes (TIL) of various tumours [1–6]. The fact that these cells are endowed with the ability to lyse autologous tumour cells has lead to their use in cancer immunotherapy trials, with encouraging results in certain instances [1].

In ovarian cancer, CTL-TIL specificity for autologous tumours has been defined as preferential lysis of autologous tumours and described as possessing a higher ability to lyse autologous than allogeneic tumours, non-malignant targets or lymphokine activated killer (LAK) cell defined targets such as Daudi cells [3–6]. The ability of these CTL to lyse allogeneic tumours may reflect either recognition of common antigens in the context of common MHC class I molecules or non-specific lysis when targets with different MHC class I phenotypes are recognized by tumour reactive CTL [7].

The simultaneous recognition of both autologous and allogeneic targets [5] may suggest either that the mechanisms of recognition of these targets by tumour reactive CTL may be distinct or antigens on these targets may be held in common and recognized in both MHC restricted and unrestricted fashion. Since T cell receptors (TCR) can recognize epitopes on peptides bound to and presented by MHC or conformational changes induced by the antigen in the MHC (the altered self-recognition hypothesis) [8], this raises the question of the relationship among the various types of cytotoxicity expressed by tumour reactive CTL as a function of antigen processing and presentation.

An analysis of this relationship would require that antigens recognized by these CTL are known; thus the effects of antigen presentation in various forms associated with different HLA molecules can be investigated. Unfortunately, there is limited knowledge of the nature, presentation and recognition of tumour antigens by T cells.

Recently, Finn and collaborators provided evidence for shared CTL recognized tumour antigens (epitopes) on tumours of different origin. They have identified the core peptide of the tandem repeat of MUC1, a polymorphic epithelial mucin (PEM) expressed on breast and pancreatic cancers as the target T cell epitope [9–10].

The interesting aspect of PEM as potential tumour antigens rests in their structure, which is simpler than that of gel forming mucins and

317

contains relatively short oligosaccharides. The apomucin (peptide core) is in general rich in proline, serine and threonine. These residues provide the sites for O-glycosidically linked oligosaccharide side chains. Recently cDNAs encoding four mucin core peptides (MUC1, MUC2, MUC3 and MUC4) have been isolated from human tissues. Comparison of amino acid sequences has revealed significant differences between mucins and it appears that each mucin gene encodes a characteristic core peptide that forms a tandem repeat. In addition, the polypeptide core varies in length in different individuals, hence the designation 'polymorphic' [11–13].

Both the presentation of the core peptide as a tandem repeat with a different sequence in different organs and its exposure as a consequence of incomplete glycosylation in tumour cells results in epitopes exposed for binding and recognition by T cells.

From target inhibition studies with mucin specific monoclonal antibodies (MAb) it was found that the likely T cell epitope on MUC1 is within, or adjacent to, the epitope PDTR recognized by the SM3 MAb. This epitope is not expressed on normal epithelial cells [9,10].

Recently, Finn and collaborators have shown that tumour reactive CTL isolated from patients with breast and pancreatic cancer lysed in a non-MHC restricted fashion ovarian tumours that possibly expressed MUC1 [9,10]. These findings raise the question of whether tumour reactive T cells isolated from ovarian cancer patients can recognize the MUC1 core peptide epitopes.

31.2 MATERIALS AND METHODS

31.2.1 TUMOURS AND TARGET CELL LINES

Ovarian tumour cell lines were: CaOV3 (HLA-A28, 29, B48, w61), MDAH 2774 (HLA-A3, 24, B45, w57), SKOV3 (HLA-A3, B18, (w6), 35(w6), Cw5).

Pancreatic tumour cell lines were HT29, Capan (HLA-A2, 9, B13, 17), PAN-1 (HLA-A2, 11, B39 (w6), 49 (w4)). They were maintained in culture in L-15 medium supplemented with 10% fetal calf serum (FCS) and 100 µg ml⁻¹ gentamicin as previously described [14].

Lymphoblastoid cell lines, Raji and Daudi, and the K562 cell line were maintained in RPMI-1640 medium with 10% FCS, supplemented with 100 µg ml⁻¹ L-glutamine and 100 µg ml⁻¹ gentamicin (hereafter termed complete RPMI medium).

The mucin plasmid expression vector pDKOF.MUC1 has been recently described by Jerome and collaborators [15]. B cell lines derived from healthy volunteers and transformed by Epstein–Barr virus (XxCr, LiSe and StBr) and the established Raji cell line were transfected either by lipofection or by electroporation using the plasmid pDKOF.MUC1, which contains 22 repeats of the 60-nucleotide tandem repeat MUC1 sequence gene and/or using MUC1-FS, which contains a frameshift mutation. These transfectants were maintained in complete RPMI medium supplemented with 200–800 µg ml⁻¹ of geneticin (Sigma Chemical Company, St Louis, MO) [15]. The complete HLA phenotypes of these lines are as follows: LiSe: HLA-A3, 11, B7, 12, {w4), (w6), Cw4, DR1, 4, w53, DQw1, w3 StBr: HLA-A2,3, B50, 57, (w4), (w6), Cw6, DR1.3, w52, DQ, w1.

Ovarian tumours OVA-16, OVA-14, OVA-24 and OVA-25 were stored in aliquots in liquid nitrogen in freezing medium (95% FCS, 5% dimethyl sulphoxide [DMSO]). Fibroblasts were generated by short term culture (14–28 days) of cells isolated from ovarian malignant ascites.

31.2.2 TAL CULTURES AND T CELL LINES

Lymphocytes were obtained from ovarian tumours and malignant ascites as previously described [5,6]. Lymphocytes were washed and cultured with autologous tumour cells at a responder-to-stimulator ratio of 10:1 in the presence of 25–50 U ml^{-1} of IL-2 (Cetus Corporation, Emeryville, CA) and 500 U ml^{-1} of TNF-α [Genentech Inc, San Francisco, CA) to favour the outgrowth of CD8+ T cells [5,16]. Please note that one unit of Cetus IL-2 is equivalent to six international units (IU) of IL-2 [4].

The MHC class I phenotypes of these ovarian TAL lines are as follows: TAL-14: HLA-A2, 3, 14, 44; TAL-16: HLA-A2, 19, B7, 35; TAL-24: HLA-A2, 24, B8, 51, and TIL-25: HLA-A1, B8, 38.

31.2.3 SYNTHETIC PEPTIDES

Synthetic peptide corresponding to the mammary/pancreatic PEM (MUC1) core peptide repeat residues 1–14 (PDTR-PAPGSTAPPA(C)) was designated A55 and synthetic peptide corresponding to colon PEM (MUC2) core peptide repeat residues 1–19 (PTTTPISTTTMVTPTTPTPT(C)) was designated A90 [9,10]. All peptides were prepared by the Synthetic Antigen Laboratory of the M.D. Anderson Cancer Center. A carboxyerminal Cys group was added to each peptide to allow chemical coupling. Similarly a number of mutated peptides maintaining the core of MUC1 and the epitope (A)PDTR were designed and prepared. Crude peptides were separated by reverse phase high pressure liquid chromatography (HPLC). Identity and purity of the final material were established by amino acid analysis. For peptide binding and investigation of the conformational changes in the HLA-A2 recognized epitope, MUC1 peptides were incubated with HLA-A2 transfectants (C1R:A2 line) overnight [17–19] in RPMI complete medium with 10 μg ml^{-1} of each peptide, as previously described [17,20]. Afterwards, the C1R:A2 cells were washed and reacted with MA2.1 and BB7.2 HLA-A2-specific MAb and

processed for FACS analysis as described below.

31.2.4 ANTIBODIES AND IMMUNOFLUORESCENCE

MAb against lymphocyte surface antigens OKT3-FITC, OKT4-FITC and OKT8-FITC were obtained from Ortho (Raritan, NJ); MAb anti-HLA-A2, BB7.2 and clone MA2.1 [21,22] were obtained from the American Type Culture Collection (ATCC, Rockville, MD) and (W6/32) anti-HLA-A-B-C from Dako (Dakopatts, Denmark). PEM reactive MAb SM-3 has been previously described [23]. SM-3 recognizes the epitope PDTR on the MUC-1 core peptide, does not react with the fully glycosylated MUC-1 and reacts mainly with deglycosylated MUC1 and/or carcinomas. Cells to be examined were incubated with the appropriate antibody at 4°C for 30 minutes, then washed, incubated with fluorescein isothiocyanate (FITC) conjugated F(ab)'2 fragments of goat antimouse or antirabbit IgG (Boehringer Mannheim Biochemicals, Indianapolis, IN) and examined by flow cytometry using an EPICS V Profile Analyzer (Coulter Corporation, Hialeah, FL).

31.2.5 WESTERN BLOTTING

Tumour cell lysates were analysed using 5% sodium dodecyl sulphate polyacrylamide gel electrophoresis (SDS-PAGE) [21]. The gel was fixed in 25% isopropanol:10% acetic acid overnight, then washed with TTBS (0.05% Tween 20 (Sigma) in tris-buffered saline), incubated with SM-3 MAb culture supernatant diluted 1/10 in TTBS overnight at 4°C, washed in TTBS, blocked with 1% bovine serum albumin in TTBS and incubated with the second antibody (^{125}I labelled goat antimouse IgG) for two hours at room temperature. The position of reactive bands was detected by autoradiography and comparison with molecular weight markers [25].

31.2.6 CYTOTOXICITY ASSAYS

The cytolytic activity of ovarian TAL was determined using the ^{51}Cr release assay [2,4]. Effectors were incubated with targets at different effector:target ratios for four or eight hours. Percentage cytotoxicity was determined from the formula $(E - S/T - S)\times100$, where E represents the cpm in wells containing effectors and S and T represent the cpm determined from wells containing only targets in the absence (S) or presence (T) of 0.1 N HCl. For comparative analysis of cytolytic activity, results were expressed in lytic units (LU) [4]. One LU was defined as the number of effector cells that lyse 20% of target cells in a four hour or eight hour ^{51}Cr release assay [4].

For experiments involving MUC1 and MUC2 synthetic peptides these were dissolved in phosphate buffered saline (PBS) at an initial concentration of 2 mg ml^{-1}, added to the wells in 50 μl aliquots at 50 or 100 μM final concentration and preincubated with the targets for 90 minutes before the effector cells were added [25,26]. Both peptides (A55 and A90) were used at the same concentration in the same assay [26]. For antibody inhibition experiments, the targets were preincubated with the corresponding antibodies (SM-3, W6/32) at 10 μg ml^{-1} for 30–45 minutes before the effectors were added. To investigate the blocking of cytolysis by antibodies to the TCR and CD3, effector cells were separately incubated at 4°C for 30 minutes with either anti-TCR-1 (WT31) MAb or anti-CD3 (OKT3) MAb. Cytotoxicity values were calculated in the presence and absence of inhibitory antibodies from at least two effector-to-target ratios and converted to LU.

31.3 RESULTS

31.3.1 T CELL RECOGNITION OF OVARIAN TUMOURS

One of the fundamental questions about involvement of the immune system in surveillance against emerging tumours and control of tumour progression and metastasis concerns the recognition by T cells of autologous tumours. The role of T cells in antitumour response to ovarian carcinoma is not known. When ovarian cancer evolves as an ascitic tumour, a large leukocyte infiltrate is present in the abdominal cavity associated with the ovarian tumour (tumour associated lymphocytes, TAL); however, the role of CD3+CD4+ or CD3+CD8+ cells in mediating antitumour response *in vivo* is still unclear. Our previous studies in this direction have been focused on demonstration and characterization of autotumour specific CTL, mainly in the ascites of ovarian cancer patients.

This response was demonstrated when freshly isolated ovarian TAL were cultured for several weeks in the initial presence of autologous tumour and moderate concentration of IL-2 (50–100 Cetus U ml^{-1}). In a recent study [6] we demonstrated that 5/16 TAL samples expand as predominantly CD3+CD8+ cultures endowed with the ability to lyse autologous tumours. Specificity for autologous tumours was defined as preferential killing, to indicate that these cells have the ability to show significantly higher levels of lysis against autologous tumours than against two randomly chosen and usually not HLA matched allogeneic ovarian tumours and against LAK and NK sensitive targets such as Daudi, Raji and K562 cells. Since in contrast with Daudi and K562, Raji cells express certain MHC class I antigens, this cell line is more often used as the specificity control target for the lytic function of MHC class I restricted CTL, which are part of ovarian TAL cultures. We found that autotumour specific lysis of ovarian CTL is mediated through the CD3-TCR complex. In order to better define this cytolytic function by the ovarian tumour reactive CTL, blocking experiments were performed with MAb specific for the TCR α/β, CD3, CD8 or MHC class I antigens [4,6]. These antibodies were able to significantly inhibit the lytic function of these CTL.

Since ovarian TAL in the first weeks of culture contain cells of various phenotypes and the lytic activity determined represents a cross-section of specificities against different targets, we wanted to address whether CD3+CD8+ cells can be separated from TAL cultures and expanded in the absence of cells of other phenotypes (e.g. CD4+ helper cells). To address this question we employed anti-CD4 and anti-CD8 MAb coated flasks and performed both positive selection with anti-CD8 MAb and negative selection with anti-CD4 MAb. Both CD3+CD8+ and CD3+CD4+ selected T cells of the TAL cultures were isolated with high purity (>98%) and were expanded in the presence of 50 U ml^{-1} of IL-2 supplemented with 500 U ml^{-1} TNF-α. We have recently observed that CD3+CD8+ T cells grow better in culture in the presence of IL-2 and moderate concentrations of TNF-α. This may be associated with synergism of these lymphokines in inducing a functional IL-2 response [5,16]. These lines were maintained in culture for several additional months (up to five months of continuous culture) and were tested repeatedly for ability to lyse autologous targets, allogeneic targets and K562 cells as indicators of NK function.

Representative results with four CTL lines are shown in Table 31.1. All ovarian CTL lines showed preferential lysis of autologous tumour targets compared with the Raji and K562 cells used as controls. Since these cells were isolated from TAL cultures containing, initially, variable numbers of CD8+ cells, we performed statistical analysis. The levels of lysis of autologous tumour (expressed in LU) were found to correlate with the percentage expression of CD8+ cells in the culture ($p <0.003$) and not with the percentage of total CD3+ cells ($p>0.50$) (data not shown).

These results demonstrated that CD8+ cells isolated from TAL and expanded in culture in

Table 31.1 Preferential lysis of autologous ovarian tumours by CTL-TAL lines developed from malignant ascitie.*

Sample	Target lytic activity (LU 20/10^7)		
	Autotumour	Raji	K562
TAL-16	216	60	30
TAL-24	206	6	41
TAL-30	143	60	ND
TAL-31	101	0	0

* Lytic activity of these lines was determined against all targets in the same experiment. The experiments were performed and LU were calculated as described in Section 31.2

the presence of IL-2 can efficiently lyse ovarian tumours. Following the nomenclature proposed by Whiteside and collaborators [3,5], we designate these cells as autotumour reactive. These findings raise the question of the nature of antigens recognized by autotumour reactive CTL.

31.3.2 AUTOTUMOUR REACTIVE CTL LYSE MUC1+ OVARIAN TUMOUR LINES

The current view of antigen recognition by CTL is that CTL recognize short peptides (9–11 amino acids) and that the epitope involved in TCR recognition spans 3–4 amino acids; which is in general agreement with the epitope recognized by MAb. Although B cell epitopes defined with MAb are conformational, this is still unclear for T cell epitopes. However, whilst models of peptide binding on MHC class I suggest a linear epitope, the fact that these peptides can induce conformational changes in the MHC class I α1 and α2 domains, which comprise the antigen binding pocket, suggests that if a sequence is presented to TCR under the appropriate conformation for binding and T cell activation, this can overcome the need for MHC class I binding and presentation.

With respect to recognition by CTL of tumour antigens, it is predicated that the

321

tumour antigen should be present on tumour cells but not on normal cells and the antigen concentration should be sufficiently high to compete with other peptides for presentation to TCR. Owing to the abundance on the tumour cell surface of certain proteins/glycoproteins, they should provide a sufficient number of peptides to initiate activation of a detectable number of T cells.

When these CTL were tested for target specificity, we observed that a number of lines were able to lyse autologous tumours and a small number of allogeneic targets, though to a much lesser extent. However, some of these showed the ability to lyse the ovarian tumour line CaOV3. Representative results with three such CTL-TAL lines are shown in Table 31.2. Lysis by these lines of the Daudi cells is presented for comparison, to indicate that the LAK activity of these cell lines was minimal. Also, from examination of the HLA antigen expression, the results suggested that antigen(s) expressed on the ovarian tumour line CaOV3 may be common for all these effectors but recognized in a non-MHC restricted manner. We focused on MUC1 expression on CaOV3 because these lines showed non-MHC restricted lysis of ovarian targets, suggestive of the recognition of deglycosylated MUC1 recently reported to involve non-MHC restricted antigen recognition.

To address the question of MUC1 expression on CaOV3 cells, we performed Northern and Western blot analysis with a MUC1 specific probe and MAb SM-3. Results of Western blotting are presented in Figure 31.1. The results show high levels of expression of the SM-3 epitope on CaOV3 cells. This suggests that a potentially common T cell epitope on the MUC1 molecule is present on the CaOV3 cells.

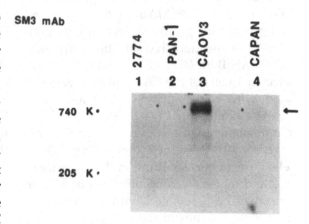

Figure 31.1 Expression of the SM-3 epitope on the CaOV3 ovarian tumour cell line. Lanes in the figure indicate: (1) 2774 cells (negative for the SM-3 epitope); (2) PAN-1 (pancreatic tumour cell line); (3) CaOV3; (4) Capan (positive control). Reactivity of the SM-3 MAb with cell lysates was determined by Western blotting as described in Section 31.2.

Table 31.2 Lysis by ovarian CTL-TAL of ovarian tumour cell line CaOV3

Sample no.	Target (LU)*		HLA compatibility**
	CaOV3	Daudi	
TAL-16	300	< 10	None
TAL-24	290	< 50	None
TAL-14	680	< 50	None

* Lysis of CaOV3 and Daudi cells was tested in the same experiment at two effector-to-target ratios in duplicate and the results were converted to lytic units (LU)
** There is no HLA-A-B-C compatibility between the effectors and targets. The MHC class I phenotypes of CaOV3 and effectors are presented in Section 31.2

31.3.3 MUC1 CORE PEPTIDE RECOGNITION BY OVARIAN CTL

To address the question of whether some of these CTL recognize a MUC1 epitope and to obtain direct proof that some T cells in these CTL lines recognize MUC1 protein, we determined their specificity in two systems:

1. EBV transformed cell lines from unrelated donors transfected with MUC1 cDNA

were used as targets, as were untransfected EBV cell lines and EBV cell lines transfected with the MUC1.FS (frame shift) mutant, the latter two being controls. These targets have recently been reported to express high levels of MUC1 and were considered superior to the CaOV3 line due to the fact that, as with all tumour cell lines, heterogeneous antigen expression and possible changes in antigen glycosylation may induce undesired variability in the assays. TAL-14, -16 and -24 show significant lysis of MUC1 cDNA transfected EBV cell lines, but not of untransfected targets or of MUC1.FS transfected targets. A representative experiment is shown in Figure 31.2. CTL-TAL-14 lysed the MUC1 cDNA transfected targets and this lysis was not inhibited by MAb W6/32 specific for MHC class I antigens, confirming that the lysis of MUC1 transfectants is non-MHC restricted. This lysis follows the predicted mechanism of recognition of the

MUC1 apoprotein by breast and pancreatic tumour cells [9,10].

2. To conclude whether the MUC1 core peptide is directly recognized by ovarian CTL-TAL, we prepared synthetic peptides that included in the sequence the core PDTR-PAPGSTAPPA. These peptides were used in cytotoxicity experiments. This core contains the epitope PDTR that is recognized by the MAb SM-3 and BC-2 [27]. The corresponding MUC2 core peptide with the sequence PTTT PISTTT MVTPTTPTPT was also prepared and used as control. These peptides were designated MUC1 (A55) and MUC2 (A90) respectively. We used at first the peptides A55 and A90 in an autologous system: CTL-TAL-16 and autologous fibroblasts (L-16). Significant lysis was observed in the presence of the A55 peptide but not in the absence of this peptide or in the presence of the A90 peptide. This suggests that within the CTL-TAL-16 line are

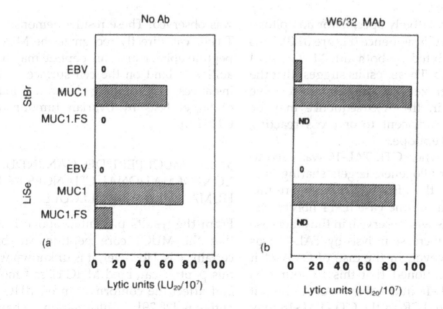

Figure 31.2 Lysis by CTL-TAL-14 of EBV-B cell lines derived from normal donors LiSe and StBr. Cytotoxicity was performed in the absence (a) or presence (b) of the MHC class I specific MAb W6/32. (EBV) control lines; MUC1 and MUC1.FS indicate the same line transfected with a plasmid containing MUC1 cDNA in the correct or incorrect (frame shift – FS) reading frame.

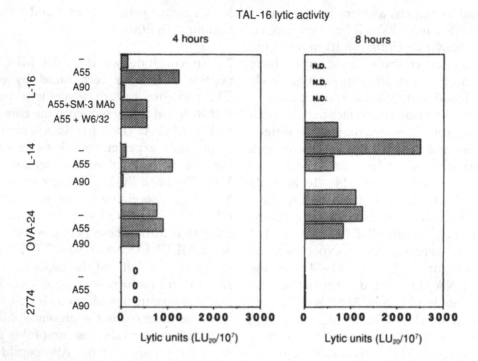

Figure 31.3 Lysis by CTL-TAL of targets pulsed with A55 and A90 peptides (L-16) indicate autologous fibroblasts. L-14 and OVA-24 are HLA-A2 compatible with L-16.

cells that are relatively specific for an epitope nested in the A55 sequence (Figure 31.3). This lysis was inhibited by both anti-MHC class I and SM-3 MAb. These results suggest that the epitope recognized by autotumour reactive CTL-TAL-16 in the A55 sequence may be either within, adjacent to or cross reacting with the SM-3 epitope.

In contrast, when CTL-TAL-16 was used to lyse two other allogeneic targets sharing only HLA-A2 with the effectors, different results were observed: in one case (L-14 fibroblasts) significant lysis was observed; in the other case (OVA-24) the increase in lysis by TAL-16 was minimal. However, in the case of OVA-24 it should be mentioned that this tumour was lysable by TAL-16 in the absence of A55 and it is possible that TCR in the CTL-TAL-16 may recognize other specificities with higher affinity. When 2774 targets of HLA incompatibility were tested using the same effectors, no lysis

was observed. These results demonstrate that T cells can directly recognize the MUC1 core peptide epitope and this peptide may have the ability to bind on the cell surface. In certain instances this binding leads to induction of target lysis by ovarian tumour reactive CTL-TAL.

31.3.4 MUC1 PEPTIDES CAN INDUCE CONFORMATIONAL CHANGES IN THE HUMAN HLA-A2 MOLECULE

From the results presented above it is clear that the MUC1 core peptide can bind to certain cells. However, it is unknown whether this peptide can bind MHC class I molecules and affect the conformation of MHC class I antigens [28,29]. Conformational changes in MHC class I may give rise to either increased recognition or lack of recognition of targets by CTL effectors. Furthermore, from the experiments presented above, when peptides were presented in the context of allo-MHC, we could not determine whether the failure of these peptides to induce lysis reflected, in fact, the lack of their ability to bind MHC class I. Recent studies have demonstrated that peptides bound to and eluted from MHC class I molecules include in their sequence certain amino acids at predetermined positions (anchors) [30]. Lack of these anchors usually results in the failure of a peptide to bind, whilst introduction of these anchors into the sequence usually gives increased peptide binding ability and correct MHC class I folding. Although there is a large body of evidence leaning in this direction from murine studies, very little is known of human HLA–peptide binding because of limited information on MHC class I anchors and allele specific conformationally dependent MAb.

To gain insight into the MUC1 peptide–HLA interaction, we have chosen as a model the HLA-A2 molecule, because both its anchors' residues are known, MAb reacting with conformationally dependent epitopes are available and initial results suggest that in some instances HLA-A2 matching between effectors and targets leads to target lysis in the presence of MUC1 peptide. Since the ideal HLA-A2 binding peptide was reported to be a nonamer (with a range 8–11 residues), we first created a set of overlapping peptides: octa- and nonamers that covered the entire MUC1 sequence. The sequence of these peptides compared with the A55 and MUC1 sequences is presented in Table 31.3 and of mutated MUC1 peptides in Figure 31.4.

To determine how these peptides affect the MHC conformation detected by serological MA2.1 and BB7.2 epitopes, we incubated these peptides overnight at 10 μg ml^{-1} final concentration with C1R:A2 cells. Cells incubated in the same conditions but without peptides were used as controls [17,18]. The HLA-A2 antigen on these cells expresses both MA2.1 and BB7.2 epitopes. The results are presented in Figure 31.4. Surprisingly, preincubation of C1R:A2 cells with peptide D133 (PDTRPAPGS) led to a significant increase in the reactivity of both MA2.1 and BB7.2 with the HLA-A2; incubation with peptide D117 (APGSTAPPAH) had essentially no effect on reactivity of these MAb. Peptide D130 (STAPPAHGV) induced an increase of MA2.1 binding, although to a lesser extent, and decreased BB7.2 binding to HLA-A2. Since D133 and D117 peptides overlap in the APGS sequence and D133 and D130 overlap only at the terminal Ser, the group PDTRP may be responsible for the induced conformational changes. Surprisingly the peptide D129 (GVTSAPDTR) was found to decrease the reactivity of both MA2.1 and BB7.2 MAb. Both D133 and D129 contain the PDTR group, but in different positions: 1–4 in D133 versus 6–9 in D129. More importantly, the peptide GVTSAPDTR was selected based on the presence of Val (P2) and Arg (P9). Since Val (P2) is an alternative anchor

Table 31.3 Sequences of MUC1 core peptide used in this study

MUC1*	PDTRPAPGSTA PPAH GVTSAPDTRPAPGSTAPPAH
D117	APGSTAPPAH
D129	GVTSAPDTR
D130	STAPPAHGV
D133	PDTRPAPGS PDTRPAPGS
A55:	PDTRPAPGSTAPPA(C)

* The sequence of MUC1 is presented as a dimer to illustrate the selection of overlapping peptides and the amino- and carboxy-terminal positioning of the group PDTR in peptides D133 and D129 respectively

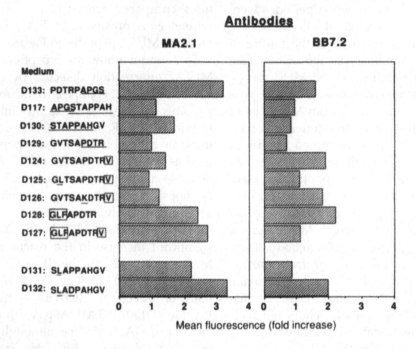

Figure 31.4 Polymorphic MAb binding profiles in the presence of MUC1 peptides for transfectants expressing the HLA-A2 molecule. The results were obtained with logarithmic amplification of fluorescence intensity expressed in channels and calculated as described in reference 28.

point for HLA-A2 binding motifs, it was expected that D129 would increased the reactivity of MA2.1 MAb with the HLA-A2.

To address this point, we added a Val (P10) to conform with the predicted anchor motif for HLA-A2. Indeed, carboxyterminal Val in peptide D124 increased the reactivity of the MA2.1 and BB7.2 with HLA-A2. Interestingly, neither a non-conservative substitution (Pro → Lys [P7]) nor a conservative one (Val → Leu [P2]) in peptides D126 and D125 respectively significantly increased the reactivity of MA2.1, although with D126, BB7.2 reacted more strongly.

Since the expected increase was not observed, this suggested that probably, as demonstrated with other HLA-A2 model peptides, residues at P3 and eventually P4 may play a role in peptide induced conformational changes of HLA-A2. To clarify this point we replaced the group GVTS with the

group GLF (D128) corresponding to the first three residues of the HLA-A2 specific influenza matrix epitope that forms the N-terminal anchor [17]. Indeed, although substituting Gly-Leu for Gly-Val can be viewed as conservative, the substitution of Phe for The should be viewed as non-conservative and apparently increased the reactivity of both MA2.1 and BB7.2.

Similarly, another MUC1 nonapeptide, D130 (STAPPAHGV with Val (P9) anchor) increased MA2.1 binding and slightly decreased BB7.2 binding. Only MA2.1 reactivity increased with the substitution of Leu for The (P2), this substitution being intended to create an anchor point. The reactivity of both MAb increased significantly (by 3.3- and 2.0-fold) when Pro (P4) was substituted with Asp. These results suggest that this substitution either created an anchor point or, if D130 and D131 peptides were contacting the HLA-

A2 molecule, affected the conformation of the epitope, making it more amenable to recognition by domain specific MAb.

These results taken together suggest that MUC1 short peptides containing amino terminal PDTR groups are capable of interacting with HLA-A2 molecules. Substitution of particular residues in anchor positions can create conformational epitopes in the MUC1 core peptide.

31.4 DISCUSSION

In this paper, we present novel and direct evidence that CTL isolated from ovarian malignant ascites can recognize epitopes on PEM core peptides. These cells lyse ovarian tumours expressing MUC1, EBV-B cell lines transfected with and expressing MUC1 cDNA and targets pulsed with synthetic peptides with sequences equivalent to MUC1. The CTL lines were derived from TAL expanded in culture in the presence of autologous tumours and low to moderate concentrations of IL-2 and TNF-α. These CTL were not stimulated with MUC1 transfected EBV-B cell lines, nor with MUC1 peptide pulsed targets. The fact that they recognize and distinguish between MUC1 and MUC2 epitopes suggests that they are antigen specific and that such epitopes can be found on autologous tumours.

Mucins are produced by many epithelial cells and their cancers. These molecules are in high molecular weight glycoproteins (HMG) that contain a large number of O-glycosidically linked sugars. Production and increased expression of these molecules has been noted in human cancers, suggesting that these molecules may play a significant role in the tumour cell expansion. High mucin production and expression have also been reported for ovarian cancers.

Furthermore, ovarian tumours are considered 'mucinous' and 'serous' according not only to their histological characteristics but also to mucin expression. Although the terminology used is still confusing and based on the fact that mucinous ovarian tumours are in the minority compared with serous tumours, it may suggest that mucin epitopes are also expressed by a smaller group of tumours.

Recent studies show that serous ovarian tumours also express PEM mucins. Most interestingly, Lloyd and colleagues [31] have recently reported that serous ovarian tumours are MUC1+ and MT334−. MT334 MAb reacts with an epitope expressed mainly on mucinous tumours. These results confirm recent studies with the MUC1 core peptide reacting MAb such as BC-2 and SM-3 [27]. The epitopes recognized by these antibodies encompass the tetrapeptide PDTR and differ at the amino terminal Ala, which is not included in the SM-3 epitope [22]. EBV-transformed B cell lines transfected with MUC1 cDNA have shown significant reactivity with BC-2 MAb [15]. This MAb has also been reported to react better than SM-3 MAb with ovarian tumours [27]. Expression of MUC1 on ovarian tumours may provide an epitope for targeted immune intervention in human cancers. The requirement for a novel tumour epitope expression on tumour cells compared with normal epithelial cells is achieved by exposing the core peptide tandem repeat to both T cells and antibodies. Exposure of this epitope is probably a consequence of incomplete or aberrant O-glycosylation in tumour cells.

With respect to tumour antigens expressed on ovarian tumour cells it should be underlined that ovarian tumours may express, in addition to mucins, other epitopes that can be recognized by T cells. Recently tumour reactive CTL from pancreatic and breast tumours were reported to recognize epitopes on PEM that are expressed on the surface of the corresponding tumour cells. Activation of PEM reactive T cells has been proposed to involve binding and engagement of CD8+ CTL by the repetitive unit of the MUC1 core. If, as suggested by MAb inhibition studies, TCR recognize the epitope PDTR, presentation of this repetitive epitope to T cells may resemble B cell stimulation by polyvalent T cell independent antigens [7,32]. The fact that these CTL can recognize a short MUC1 core peptide when probably associated with a common HLA molecule conforms to the model presentation of peptide antigens derived from endogenously synthesized and degraded proteins [32] and supports the recently proposed model of dual presentation of the MUC1 core peptide as a tumour antigen [32].

Short peptide antigens presented to T cells have been predicted to include in-sequence MHC allele specific binding motifs. The MUC1 peptide used in these experiments (PDTRPAPGSTAPPA), however, does not contain the predicted HLA-A2 strong anchor residues L/I/V (P2) and V/M/L (P9) followed by the weaker anchors K/R (P8) and eventually F (P3), in the correct positions.

Therefore it was important to address whether preincubation of HLA-A2+ targets with MUC1 peptides affects the conformation of the epitope recognized by the MA2.1 and BB7.2 MAb. These antibodies react with the α1 domain of the antigen binding pocket and the external N-terminal loop of the α2 domain [32].

HLA-A2 expressed on C1R:A2 transfectants contains mainly endogenous bound peptides [33]. Surprisingly, the peptide D133 (PDTRPAPGS) induced the highest reactivity of HLA-A2 with both MAb, compared with the other MUC1 peptides (STAPPAHGV, APGSTAPPAH and GVTSAPDTR) which together encompass the entire MUC1 core. These results clearly demonstrate that the peptide with the sequence PDTRPAPGS has the ability to interact with HLA-A2. These findings are strengthened by the observation that another peptide (GVTSAPDTR) containing the group PDTR in the positions 5–9 of the sequence failed to enhance the reactivity of MA2.1 and BB7.2 with HLA-A2. To achieve equivalent modification of these epitopes we added a carboxyterminal Val as anchor and

replaced the group GVTS with GLF. At this moment it is unclear how this peptide interacts with HLA-A2 and why the MA2.1 and BB7.2 epitopes are affected in different ways when the group PDTR is located amino or carboxyterminal in a MUC1 derived nona- or decamer.

Another important question that needs to be addressed is whether during antigen processing and presentation such peptides (of the described sequence and length) are indeed generated by endogenous antigen processing. This is an important question, because the failure to observe MHC restricted recognition of these peptides may reflect the inability of the antigen processing and transport mechanisms to load peptides of the described length and sequence on HLA-A2, or if such peptides are generated endogenously, their binding on MHC may affect the complex mechanism of assembly and transport to the cell surface.

The implications of the T and B cell recognition of tumour mucins as antigens (epitopes) generated by post-translational modifications are significant, because such antigens may either form the basis for a tumour vaccine or for novel adoptive immunotherapy protocols with mucin reacting cells and antibodies, whilst MUC1 peptide expressing EBV transfectants or MUC1 peptide pulsed cells (e.g. fibroblasts) can serve as surrogate antigens for human tumour vaccination studies.

To this end, further studies should determine the effect of the glycosylation state on T cell recognition of MUC1 and the definition of the MUC1 epitope. Such studies are in progress in our laboratory. In conclusion, our findings presented here demonstrate that PEM should be considered as a potential target antigen for T cells on ovarian tumours.

ACKNOWLEDGEMENTS

We thank Dr David Lawlor (Department of Immunology) for fruitful discussions and advice with anti-HLA-A2 MAbs, Mr Kevin Flynn for revising and editing this paper and Ms Susan Walker and Ms Donna Williams for secretarial assistance.

This work was supported by NIH-NCI grants CA-57923 (CGI), O.K CA-56103 (OJF) and peptide synthesis was supported in part by core-grant CA 16672.

REFERENCES

1. Topalian, S.L., Solomon, D., Avis, F.P. *et al.* (1988) Immunotherapy of patients with advanced cancer using tumour infiltrating lymphocytes and recombinant interleukin-2: a pilot study. *J. Clin. Oncol.*, **6**, 839–53.

2. Itoh, K., Platsoucas C.D. and Balch, C.M. (1988) Autologous tumour-specific cytotoxic T lymphocytes in the infiltrate of human metastatic melanomas. *J. Exp. Med.*, **168**, 1419–41.

3. Heo, D.S., Whiteside, T.L., Kanbour, A. and Herberman, R.B. (1988) Lymphocytes infiltrating human ovarian tumours. I. Role of Leu-19 (NKH1)-positive recombinant IL-2 activated cultures of lymphocytes infiltrating human ovarian tumours. *J. Immunol.*, **140**, 4042–9.

4. Ioannides, C.G., Freedman,R.S., Platsoucas, C.D. *et al.* (1991) Cytotoxic T cell clones isolated from ovarian tumour infiltrating lymphocytes recognize multiple antigenic epitopes on autologous tumour cells. *J. Immunol.*, **146**, 1700–7.

5. Vaccarello, L., Wang, Y. and Whiteside, T.L. (1986) Sustained outgrowth of autotumour-reactive T lymphocytes from human ovarian carcinomas in the presence of tumour necrosis factor α and IL-2. *Hum. Immunol.*, **28**, 216–27.

6. Ioannides, C.G., Platsoucas, C.D., Rashed, S. *et al.* (1991) Tumour cytolysis by lymphocytes infiltrating ovarian malignant ascites. *Cancer Res.*, **51**, 4257–65.

7. Ioannides, C.G. and Whiteside, T.L. (1993) T cell recognition of human tumours: implications for molecular immunotherapy of cancer. *Clin. Immunol. Immunopathol.*, **66**, 91–106.

8. Jorgenson, J.L., Esser, U., St Groth, B.F. *et al.* (1992) Mapping T cell receptor–peptide contacts by various peptide immunization of single chain transgenics. *Nature*, **355**, 224–8.

9. Jerome, K.R., Barnd, D.L., Bendt, K.M. *et al.* (1991) Cytotoxic T-lymphocytes derived from patients with breast adenocarcinoma recognize an epitope present on the protein core of a mucin molecule preferentially expressed by malignant cells. *Cancer Res.*, **51**, 2908–16.

10. Barnd, D.L., Lan, M.S., Metzgar, R.S. and Finn, O.J. (1989) Specific major histocompatibility complex-unrestricted recognition of tumour-associated mucins by human cytotoxic T cells. *Proc. Natl. Acad. Sci. USA*, **86**, 7159–63.

11. Zotter, S., Hageman, P.C., Lossnitzer, A. *et al.* (1988) Tissue and tumour distribution of human polymorphic epithelial mucin. *Cancer Rev.*, **11–12**, 55–101.

12. Gendler, S., Papadimitriou, J., Duhig, T. *et al.* (1988) A highly immunogenic region of a human polymorphic epithelial mucin expressed by carcinomas is made up of tandem repeats. *J. Biol. Chem.*, **263**, 1282–3.

13. Papadimitriou, J.T. and Gendler, S. (1988) Molecular aspects of mucins. *Cancer Rev.*, **11–12**, 11–24.

14. Ioannides, C.G., Platsoucas, C.D., Kim, Y.P. *et al.* (1990) T cell functions in ovarian cancer patients treated with viral oncolysates: increased helper activity to immunoglobins production. *Anticancer Res.*, **10**, 645–54.

15. Jerome, K.R., Bu, D. and Finn, O. (1992) Expression of tumour associated epitopes on Epstein–Barr virus-immortalized B-cells and Burkitt's lymphomas transfected with epithelial mucin complementary DNA. *Cancer Res.*, **52**, 5985–90.

16. Ioannides, C.G., Fisk, B., Tomasovic, B. *et al.* (1992) Induction of IL-2 receptor by TNF-α on cultured ovarian tumour associated lymphocytes. *Cancer Immunol. Immunother.*, **35**, 83–91.

17. Catipovic, B., Dal Porto, J., Mage, M. *et al.* (1992) Major histocompatibility complex conformational epitopes are peptide specific. *J. Exp. Med.*, **176**, 1611–18.

18. Parker, K.C., Bednarek, M.A., Hull, L.K. *et al.* (1992) Sequence motifs important for peptide binding to the human MHC class I molecule, HLA-A2, *J. Immunol.*, **149**, 2580–7.

19. Gammon, M.C., Bednarek, M.A., Biddison, W.E. *et al.* (1992) Endogenous loading of HLA-A2 molecules with an analog of the influenza

virus matrix protein-derived peptide and its inhibition by an exogenous peptide antagonist. *J. Immunol.*, **148**, 7–12.

20. Bluestone, J.A., Jameson, S., Miller, S. and Dick, R. (1992) Peptide induced conformational changes in class I heavy chains alter major histocompatibility complex recognition. *J. Exp. Med.*, **176**, 1757–61.

21. McMichael, A.J., Parham, P., Rust, N. and Brodsky F.M. (1980) A monoclonal antibody that recognizes an antigenic determinant shared by HLA-A2 and B-17. *Hum. Immunol.*, **1**, 121–31.

22. Salter, R.D., Clayberger, C., Lomen, C.E. *et al.* (1987) *In vitro* mutagenesis at a single residue introduces B and T cell epitopes into a class I HLA molecule. *J. Exp. Med.*, **166**, 283–8.

23. Layton, G.T., Devine, P.L., Warren, J.A. *et al.* (1990) Monoclonal antibodies reactive with the breast carcinoma-associated mucin core protein repeat sequence peptide also recognize the ovarian-associated sebaceous gland antigen. *Tumour Biol.*, **11**, 274–86.

24. Ioannides, C.G., Itoh, K., Fox, F.E. *et al.* (1987) Identification of a second T cell antigen receptor in human and mouse by antipeptide gamma chain specific monoclonal antibody. *Proc. Natl. Acad. Sci. USA*, **84**, 4244–8.

25. Matsushita, Y., Cleary, K.R., Ota, D.M. *et al.* (1990) Sialyl-dimeric Lewis-X antigen expres- sed on mucin-like glycoproteins in colorectal cancer metastases. *Lab. Invest.*, **63**, 780–91.

26. Townsend, A.R.M., Rothbard, J., Gotch, F.M. *et al.* (1986) The epitopes of influenza nucleoprotein recognized by cytotoxic T-lymphocytes can be defined with short peptides. *Cell*, **44**, 959–68.

27. McGuckin, M.A., Wright, G. and Ward, B.G. (1990) Expression of a polymorphic epithelial mucin antigen defined by the monoclonal antibody BC2 in ovarian carcinoma. Use of the BC2 antibody for the detection of micrometastasis. *Am. J. Pathol.*, **96**, 46–52.

28. Lie, R., Myers, N.B., Gorka, J. *et al.* (1990) Pepitide ligand-induced conformation and surface expression of the class I MHC molecule. *Nature*, **344**, 439–41.

29. Guo, H.C., Jardetzky, T.S., Garrett, T.P.J. *et al.* (1992) Different length peptides bind to HLA-Aw68 similarly at their ends but bulge out in the middle. *Nature*, **360**, 364–9.

30. Falk, K., Rotzschke, O., Stevanovic, S. *et al.* (1991) Allele-specific motifs revealed by sequencing of self-peptides eluted from MHC molecules. *Nature*, **351**, 290–6.

31. Lloyd, K.O. (1992) Ovarian Cancer Mucins. Second International Workshop on Carcinoma-associated Mucins, Robinson College, Cambridge, August 2–6.

32. Finn, O.J. (1992) Antigen-specific, MHC-unrestricted T cells. *Biotherapy*, **4**, 1239–49.

33. Henderson, R.A., Michel, H., Sakaguchi, K. *et al.* (1992) HLA-A2.1-associated peptides from a mutant cell line: a second pathway of antigen presentation. *Science*, **255**, 1264–6.

Chapter 32

Use of bifunctional monoclonal antibodies for retargeting human lymphocytes against ovarian carcinoma cells

M.I. COLNAGHI

32.1 INTRODUCTION

Over the past years intense efforts have been made to identify tumor specific or tumor associated markers which could be immunogenic in humans and animals. A considerable amount of data, which at least proves the existence of tumor associated antigens in humans, has been collected. Immunological techniques applied to diagnosis in oncology have allowed improvement, both in terms of sensitivity and specificity, in the area of pathology as well as in the laboratory and in nuclear medicine. More recently, the use of monoclonal antibodies (MAbs) derived by somatic hybridization [1] has allowed further improvement of results obtained with conventional antisera and opened new pathways in the field of research. In fact, these reagents possess a peculiar characteristic, that is, monospecificity, which makes them particularly suitable for immunological applications where the target of the immune response, the putative tumor antigen, is often undefined, possibly poorly immunogenic and difficult to identify.

Theoretically, in the perspective of clinical applications, the specificity of the MAbs should be restricted to tumor cells only. However,

some reagents with a reactivity which was not so restricted were found to be suitable for several *in vitro* diagnostic approaches, such as immunohistochemistry and immunocytology, as well as for some kinds of *ex vivo* therapeutic approaches, such as bone marrow purging in the perspective of autologous bone marrow transplants after high dose chemo- or radiotherapy, provided they were selected on a basis of operational tumor specificity.

On the contrary, the successful application of MAbs in *in vivo* cancer therapy is still limited by several different problems. Besides the tumor restricted specificity, essential to avoid systemic effects which hamper the results of conventional therapy, many other factors such as the binding kinetics and affinity of the MAbs, the heterogeneous expression of MAb recognized determinants on tumor cells, the possible presence in the blood of the relevant antigen and the fate of the antigen–antibody complex after MAb binding at the cell surface can all deeply affect the MAb's therapeutic efficiency.

MAbs used as carriers of therapeutic agents must fulfil several essential requirements. The first one is tumor specificity and so far only a few of the reported MAbs directed against solid tumors seem to be suitable reagents [2–5].

A second problem concerns the inability of a single MAb to react with all cells within a single tumor. This is due to tumor heterogeneity which derives from the coexistence within a tumor of cells with distinct phenotypes. In fact, within the same tumor cell population it is possible to find cells with different metastatic potentials, with different patterns of susceptibility to drug therapy and which are antigenically heterogeneous.

Research today focuses on developing new approaches aimed at generating MAbs directed against appropriate targets with tumor restricted distribution and homogeneous expression. Recently some particular cell surface molecules, such as receptors involved in signal transduction, have been suggested as appropriate targets. The results of several studies in these fields, including those which demonstrated homologies between oncogene products and this type of receptor, as well as those which showed a large quantitative difference in their expression in tumors as compared to normal cells, provide support for the exploitation of these molecules as targets for antibody driven therapy, despite their expression which is not restricted to tumor cells.

Another problem regards the origin of the antitumor MAbs which are available today, the majority of which were raised in mouse species. One major side effect of the *in vivo* administration of these murine derived reagents is the sensitization of the patients against the foreign proteins, which can lead to the production of human antimurine antibodies (HAMA) [6,7], with the consequent complete abrogation of the MAbs therapeutic effect and which may even be harmful to the patients. Several approaches have been tried to prevent or reduce HAMA development. Theoretically, human MAbs seem to offer a solution to this problem but the production of human MAbs is somewhat difficult and

limited. Controversial data are available concerning the use of MAb fragments. Large quantities of MAbs are required to achieve tolerance and immunosuppressive drugs are required to prevent T helper or B cell activity. All these approaches, however, proved to be disappointing. The application of recombinant DNA techniques and the creation of murine variable/human constant chimeric immunoglobulins, which incorporate the specificity of a murine MAb in a human antibody [8], seem to offer an alternative suitable approach to prevent HAMA production.

MAbs which possess all the requirements (in terms of tumor restricted specificity, homogeneous reactivity, non-immunogenicity) as suitable carriers can be exploited to deliver in a selective manner to cancer cells the toxic potential of various types of substances or of cytotoxic cells. Up-to-date cellular adoptive cancer immunotherapy was mainly carried out by using *in vitro* activated lymphocytes which display antitumor activity, such as LAK cells or TILs [9]. Several limitations, depending on the effector cells used, affect the efficacy of these procedures. As far as LAK cells are concerned, the ability to traffic to the tumor site is one of the major problems together with the need to use IL-2 in order to maintain the antitumor activity. TILs, which seem to have higher tumor specificity and to recirculate better than LAK, are, however, difficult to obtain. A new approach to generate efficient antitumor cell mediated cytotoxicity is based on the exploitation of bispecific MAbs (BiMAbs) for retargeting effector lymphocytes, regardless of their specificity, on tumor cells.

To this end two parental MAbs are required, an adequate antitumor MAb and a MAb able to recognize on effector cells an activating molecule such as, in the case of T cells, the CD3 structure of the TCR complex. The recognition by BiMAbs of triggering surface molecules on the effector cells is crucial for inducing the eventual cytotoxic effect. In addition, due to the requirement of cross-linkage, which only occurs at the tumor site, for obtaining activation [10], operational tumor specific killing can be obtained. The bifunctional reagents can be raised from hybrid hybridomas generated by somatic fusion of the two relevant hybridomas producing the parental MAbs (hybrid MAbs) or through chemical linkage of the two parental MAb molecules (heteroconjugates) [11–13].

The efficiency and specificity of this approach mainly depend on the characteristics of the BiMAb and the effector cells. Due to the instability of the artificial disulphide bridge between the two molecules of the bifunctional antibody, heteroconjugates seem to be less adequate than natural hybrid reagents for *in vivo* therapy [14]. The use of constructs, consisting of the two parental Fab' fragments joined via a stable thioether linkage, seems to overcome this problem [15].

For the relevant *in vitro* studies CTL from T cell clones have mainly been used. Peripheral blood mononuclear cells (PBMCs) from healthy donors (HD) have also been reported to exert a heteroconjugate mediated cytotoxicity, provided that they were previously fractionated and briefly exposed to IL-2 [12] or stimulated by an anti-CD3 antibody [16].

We recently reported that properly activated PBMCs, from both HD and cancer patients, can be efficiently retargeted by an anti-ovarian carcinoma/anti-CD3 bifunctional MAb on ovary tumor cells on which they exert a specific antibody mediated cytotoxic effect [14,17].

To obtain the suitable antitumor MAb we adopted a particular immunization procedure based on the observation that the majority of the available MAbs, which were of murine origin, recognized similar structures: high molecular weight molecules, such as glycoproteins and mucins, present on tumors but also on certain normal cells. This similarity of the MAb recognized antigens on tumor cells suggested that the available MAbs were induced by antigens which were immunodominant for the immune system of mice sensitized with human tumors. In order to retrieve immune responses against possible, still undiscovered, less immunogenic but tumor restricted antigens, we immunized the animal donor of the spleen cells to be hybridized with an ovarian tumor which was completely unreactive with our already available MAbs (first generation reagents). In this way, we obtained a second generation of MAbs and then, using the same criteria and a long lasting immunization procedure, a third generation was produced.

Among the products of this final generation we identified one MAb, designated MOv18, which showed proper tumor restricted specificity for ovarian carcinomas [4]. Conjugated with fluorescien isothiocyanate, it showed homogeneous positive staining in 100% of non-mucinous carcinomas, whereas only 2% of non-ovarian tumors were found to react with the MAb. Moreover, the normal tissues tested were unreactive. MOv18 is of IgG1k isotype and the recognized molecule is a membrane glycoprotein of 38 kd molecular weight which is stable on the cell surface of ovarian carcinoma cells. The cloning of the relevant gene demonstrated that the coded protein is a folate binding protein [18]. MOv18 shows a good affinity constant of the order of $2 \times 10^9 \, M^{-1}$.

In order to evaluate the suitability of MOv18 for therapeutic approaches, its biodistribution in 30 ovarian carcinoma patients was analysed by immunoscintigraphy [19,20]. The results demonstrated MAb localization and positive imaging with good sensitivity (73%) and very high specificity (100%). The immunoscintigraphic negativity in the case of diaphragmatic lesions in different patients could be attributed to the minimal size of the lesions. The other non-localized lesions were in the liver where the difficulty of obtaining images of metastases is already a well-known finding, as observed previously with other

MAbs. It is, however, noteworthy that in these patients the radioactive concentration in the liver seemed to be lower than observed in previous studies with other MAbs.

Altogether, the results of our studies suggested that MOv18 could be an appropriate candidate for a particular therapeutic approach and it was therefore selected for generating bifunctional MAbs, together with a second parental reagent, an anti-CD3 MAb [11].

The bispecificity of the reagents was obtained either by chemical cross-linkage [14] or by using cell fusion techniques [11,17], thus obtaining in the first case a heteroconjugate and in the second one a hybrid MAb. Both of them showed a pattern of reactivity on tumor cells analogous to that of the native MOv18 MAb and a similar ability to bind to cells expressing the CD3 molecule.

As shown in Figure 32.1, the BiMAb efficiently mediated target cell lysis by CTL from T clones or from activated PBMCs from HD. No lysis was induced by CTL and PBMCs alone or by CTL in the presence of the relevant parental MAbs. The cytotoxicity on the human ovarian carcinoma cell line OVCA432 was MAb concentration related with a maximum activity (70–90%) at 20 pM and a specific lysis of over 30% was still observed at 1 pM. The control MEWO melanoma cell line was unaffected.

The efficient specific lysis promoted also by F(ab')2 fragments obtained from the BiMAb excluded Fc receptor mediated lysis in the system studied [14]. Targeted T cells act against tumor cells in at least two ways, by lysing them directly and by releasing factors that eventually result in tumor cell death [21].

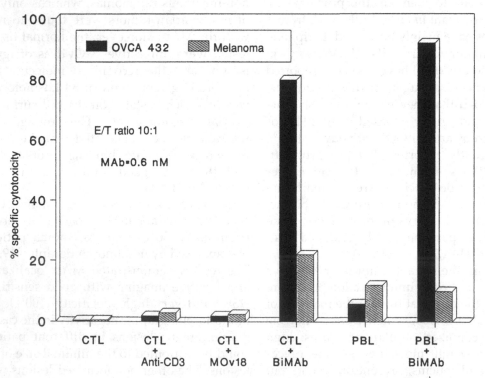

Figure 32.1 BiMAb dependent lysis of human tumor cell lines by human T cells. The BiMAb was used at a final concentration of 0.6 nM in either the absence or presence of CTL or activated PBL.

In vitro PBMC preactivation was required to deliver the second signal to the effector cells. The adequate activation protocol for uncloned resting PBMCs of HD, as well as ovarian carcinoma patients, includes two-day stimulation with PHA followed by 6–8 days of culture with a low dose of IL-2. The PBMCs maintained in parallel for eight days with the same low dose of IL-2 only were unable to exert any BiMAb mediated cytotoxic effect on the tumor cells. The BiMAb mediated cytotoxic effect correlated with the relevant antigen expression on tumor target cells [17].

In vivo preclinical studies confirmed the efficacy of this approach [22]. Human PBMCs armed with bifunctional F(ab')2 were injected into nude mice bearing an intraperitoneal transplant of a human ovarian carcinoma line which expressed the MOv18 recognized epitope. The therapeutic treatment was shown to protect 80% of the treated animals in a short term experiment. In long term experiments 150 days after treatment, 30% of the animals treated with the armed lymphocytes were still alive, whereas all of the control mice were dead. This difference is statistically significant. Clinical results of a study of glioma therapy by this approach have also been reported [23]. On the basis of these preclinical and clinical results a multicentric clinical trial, using the hybrid MOv18/anti-CD3 BiMAb, called OC/TR, which includes a phase I–II and a phase II study, has been started in the Netherlands and Italy [24].

At the National Cancer Institute of Milan a total of 13 patients have been entered to the study to date. Eligible patients have advanced cancer (FIGO stage III and IV) with tumor dissemination restricted to the abdomen, which makes these patients good candidates for intraperitoneal (IP) treatment.

Figure 32.2 outlines the general scheme of the study and Figure 32.3 the scheme of the phase I–II toxicity study which included four

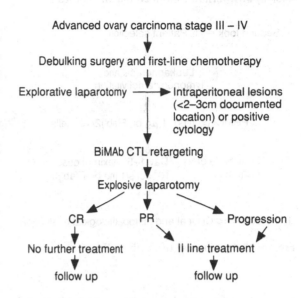

Figure 32.2 BiMAb CTL retargeting: outline of the INT study.

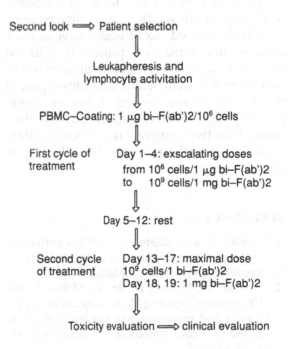

Figure 32.3 Clinical trial: phase I-II.

335

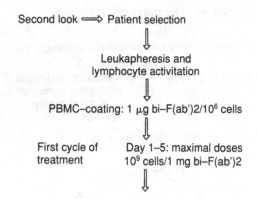

Second look ⟹ Patient selection

Leukapheresis and
lymphocyte activitation

PBMC–coating: 1 μg bi–F(ab')2/10⁶ cells

First cycle of   Day 1–5: maximal doses
treatment   10⁹ cells/1 mg bi–F(ab')2

Third look ⟹ Clinical and histopathological evaluation

Figure 32.4   Clinical trial: phase II.

patients evaluated in Milan and 10 Dutch patients. Of the four Italian patients, one had complete clinical remission lasting 12 months, one patient showed stable disease, whereas the other two patients had progressive disease.

Figure 32.4 reports the details of the phase II Milan study in which, to date, nine patients have been entered, six of whom have already undergone a third look procedure. Clinical and pathological evaluation demonstrated two complete remissions and three partial remissions. In one patient, however, unexpected progression was observed. The duration of the two complete responses is to date 16 and 13 months respectively. All patients are still being followed up.

REFERENCES

1. Kohler, G. and Milstein, C. (1975) Continuous cultures of fused cells secreting antibody of predefined specificity. *Nature*, **246**, 495–7.
2. Colcher, D., Milenic, D., Roselli, M. *et al.* (1989) Characterization and biodistribution of recombinant and recombinant/chimeric constructs of monoclonal antibody B72.3. *Cancer Res.*, **49**, 1738–45.
3. Liu, A.Y., Robinson, R.R., Hellström, K.E. *et al.* (1987) Chimeric mouse–human IgG1 antibody that can mediate lysis of cancer cells. *Proc. Natl. Acad. Sci. USA*, **84**, 3439–43.
4. Miotti, S., Canevari, S., Ménard, S. *et al.* (1987) Characterization of human ovarian carcinoma-associated antigens defined by novel monoclonal antibodies with tumor-restricted specificity. *Int. J. Cancer*, **39**, 297–303.
5. Wilson, B.S., Imai, K., Natali, P.G. and Ferrone, S. (1981) Distribution and molecular characterization of a cell surface and a cytoplasmic antigen detectable in human melanoma cells with monoclonal antibodies. *Int. J. Cancer*, **28**, 293–300.
6. Dillman, R.O. (1990) Human antimouse and antiglobulin responses to monoclonal antibodies. *Immunoconj. Radiopharm.*, **3**, 1–15.
7. Adair, J.R. (1992) Engineering antibodies for therapy. *Immunol. Rev.*, **130**, 5–400.
8. Orlandi, R., Gussow, D.H., Jones, P.T. and Winter, G. (1989) Cloning immunoglobulin variable domains for expression by the polymerase chain reaction. *Proc. Natl. Acad. Sci. USA*, **86**, 3833–7.
9. Rosenberg, S.A. (1992) The immunotherapy and gene therapy of cancer. *J. Clin. Pathol.*, **10**, 180–99.
10. Roosnek, E. and Lanzavecchia, A. (1989) Triggering T cells by otherwise inert hybrid anti-CD3/anti-tumor antibodies requires encounter with the specific target cell. *J. Exp. Med.*, **170**, 297–302.
11. Lanzavecchia, A. and Scheidegger, D. (1987) The use of hybrid hybridomas to target human cytotoxic T lymphocytes. *Eur. J. Immunol.*, **17**, 105–11.
12. Perez, P., Hoffman, R.W., Titus, J.A. and Segal, D.S. (1986) Specific targeting of human peripheral blood T cells by heteroaggregates containing anti-T3 cross linked to anti-target antibodies. *J. Exp. Med.*, **163**, 166–78.
13. Staerz, U. and Bevan, M.J. (1986) Hybrid hybridoma producing a bispecific monoclonal antibody that can focus effector T-cell activity. *Proc. Natl. Acad. Sci. USA*, **83**, 1453–7.
14. Mezzanzanica, D., Canevari, S., Ménard, S. *et al.* (1988) Human ovarian carcinoma lysis by cytotoxic T cells targeted by bispecific monoclonal antibodies: analysis of the antibody components. *Int. J. Cancer*, **41**, 609–15.

15. Glennie, M.J., McBride, H.M., Worth, A.T. and Stevenson, G.T. (1987) Preparation and performance of bispecific F(ab')2 antibody containing thioether-linked Fab' fragments. *J. Immunol.*, **139**, 2367–75.

16. Jung, G., Honsik, C.J., Reisfeld, R.A. and Muller-Eberhard, H.J. (1986) Activation of human peripheral blood mononuclear cells by anti-T3: killing of tumor target cells coated with anti-target–anti-T3 conjugates. *Proc. Natl. Acad. Sci. USA*, **83**, 4479–83.

17. Pupa, S.M., Canevari, S., Fontanelli, R. *et al.* (1988) Activation of mononuclear cells to be used for hybrid monoclonal antibody-induced lysis of human ovarian carcinoma cells. *Int. J. Cancer*, **42**, 455–9.

18. Coney, L.R., Tomassetti, A., Carayannopoulos, L. *et al.* (1991) Cloning of a tumor-associated antigen: MOv18 and MOv19 antibodies recognize a folate-binding protein. *Cancer Res.*, **51**, 6125–32.

19. Buraggi, G.L., Crippa, F., Landoni, L. *et al.* (1988) A new monoclonal antibody (MOv18) against ovarian cancer for imaging and therapy. In *Radioactive Isotopes in Clinical Medicine and Research*, (eds. R. Hoffer and H. Bergman), Schattauer, Stuttgart, pp. 57–62.

20. Crippa, F., Buraggi, G.L., Di Re, E. *et al.* (1991) Radioimmunoscintigraphy of ovarian cancer with the MOv18 monoclonal antibody. *Eur. J. Cancer*, **27**, 724–9.

21. Segal, D.M., Qian, J., Titus, J.A. *et al.* (1992) Targeted cytokine production. *Int. J. Cancer*, **52** (Suppl.), 36–8.

22. Mezzanzanica, D., Neblock, D.S., Garrido, M.A. *et al.* (1990) *In vivo* retargeting of human T cells against human ovarian carcinoma by bifunctional F(ab')2 antibodies. *Antib. Immun. Radiopharm.*, **3**, 81

23. Nitta, T., Sato, K., Yagita, H. *et al.* (1990) Preliminary trial of specific targeting therapy against malignant glioma. *Lancet*, **335**, 368–71.

24. Bolhuis, R.L.H., Lamers, C.H.J., Goey, H.S. *et al.* (1992) Adoptive immunotherapy of ovarian carcinoma with Bs-MAb targeted lymphocytes. A multicenter study. *Int. J. Cancer*, **7**, 78–81.

Chapter 33

Active specific immunotherapy (ASI). An immunological approach to ovarian cancer treatment

G.D. MACLEAN and B.M. LONGENECKER

33.1 INTRODUCTION

The response rate of ovarian cancer to platinum based (cisplatin and carboplatin) chemotherapies has given cause for optimism in the management of metastatic ovarian cancer, but we are still faced with the challenge that more than 50% of these patients have died within five years of diagnosis and commencing chemotherapy. Alternative second line cytotoxic therapies have not significantly influenced the survival of women with residual or relapsing metastatic ovarian cancer. What can we offer the young woman who has been treated with cisplatin or carboplatin and who is at high risk of relapse because of bulky or high grade disease at presentation or because of a persisting elevated serum CA125 antigen level?

'Biomodulation' [1] presents an exciting possibility to be explored in the 1990s. 'Biomodulation' includes those therapeutic measures designed to affect either the host or the tumour, to modify the host–tumour relationship, to increase the likelihood of control of the tumor. One aspect of biomodulation that we are developing is called active specific immunotherapy (ASI). ASI involves actively immunizing the host or the patient with a specified antigen to induce an immune response to

that specific antigen. Can this immune response eradicate or control a cancer?

A decade ago Old [2], acknowledging the potential of immunotherapy, pointed to the need to identify cancer associated antigens which could be used in ASI and which would be essential for monitoring a specific immune response to a cancer. As Old stated, the 'basic tenet in the field ... is that cancer cells are antigenically distinguishable from their normal progenitors, whether this leads to immune recognition or not.' Old also reminded us that 'a far more detailed knowledge of surface antigens of tumour cells will be necessary before we can begin to assess the possibility of immunological control of cancer' [2].

A few years later Hakomori summarized recent findings of aberrant glycosylation in cancer cells, resulting in changes in the cell surface glycoproteins and glycolipids [3]. Hakomori postulated that the aberrant glycosylation is probably the result of altered gene regulation or the effect of oncogenes. Since that time we have come to learn much about the mucins expressed by and shed by cancer cells. Mucins consist of peptide backbones with multiple carbohydrate branches. Mucins extend from within the cell cytoplasm through the cell membrane to a significant distance from the cell surface. Mucins are expressed abundantly by normal cells but because of aberrant glycosylation, cancer mucins are different, with exposure of peptide sequences and carbohydrates that are concealed in the fully glycosylated normal mucins [4]. These changes in cancer mucins are apparent to the immune system and the new or revealed epitopes may form the cancer associated antigens that would be appropriate targets for immunotherapy.

If these cancer associated epitopes are 'foreign' and recognizable by the immune system, why do they not induce a protective immune response against the cancer? Our hypothesis has been that cancer mucin epitopes can induce suppressor activity; actively suppressing an immune response to a cancer. We also propose that this antigen specific immune suppression can be inhibited, allowing for active immunization against the cancer.

Studies with monoclonal antibodies have highlighted the potential of using cancer associated antigens both as serum tumor markers for monitoring disease and as targets for radiolabelled monoclonal antibodies for *in vivo* localization of metastatic disease. We initially developed synthetic mimics of cancer associated carbohydrates for development of such monoclonal antibodies [5,6]. However, with the realization of the potential of biomodulation, and more specifically ASI, we have continued to develop synthetic carbohydrates and synthetic peptides so that these can be incorporated into appropriate formulations (or 'vaccines') for active specific immunotherapy of human adenocarcinomas. We have also been able to use these synthetic antigens to probe the effect mucin epitopes might have in suppressing an immune response to a cancer [7].

33.2 ANIMAL MODELS

We have previously described the results of our animal model studies designed not only to develop formulations for ASI in humans but also to address key questions that challenge the progress of ASI. Our first animal model utilized the murine mammary adenocarcinoma, TA3Ha. This metastasizing breast cancer is rapidly lethal, killing mice in approximately 20 days. We demonstrated that low doses of soluble cancer mucin (epiglycanin) injected into the mice (mimicking low doses of antigen shed by a growing cancer) induced a state of active immune suppression, hastening the death of the mice from subsequent inoculations of TA3Ha.

Preliminary experiments with cyclophosphamide showed that this cytotoxic drug could restore a cellular immune response to a specific cancer associated epitope. While cyclophosphamide on its own had no impact on the survival of the mice, cyclophosphamide could be used to inhibit *in vivo* suppressor activity and when followed by ASI using a synthetic carbohydrate (the TF antigen) on an appropriate carrier molecule (KLH) with an appropriate immune adjuvant (a RIBI formulation, like DETOX™ as used in humans), more than 90% of the mice were alive and well at 120 days [8].

These results prompted us to develop clinical trials using our ASI formulations with synthetic mimics of natural cancer associated antigens. The clinical strategy would also use a low dose of cyclophosphamide administered three days prior to the first ASI treatment, with the hope of inhibiting the suppressor activity believed to be induced by the adenocarcinoma mucin antigens.

33.3 FIRST CLINICAL TRIAL WITH A SYNTHETIC ASI FORMULATION IN PATIENTS WITH METASTATIC OVARIAN CANCER

We have previously reviewed [9] the relevance of the Thomsen–Friedenreich (TF) antigen expressed by the majority of adenocarcinomas, including ovarian cancers. First discovered as a laboratory hemagglutination phenomen, TF was described as a cancer associated epitope by Springer [10]. TF is described as β-D-Gal-(1-3)-α-GalNAc-R. Its monosaccharide precursor, Tn, is also a cancer associated epitope. Springer claimed that the ratio of expression of Tn to TF was indicative of the aggressiveness of a cancer. Since then many papers have described the aggressiveness of various cancers in terms of the expression or lack of expression of TF on the cell surface. The sialylated form of Tn, STn (sialyl Tn), is also now appreciated as an important cancer associated epitope [11].

The first clinical trial of a synthetic antigen in active specific immunotherapy used synthetic TF conjugated to the protein carrier keyhole limpet hemocyanin (KLH), with DETOX adjuvant, with a single pretreatment of low dose cyclophosphamide administered intravenously three days prior to ASI.

In this phase I study we demonstrated that the TF formulation was very well tolerated with minimal toxicity. Most patients developed first an IgM and then an IgG response specific to the TF epitope, in a classic immunological fashion [12]. The specificity of the immune response induced by the ASI was confirmed using two assays – a solid phase antigen assay and a hapten inhibition assay (using various synthetic haptens). Two patients developed IgG anti-TF titres of only 1:80, but three patients developed titres up to 1:5120 or 1:10240. The anti-TF response was also associated with reactivity with cancer cells *in vitro*, with complement dependent cytotoxicity. Several patients had transient decreases in serum CA125 antigen level concomitant with the rising anti-TF titres. Whether this represented response to the ASI or whether this simply indicated interference of the anti-TF with the CA125 assay was not

clear. For example, there may be TF on the CA125 glycoprotein. However, the only patient who did not develop a rising anti-TF titre had a steadily rising serum CA125 level. Two patients developed initial IgG responses (rather than the initial IgM response) suggesting they had been primed previously to the TF epitope, perhaps by the natural cancer antigen. At the time of this phase I study other immunological assays were being developed trying particularly to assess specific cellular immune responses, with the understanding that cellular immune responses may be more relevant to cancer cell cytotoxicity.

We have to be very cautious in interpreting pilot studies which are non-randomized. However, two patients with widespread metastatic ovarian cancer who commenced ASI with the TF formulation in November of 1990 remain alive and well in April of 1993 (both developed high titres of anti-TF). One of these has had intermittent relapses which have responded dramatically (clinically, radiologically and by serum CA125) to low dose carboplatin – 100 mg m^{-2} weekly, for six weeks. Interestingly she also had a decrease in serum CA125 levels during ASI. Crum's recent report [13] of the immunomodulatory effect of low dose cisplatin supports our contention that the efficacy of the low dose carboplatin (in a patient previously treated with conventional cisplatin and carboplatin chemotherapies) may be a biomodulatory effect rather than a cytotoxic effect.

Nevertheless, it is difficult to be confident that ASI can control widespread bulky metastatic disease, particularly following multiple chemotherapies which may adversely affect the immune system. Our subsequent phase I and II studies (with our synthetic mimics of cancer associated antigens) have been directed more at patients with low volume metastatic disease or early metastatic disease.

33.4 THE RELEVANCE OF SIALYL Tn (STn) IN ASI

Tn is the monosaccharide precursor of the TF disaccharide. Sialyl Tn, or sialylated Tn, is commonly expressed by many adenocarcinomas and is seldom found on normal tissues. STn appears to be the epitope identified by the monoclonal antibody B72.3 first described by Nuti *et al.* (14), an antibody that has subsequently been studied extensively *in vitro* and *in vivo* for its potential for immunodiagnosis. Recent studies by Itzkowitz in colon cancer [11], Kobayashi in ovarian cancer [15] and Miles in breast cancer [16] have demonstrated that the expression of STn is associated with a poor prognosis compared with STn negative cancers. Is STn a marker of more aggressive cancer cells in several common adenocarcinomas, including ovarian cancer? STn would thus appear to be a good target for immunotherapy but the concern is raised that cancers are heterogeneous with respect to expression of STn.

Cancer heterogeneity is the main reason that our program is developing multiepitope 'vaccines' for ASI. STn could be an important component of such a formulation but the question was still asked whether it was foolish to include an immunogen where its natural epitope is heterogeneously expressed. However, rather than rejecting STn for ASI because it is not expressed on all cancer cells, we have wondered whether there is a difference in behavior between STn positive and STn negative cancer cells and whether there is merit in targeting a therapy specifically to STn positive cells. The findings noted above suggest that STn may be a marker for those cells which are more aggressive. Indeed, STn may even be related to the actual process of metastasis. Thus, an anti-STn immune response may be important in controlling the more aggressive cells within an adenocarcinoma.

Our first study with a synthetic STn formulation was in patients with metastatic breast cancer [17]. While three patients had widespread metastatic breast cancer and progressed despite ASI, two patients achieved partial responses with ASI and five patients had disease stability following ASI. Although the mean time to progression has been a somewhat disappointing six months, one patient with pulmonary metastases remains stable 22 months after entry into the ASI program (with no therapy subsequent to the ASI treatments). One young woman who entered the ASI program with internal mammary lymphadenopathy was stable until she developed cervical lymphadenopathy (confirmed by needle aspirate). She had a dramatic response to low dose chlorambucil chemotherapy (10 mg p.o. daily for seven days, repeated at 28 day intervals, $\times$ 3–4). This again raises the question whether the low dose chemotherapy effect was due to cytotoxicity (possibly influenced by the ASI) or whether the low dose chlorambucil was biomodulatory enhancing the immune response induced by the ASI.

Two patients achieved mixed responses with reduction in size of at least one metastatic lesion, with stability or progression of other metastatic lesions. Biopsies with immunohistological analysis would be necessary for confirmation, but our hypothesis is that these mixed responses reflect the importance of tumor heterogeneity and the need for multiepitopic formulations.

Again, this study showed the relative safety of ASI. All patients developed typical delayed type hypersensitivity reactions at the treatment sites and five of the patients developing small fluctant ulcerating granulomas which healed uneventfully. Two patients had vomiting after the cyclophosphamide (despite metoclopramide being used as a prophylactic antiemetic) and five had nausea for at least the first day following the cyclophosphamide.

All patients have developed at least a humoral immune response specific for the synthetic STn epitope, with *in vitro* studies showing this immune response is capable of complement dependent cytotoxicity of tumor cells. Ongoing studies are assessing the specificity of the cellular immune response following ASI.

33.5 THE FUTURE OF ASI IN OVARIAN CANCER

As part of ongoing phase II studies seeking clinical efficacy, one study will assess STn-KLH with DETOX in patients with ovarian cancer following primary therapy with cisplatin or carboplatin. Patients are stratified according to disease burden, including a group of patients who have no detectable residual disease following chemotherapy but who have elevated serum CA125 antigen levels. Is there a future for STn ASI formulations or multiepitopic formulations including STn in the treatment of patients with ovarian cancer? Current animal model studies suggest that a synthetic mimic of Taylor's 'MUC1' mucin peptide antigen [18] may be an important component of future formulations for clinical studies. Can ASI as adjuvant immunotherapy or as an adjunct to current chemotherapy increase the survival of patients with metastatic or micrometastatic disease?

Current studies are addressing some important questions, including:

1. What is the optimum dose? In chemotherapy we have tended to think that 'a bigger dose must be better.' From preliminary animal studies it appears that a lower dose of ASI may be better in terms of survival (Itzkowitz, personal communication) and this would correlate with current immunological theory where lower doses are more likely to induce cellular immune

responses than higher doses which are more likely to induce humoral immune responses.
2. What is the optimum schedule of ASI administration?
3. What is the role, if any, and what is the best means of administration of cyclophosphamide with ASI (in relation to the theory of trying to overcome the immune suppression induced by cancer mucins)?
4. What are the roles of other biomodulators in enhancing a protective immune response against the cancer? In addition to such agents as interferon we should give consideration to the potential of low dose chlorambucil or low dose carboplatin as biomodulators, particularly in patients receiving ASI for metastatic ovarian cancer.

33.6 THE FUTURE

Fifteen years ago many became optimistic that the answer to the question of management of metastatic ovarian cancer would be found in manipulating the dose or scheduling of cisplatin or one of its analogs. Dramatic response rates and apparent prolonged survival in some patients encouraged us. That hope has not yet materialized, although it is clear that platinum based chemotherapy has an important role in management of ovarian cancer.

Perhaps what is needed is not an alternative chemotherapy or a bigger dose of chemotherapy but a different approach to the patient who is at high risk of relapse following platinum based chemotherapy. We believe that ASI and biomodulation hold hope in the management of ovarian cancer. Current studies are exploring the potential of synthetic ASI formulations in an attempt to immunize patients against their cancers. In particular, ASI may have real promise when used in a truly adjuvant setting for patients at high risk of residual micrometastatic disease following primary surgery and/or chemotherapy. The exciting aspect of biomodulation is that this field is in its infancy and there is much yet to discover about the potential for modifying the host immune response to a cancer. Patients find this approach particularly appealing both because they can relate to efforts to stimulate the body to respond to a cancer and because the toxicity of ASI is considerably less than our current 'standard' chemotherapies.

Preliminary data on our initial pilot studies using novel 'vaccine formulations' have been presented, but as we search for better ways to use these formulations and a better understanding of the immune response to cancer associated antigens, we are mindful of Edward de Bono's caution: 'Unfortunately we cannot be aware of what we are not aware' [19]. Rather than arguing why ASI will not be effective, at this stage we would prefer to explore how ASI might become part of an effective combined modality therapy strategy for the treatment of metastatic ovarian cancer.

REFERENCES

1. Mitchell, M.S. (1992) Biomodulators in cancer treatment. *J. Clin. Pharmacol.*, **32**, 2–9.
2. Old, L.J. (1981) Cancer immunology: the search for specificity. G.H.A. Clowes Memorial Lecture. *Cancer Res.*, **41**, 361–75.
3. Hakomori, S. I. (1985) Aberrant glycosylation in cancer cell membranes as focused on glycolipids: overview and perspectives. *Cancer Res.*, **45**, 2405–14.
4. Hanisch, F.G., Uhlenbruek G., Egge, H. *et al.* (1989) A B72.3 second-generation monoclonal antibody (CC49) defines the mucin-carried carbohydrate epitope Galβ(1-3)[NeuAcα(2-6)]GalNAc. *J. Biol. Chem.*, **370**, 21–6.
5. Longenecker, B.M., Willans, D.J., MacLean, G.D. *et al.* (1987) Monoclonal antibodies and synthetic tumor-associated glycoconjugates in the study of the expression of Thomsen-Friedenreich-like and Tn-like antigens on human cancers. *J. Natl. Cancer Inst.*, **78**, 489–96.
6. MacLean, G.D., McEwan, A., Noujaim A.A. *et al.* (1991) Two novel monoclonal antibodies have potential for gynecologic cancer imaging. *Antibody Immunocon. Radiopharm.*, **4**, 297–308.
7. Fung, P.Y.S. and Longenecker, B.M. (1991) Specific immunosuppressive activity of epiglycanin, a mucin-like glycoprotein secreted by a murine mammary adenocarcinoma (TA3-HA). *Cancer Res.*, **51**, 1170–6.
8. Fung, P.Y.S., Madej, M., Koganty, R. *et al.* (1990) Active specific immunotherapy of a murine mammary adenocarcinoma using a synthetic tumor-associated glycoconjugate. *Cancer Res.*, **50**, 4308–14.
9. MacLean, G.D. and Longenecker, B.M. (1991) Clinical significance of the Thomsen-Friedenreich antigen. *Semin. Cancer Biol.*, **2**, 433–9.
10. Springer, G.F. (1984) T and Tn, General carcinoma autoantigens. *Science*, **244**, 1198–206.
11. Itzkowitz, S.H., Bloom, E.J., Kokal, W.A. *et al.* (1990) Sialosyl-Tn. A novel mucin antigen associated with prognosis in colorectal cancer patients. *Cancer*, **66**, 1960–6.
12. MacLean, G.D., Bowen-Yacyshyn, M.B., Samuel, J. *et al.* (1992) Active immunization of human ovarian cancer patients against a common carcinoma (Thomsen–Friedenreich) determinant using a synthetic carbohydrate antigen. *J. Immunother.*, **11**, 292–305.
13. Crum, E. (1993) Effect of cisplatin upon expression of *in vivo* immune tumor resistance. *Cancer Immunol. Immunother.*, **36**, 18–24.
14. Nuti, M., Teramoto, Y.A., Mariani-Costantini, R. *et al.* (1982) A monoclonal antibody (B72.3) defines patterns of distribution of a novel tumor-associated antigen in human mammary carcinoma cell populations. *Int. J. Cancer*, **29**, 539–45.
15. Kobayashi, H., Terao, T., Kawashima Y. *et al.* (1992) Serum sialyl Tn as an independent predictor of poor prognosis in patients with epithelial ovarian cancer. *J. Clin. Oncol.*, **10**, 95–101.
16. Longenecker, B.M., Reddish, M., Miles, D. *et al.* (1993) Synthetic tumor associated sialyl-Tn antigen as an immunotherapeutic cancer vaccine. *Vaccine Res.*, in press.

17. MacLean, G.D., Reddish, M., Koganty, R.R. *et al.* (1993) Immunization of breast cancer patients using a synthetic sialyl-Tn glycoconjugate plus Detox adjuvant. *Cancer Immunol. Immunother.*, **36**, 215–22.

18. Ding. L, Lalani, E., Reddish, M. *et al.* (1992) Immunogenicity of synthetic peptides related to the core peptide sequence encoded by the human MUC1 gene: effect of immunization of the growth of murine mammary adenocarcinoma cells transfected with the human MUC1 gene. *Cancer Immunol. Immunother.*, **36**, 9–17.

19. De Bono, E. (1971) *Practical Thinking*, Penguin Books, Harmondsworth, Chapter 7.

Chapter 34

Antibody targeting of ovarian cancer: recombinant single-chain fragments and the role of internalization

M.A. BOOKMAN, B.J. GIANTONIO and J. SCHULTZ

34.1 INTRODUCTION

Among the factors that have hindered development of antibody based therapy are the heterogeneity of tumor antigen expression, the limited penetration of bulk tumor masses by macromolecules, cross reactivity between tumor and normal host antigens and unfavourable patterns of antibody internalization [1]. With greater understanding of these obstacles and the ability to engineer changes within the antibody molecule itself, there has been renewed enthusiasm for development and evaluation of immunoconjugates. Improved molecular and functional characterization of tumor antigens has influenced the design of targeting strategies and contributed to the analysis of normal tissue distribution and potential for host toxicity. Furthermore, the choice of specific radionuclide, toxin or drug conjugate has been influenced by increased knowledge of antibody internalization and processing pathways. Thus, a new generation of reagents is being prepared for clinical trial that takes full advantage of past experiences and recent advances in molecular and cellular biology.

34.2 CHOICE OF REAGENTS

We have been evaluating c-erbB2 as a target antigen for therapy of ovarian and breast carcinoma. This transmembrane growth factor receptor has tyrosine kinase activity and extensive homology to the epidermal growth factor receptor (EGFR). Increased cell surface expression of c-erbB2 is common among adenocarcinomas from multiple sites, including breast and ovary [2]. Although the differentiation and growth regulatory functions of c-erbB2 have not been fully elucidated, increased expression has been correlated with adverse prognosis in patients with breast and advanced ovarian cancer [3]. A variety of monoclonal antibodies has been described with reactivity against the extracellular domain of c-erbB2. A subset of these antibodies is capable of direct receptor activation [4], blockade of ligand binding or inhibition of tumor growth in vivo [5]. However, the majority of native antibodies has only limited potential for sustained tumor growth regulation and therapeutic studies have focused on antibodies conjugated to radionuclides, drugs or toxins.

The choice of therapeutic conjugate is influenced by several factors, including antigen density, antigenic heterogeneity, kinetics of internalization and intracellular routing. Receptor mediated endocytosis is usually followed by lysosomal acidification, reduction and proteolysis. Intracellular processing has the undesirable effect of accelerated release of free radionuclide from commonly used reagents such as ^{131}I or ^{90}Y [6], resulting in decreased tumor exposure and increased potential for systemic toxicity. Thus, slowly internalized antibodies that tend to remain at the cell surface would be preferred for radionuclide studies, particularly in combination with strategies that would increase tumor localization and retention. Conversely, internalization and processing are absolutely necessary for the activity of ribosomal toxins such as ricin A-chain (RA) or *Pseudomonas* exotoxin (PE), chromosomal damage mediated by ^{125}I Auger electrons [7] and cytotoxicity of doxorubicin conjugates [8,9].

Reagents that depend on lysosomal processing are restricted to killing target cells with accessible surface antigens that lead to internalization. Specifically, there are no mechanisms for toxin mediated killing of adjacent antigen negative cells within a single tumor site. However, β-emitting isotopes such as ^{131}I or ^{90}Y are capable of irradiating antigen negative tumor cells within an effective radius of several millimeters. Thus, the optimal antigen–antibody profiles for radioconjugates and intracellular toxins vary considerably (Table 34.1).

34.3 INTERNALIZATION KINETICS AND IMMUNOTOXIN ACTIVITY

Internalization of surface antigens varies in accordance with their function and also as a consequence of ligand or antibody interactions, each of which may influence targeting strategies. For example, the transferrin receptor (TFR) is the primary means for cellular iron uptake and is efficiently internalized via clathrin coated pits followed by removal of iron-transferrin and recycling of unbound receptor to the cell surface. In contrast, β2-microglobulin, a glycoprotein associated with the class I major histocompatability complex, is slowly internalized as a consequence of normal membrane turnover and is not recycled. Signal transduction molecules, such as EGFR, are slowly internalized at baseline but more rapidly internalized following ligand binding and receptor activation. Once internalized EGFR is routed to the acidic lysosomal compartment where it undergoes proteolytic degradation without surface recycling of receptor protein.

The intracellular routing of c-*erb*B2 is similar to EGFR, without evidence of receptor recycling. Consequently, we were concerned that anti-c-*erb*B2 antibodies might not make highly effective immunotoxins. Therefore, a number of different immunotoxins were prepared by conjugation of recombinant RA to three anti-c-*erb*B2 IgG1 monoclonal antibodies and their Fab fragments (520C9, 741F8,

Table 34.1 Comparison of radionuclide and toxin conjugates

Radionuclides
  Uniform tumor antigen expression not required
  Internalization and processing undesirable
  Potential bystander toxicity to antigen negative tissues
  Limited radionuclide half life
  Conjugation or chelation required immediately prior to use
  Potential for radiation induced damage to antibody

Toxins
  Uniform tumor antigen expression required
  Internalization and processing required
  Potential toxicity to antigen positive non-tumor tissues
  Increased immunogenicity of xenobiotic toxins
  Favorable long term stability of conjugates *in vitro*

454C11; Cetus Oncology, Emeryville, CA). Functional comparisons were made with an anti-TFR immunotoxin (454A12-rRA, Cetus Oncology) and an isotype-matched control non-reactive immunotoxin (MOPC21-rRA, Cetus Oncology). Protein synthesis inhibition was measured by [³H]-leucine incorporation at 18 hours and cell growth inhibition measured by MTT tetrazolium dye conversion at 4–8 days. When tested against cell lines with high level expression of c-*erb*B2 (e.g. SKBR3), the anti-TFR immunotoxin was 2–3 logs more potent than anti-c-*erb*B2 (data not shown). Cell lines with intermediate (e.g. SKOV3) or low level expression of c-*erb*B2 (e.g. OVCAR3) were relatively insensitive to c-*erb*B2 specific immunotoxin, which appeared only slightly more toxic than the non-reactive control (MOPC21-rRA). Divalent IgG and (Fab')2 reagents were comparable to monovalent Fab reagents (Figure 34.1), while mixtures of different anti-c-*erb*B2 IgG immunotoxins were additive but not synergistic in their activity. These data suggested that antigen internaliza-

tion kinetics may help predict immunoconjugate efficacy.

To evaluate the relationship between internalization kinetics and immunotoxin activity, we developed flow cytometric assays for monitoring internalization on SKBR3, which expresses both c-*erb*B2 and TFR at high levels. After binding of phycoerythrin conjugated rat antimouse κ secondary antibody, internalized antibody was distinguished from surface bound antibody by resistance to acid washing at pH 3, which removed 100% of residual surface bound antimouse κ. For example, after 45 minutes at 37°C, there was 86% internalization of anti-TFR compared to only 12% for anti-c-*erb*B2 (Figure 34.2). Time course studies revealed that the majority of anti-TFR internalization occurred within 10 minutes. Incubations for as long as six hours showed only a maximum of 25–30% internalization for anti-c-*erb*B2. Companion flow cytometric studies of surface antibody density confirmed that the majority of antibody remained at the cell surface, with less than 30% internalization

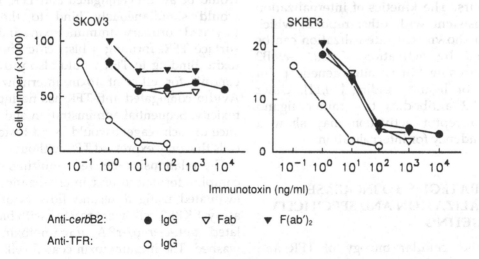

Figure 34.1 Activity of anti-c-*erb*B2 and anti-TFR rRA immunotoxins *in vitro*. Conjugates were prepared using anti-c-*erb*B2 520C9 and anti-TFR 454A12 (Cetus Oncology) and continuously incubated with either SKOV3 (ovarian cancer, intermediate c-*erb*B2 expression) or SKBR3 (breast cancer, high c-*erb*B2 expression) for six days in 96-well tissue culture plates. Viable cell number was determined by conversion of MTT dye and measured on a plate spectrophotometer.

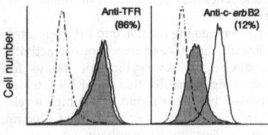

Figure 34.2 Internalization of antibodies bound to cell surface receptors. Monoclonal IgG1 antibodies directed against TFR (454A12) and c-*erb*B2 (741F8) were incubated with SKBR3 cells and stained with monoclonal phycoerythrin conjugated rat antimouse κ. Initial surface staining (solid line) was uniformly bright for both primary antibodies. Cells were then incubated for 45 minutes and acid-washed (at pH3) to remove residual non-internalized surface bound antibody. Internalized (i.e. acid resistant) staining after incubation at 37°C (shaded area) reached 86% for TFR compared to only 12% for c-*erb*B2. No internalization occurred at 4°C (dashed line).

at six hours. The kinetics of internalization were consistent with other reports, which have also shown that internalization can be accelerated by activation of the c-*erb*B2 protein tyrosine kinase after genetic point mutation or ligand binding [10,11]. Other anti-c-*erb*B2 antibodies that mimic ligand induced receptor activation may show a greater tendency for internalization.

34.4 STRATEGIES TO INCREASE INTERNALIZATION AND SPECIFICITY OF TARGETING

The distinct cellular biology of TFR and c-*erb*B2 prompted us to consider the benefits of a hybrid reagent that would target both antigens. Most tumor associated antigens are not truly tumor specific and they can also be identified on various normal host tissues. In particular, both c-*erb*B2 and TFR are products of normal genes found at low levels on many glandular or epithelial cells, with increased expression on a subset of adenocarcinomas. Simultaneous targeting of both antigens on the same cell would potentially increase the specificity and avidity for tumor tissue. However, simultaneous targeting would not prevent delivery of toxic reagents to cells expressing only one of the target antigens. This would pose a significant problem with TFR, which is widely expressed by normal cells. For example, a phase I clinical trial of anti-TFR immunotoxin found central nervous system toxicity to be dose-limiting due to hemorrhagic capillary necrosis [12].

We hypothesized that sequential construction of bifunctional complexes *in situ* would provide a means to limit toxicity only to cells that expressed both antigens (Figure 34.3). The primary reagent would be a biotinylated anti-c-*erb*B2 rRA immunotoxin, which would bind to tumor cells without significant internalization or toxicity. The secondary reagent would be avidin conjugated anti-TFR, which would simultaneously bind to the biotinylated primary immunotoxin and cell surface TFR, forming a bispecific immunotoxin. Binding to TFR would also provide a conduit for efficient toxin internalization. Avidin conjugated anti-TFR has no intrinsic toxicity. Sequential administration and clearance of each reagent would avoid toxicity to cells that only expressed TFR without c-*erb*B2.

The relationship between multimolecular complex formation and internalization was evaluated using a second flow cytometric assay. SKBR3 cells were reacted with biotinylated anti-c-*erb*B2-rRA immunotoxin and washed. The immunotoxin coated cells were then split into two groups for incubation with either avidin conjugated anti-TFR or a mixture of avidin and non-conjugated anti-TFR followed by staining for residual surface

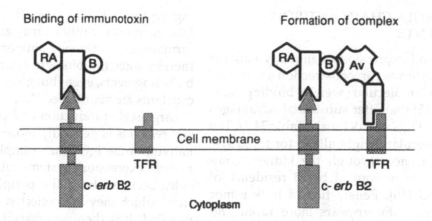

Figure 34.3 Formation of multimolecular complexes for promotion of internalization. Biotinylated (B) anti-c-*erb*B2 antibody conjugated to ricin A-chain (RA) is bound to the extracellular domain of c-*erb*B2 (step 1). After allowing time for clearance of excess unbound antibody, streptavidin (Av) conjugated anti-TFR antibody is bound to cell associated TFR (step 2). High affinity non-covalent associations between biotin and streptavidin lead to the formation of multimolecular complexes at the cell surface that may promote internalization via TFR.

bound rRA. Only the avidin conjugated anti-TFR complexes resulted in significant internalization, as reflected by decreased staining for residual surface bound rRA (Figure 34.4). This supports the hypothesis that internalization can be accelerated by formation of complexes between antigens with diverse functions. Functional confirmation using tumor growth inhibition assays and electron microscopy to visualize colloidal gold-labeled antibodies is in progress.

Sequential multimolecular targeting also offers the potential for amplified localization of therapeutic conjugates within tumor sites through multivalent high affinity biotin–avidin linkages. For example, preliminary clinical studies have successfully used sequential administration of biotinylated anti-CEA antibodies, avidin and biotinylated radionuclides [13]. A further potential advantage of these strategies would be *in situ* formation of high molecular weight multivalent complexes, thereby increasing retention of conjugates at tumor sites due to increased avidity and decreased diffusion mobility.

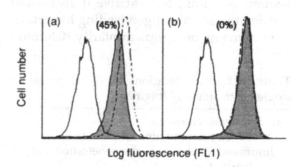

Figure 34.4 Promotion of internalization using multimolecular complexes. SKBR3 cells were coated with biotinylated anti-c-*erb*B2-rRA immunotoxin (520C9-rRA), washed and secondarily coated with either streptavidin conjugated anti-TFR (454A12) antibody (a), or a mixture of streptavidin and anti-TFR (b). After incubation for 60 minutes, each cell population was stained for residual surface bound rRA and examined by flow cytometry. Cells incubated at 4°C showed bright surface staining (dashed line) with both sets of reagents. Cells incubated at 37°C (shaded area) showed no change in surface staining in the absence of complexes (b) and a 45% decrease in surface staining in the presence of complexes (a), consistent with internalization. Unstained controls are illustrated by the solid line.

34.5 SINGLE-CHAIN ANTIBODY FRAGMENTS

Cloning and expression of antibody variable domains allows for construction of single-chain low molecular weight binding sites (sFv) [14,15] that offer substantial advantages over native IgG monoclonals (Table 34.2). The lower molecular weight allows for rapid systemic clearance through the kidney, compared to the prolonged blood residence of native IgG [16]. Penetration of bulk tumor masses with sFv appears more rapid and uniform than IgG or Fab [17]. In addition, immunogenicity is substantially reduced by elimination of constant domains from both the heavy and light chains. Further reductions in immunogenicity can be achieved by substitution of human immunoglobulin framework sequences for residual murine sequences within the variable domains but outside the actual antigen binding hypervariable domains or complementarity determin-

Table 34.2 Considerations for development of single-chain antibody fragments

Rapid systemic clearance
  Improved tumor to normal tissue ratios
  Improved kinetics of tumor penetration and
    distribution
  Low percent injected dose (~1–2%) per gram of
    tumor tissue
  Requirement for higher cumulative dosage
  Increased renal exposure and potential for
    toxicity

Molecular engineering
  Difficulties with large scale production,
    refolding and purification
  Favorable decreased immunogenicity,
    particularly with human sequences
  Decreased avidity of monovalent sFv
  Propensity for non-covalent protein
    interactions
  Construction of multivalent sFv
  Construction of chimeric multifunctional
    proteins

ing region (CDR). However, some human framework substitutions may alter CDR conformation or influence antigen contact and thereby alter the biological activity of antibody fragments, even though antigen binding constants are maintained [18].

Large-scale production and purification of sFv reagents is generally more difficult than native murine IgG. For example, with some *E. coli* expression systems, nascent molecules accumulate in the periplasmic space, from which they are collected and partially purified. It is then necessary to refold each molecule to recover antigen binding activity, which may require denaturation–renaturation conditions, associated with significant reduction in yield. Properly folded active material must then be separated from residual inactive material, often through antigen chromatography. This further requires a purified or recombinant source of antigen that can be recycled on the affinity column. If alternative *E. coli*, yeast, insect or mammalian cell expression systems are utilized, it is possible to take advantage of secretion pathways where the nascent protein chains are spontaneously folded as they are synthesized and transported across cellular membranes. Each of these systems requires considerable expertise for large-scale production of sufficient purified material suitable for preclinical and clinical testing.

Although the small size and rapid renal clearance of sFv would appear advantageous, these factors pose unique problems with regard to therapeutic drug delivery. Preliminary animal experiments have documented favorable tumor to normal tissue ratios that greatly exceed values obtained with IgG. However, the kidney is rapidly exposed to high levels of sFv due to glomerular filtration and clearance, with increased potential for end-organ toxicity.

Importantly, the percent of injected dose per gram of tumor tissue has been typically one log less than that reported with native

IgG. In addition, sFv reagents are monovalent with inherent decreased antigen avidity compared to divalent IgG. This decreased avidity, together with the rapid reduction in systemic concentrations favors a situation where sFv detaches from the tumor and is rapidly cleared. Delivery of therapeutic concentrations of radionuclides or toxins under these circumstances may require novel scheduling and high cumulative doses in accordance with pharmacokinetic modeling.

Recombinant technology also allows for construction of chimeric or hybrid molecules with more than one functional domain [19,20]. Chimeric proteins with anti-c-*erb*B2 reactivity and modified *Pseudomonas* exotoxin have been evaluated *in vivo* using nude mice bearing human tumor xenografts [21]. In one model, antitumor effects were observed after a seven day continuous infusion of the chimeric toxin molecule [22], emphasizing the pharmacokinetic consequences of low molecular weight reagents.

Construction of dimeric sFv would provide another means to increase binding avidity and potentially increase tumor retention of injected reagents. Homodimers have been formed from disulfide or chemically linked sFv-Cys (sFv′) monomers [23]. Bis-maleimidohexane chemically linked (sFv′)₂ dimers appear stable *in vivo*, although dimers and sFv′ sulfhydryl blocked monomers tend to form non-covalent associations with serum proteins that could alter biodistribution and pharmacokinetics [24].

Evaluation of disulfide linked anti-c-*erb*B2 (sFv′)2 homodimers in tumor bearing scid mice revealed tumor uptake (1% injected dose g^{-1} at 24 hours) that was comparable to monovalent glutathionyl blocked sFv′ [25]. The ability of each sFv′ monomeric subunit to simultaneously and independently bind soluble c-*erb*B2 extracellular domain was verified by equilibrium centrifugation analysis. Chemically linked (sFv′)₂ homodimers prepared with bis-maleimidohexane and disul-

fide linked homodimers with a long flexible peptide spacer showed somewhat greater localization (1.6–1.8% injected dose g^{-1} at 24 hours) compared to the disulfide linked reagents with a short spacer. However, a slight prolongation of systemic clearance seen with the higher molecular weight dimers may contribute to the observed increase in tumor localization. The optimal reagent for tumor targeting remains to be established, but plans would tentatively favor an (sFv′)₂ dimer with a flexible spacer, rather than sFv′ monomer.

Although these results are encouraging, it has been more difficult to verify that dimeric sFv′ can actually bind to native antigen in a divalent fashion. Steric constraints may prevent divalent binding to cell associated antigen *in situ*, in contrast to assays with soluble extracellular domains *in vitro*. We compared various monomeric and dimeric sFv′ for their ability to inhibit binding of biotinylated native IgG on intact SKBR3 cells using a flow cytometric assay (Figure 34.5). Within the limits of the assay, it was not possible to discern any difference between the various sFv′ species, which appeared similar to Fab on a molar basis and somewhat less avid than native IgG. This suggested that the dimeric (sFv′)₂ reagents might only bind antigen using one site at a time due to steric constraints or that non-covalent interactions between sFv′ monomers resulted in the formation of functional dimers indistinguishable from chemically linked dimers, but less avid than native IgG.

Several species of sFv produced thus far have been reported to spontaneously form non-covalent dimers *in vitro*. Dimerization most likely occurs with an end-to-end orientation that would limit mobility of each subunit for antigen binding. Addition of flexible peptide spacers may fail to change subunit orientation, as the spacers could be wrapped around the sFv subunits rather than extended between them. Experiments with rigid spacer elements or sFv that contain spe-

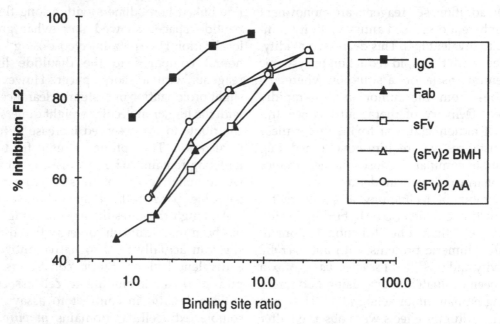

Figure 34.5 Competitive binding assay with monomeric and dimeric sFv. SKBR3 cells were incubated with biotinylated 741F8-IgG (1 μg 10⁻⁶ cells) together with non-biotinylated competing reagents at 37°C for 15 minutes. The cells were then washed and stained with streptavidin–phycoerythrin in preparation for flow cytometry. The percent inhibition of scaled mean fluorescence is plotted as a function of increasing binding site ratios between the test reagents and control Biot-741F8-IgG. Monovalent Fab fragments were prepared by enzymatic digestion and column chromatography: sFv refers to sFv' blocked monomer; (sFv)₂ BMH refers to a thioether-linked sFv' dimer; (sFv)₂ AA refers to a disulfide-linked sFv' dimer with an oligopeptide spacer. Note that native divalent IgG was more effective at competition compared to the monovalent Fab, even though the data were adjusted for number of binding sites and molecular weight. The sFv' monomer compared favorably to Fab. Both of the sFv' dimers were similar to sFv' monomer and Fab, rather than IgG.

cific amino acid substitutions to diminish spontaneous self-association are required to resolve the significance of these interactions *in vitro* and *in vivo*.

34.6 CONCLUSIONS

Strategies for improved antibody targeting of ovarian cancer continue to evolve. Many tumor associated antigens have been well characterized with regard to heterogeneity, structure, function and normal tissue distribution permitting a more rational choice of specific targets. Kinetics of antibody internalization and intracellular processing can

also influence the choice of therapeutic reagents for clinical evaluation. Molecular genetic techniques have been devised for construction of low molecular weight antibody fragments with decreased immunogenicity, improved tumor penetration and greater specificity of uptake. Chimeric single-chain proteins, multivalent binding sites and use of biotin–avidin linkage *in vivo* offer new possibilities for amplification of tumor localization and effectiveness.

ACKNOWLEDGEMENTS

The authors thank their NCDDG collaborators at Cetus Oncology (L.L Houston, J. Apell,

A. Laminet), Creative BioMolecules (J.S. Huston, H. Oppermann, J.E. McCartney, M.-S. Tai), Boston Biomedical Research Institute (W.F. Stafford III, S. Liu), and Fox Chase Cancer Center (L.M. Wiener, G.P. Adams) for sharing reagents, preliminary results and expertise.

This work was supported in part by National Cancer Institute Co-operative Drug Discovery Group (NCDDG) grant UO1 CA51880.

REFERENCES

1. Bookman, M.A. (1993) Biologic therapy in the management of refractory ovarian cancer. *Gynecol. Oncol.*, **51**, 113–26.

2. Slamon, D.J., Godophin, W., Jones, L.A. *et al.* (1989) Studies of HER-2/neu proto-oncogene in human breast and ovarian cancer. *Science*, **244**, 707–12.

3. Berchuck, A., Kamel, A., Whitaker, R. *et al.* (1990) Overexpression of HER-2/neu is associated with poor survival in advanced epithelial ovarian cancer. *Cancer Res.*, **50**, 4087–91.

4. Drebin, J.A., Link, V.C., Stern, D.F. *et al.* (1985) Down-modulation of an oncogene protein product and reversion of the transformed phenotype by monoclonal antibodies. *Cell*, **41**, 695–706.

5. Drebin, J.A. Link, V.C., Greene, M.I. (1988) Monoclonal antibodies specific for the *neu* oncogene product directly mediate anti-tumor effects *in vivo*, *Oncogene*, **2**, 387–94.

6. Stewart, J.S.W., Hird, V., Snook, D. *et al.* (1990) Intraperitoneal yttrium-90-labeled monoclonal antibody in ovarian cancer. *J. Clin. Oncol.*, **8**, 1941–50.

7. Woo, D.V., Li, D., Mattis, J.A. and Steplewski, Z. (1989) Selective chromosomal damage and cytotoxicity of ^{125}I-labeled monoclonal antibody 17-la in human cancer cells. *Cancer Res.*, **49**, 2952–8.

8. Braslawsky, G.R., Kadow, K., Knipe, J. *et al.* (1991) Adriamycin(hydrazone)-antibody conjugates require internalization and intracellular acid hydrolysis for antitumor activity. *Cancer Immunol. Immunother.*, **33**, 367–74.

9. Trail, P.A., Willner, D., Lasch, S.J. *et al.* (1993) Cure of xenografted human carcinomas by BR96-doxorubicin immunoconjugates. *Science*, **261**, 212–5.

10. Van Leeuwen, F., van de Vijver, M.J., Lomans, J. *et al.* (1990) Mutation of the human *neu* protein facilitates down-modulation by monoclonal antibodies. *Oncogene*, **5**, 497–503.

11. Huang, S.S., Koh, H.A., Konish, Y. *et al.* (1990) Differential processing and turnover of the oncogenically activated *neu/erb* B2 gene product and its normal cellular counterpart. *J. Biol. Chem.*, **265**, 3340–6.

12. Bookman, M.A. (1992) Immunotoxin therapy in ovarian cancer. In *Ovarian Cancer 2: Biology, Diagnosis and Management*, (eds P. Mason, F. Sharp and W. Creasman), Chapman & Hall, London, pp. 153–60.

13. Paganelli, G., Magnani, P., Zito, F. *et al.* (1991) Three-step monoclonal antibody tumor targeting in carcinoembryonic antigen-positive patients. *Cancer Res.*, **51**, 5960–6.

14. Huston, J.S., Levinson, D., Mudgett-Hunter, M. *et al.* (1988) Protein engineering of antibody binding sites: recovery of specific activity in an anti-digoxin single-chain Fv analogue produced in E. coli. *Proc. Natl. Acad. Sci. USA*, **85**, 5879–83.

15. Skerra, A. and Pluckthun, A. (1988) Assembly of a functional immunoglobulin Fv fragment in *Escherichia coli. Science*, **240**, 1038–41.

16. Milenic, D.E., Yokota, T., Filpula, D.R. *et al.* (1991) Construction, binding properties, metabolism, and tumor targeting of a single-chain Fv derived from the pancarcinoma monoclonal CC49. *Cancer Res.*, **51**, 6363–71.

17. Yokota, T., Milenic, D.E., Whitlow, M. and Schlom, J. (1992) Rapid tumor penetration of a single-chain Fv and comparison with the immunoglobulin forms. *Cancer Res.*, **52**, 3402–8.

18. Kelley, R.F., O'Connell, M.P., Carter, P. *et al.* (1992) Antigen binding thermodynamics and antiproliferative effects of chimeric and humanized anti-p185[HER2] antibody Fab fragments. *Biochemistry*, **31**, 5434–41.

19. Chaudhary, V.K., Queen, C., Junghans, R.P. *et al.* (1989) A recombinant immunotoxin consisting of two antibody variable domains fused to Pseudomonas exotoxin. *Nature*, **339**, 394–7.

20. Tai, M.-S., Mudgett-Hunter, M., Levinson, D. *et al.* (1990) A bifunctional fusion protein containing Fc-binding fragment B of staphylococcal protein A amino terminal to anti-digoxin single-chain Fv. *Biochemistry*, **29**, 8024–30.

21. Batra, J.K., Kasprzyk, P.G., Bird, R.E. *et al.* (1992) Recombinant anti-*erb*B2 immunotoxins containing *Pseudomonas* exotoxin. *Proc. Natl. Acad. Sci. USA*, **89**, 5867–71.

22. Wels, W., Harwerth, I.-M., Mueller, M. *et al.* (1992) Selective inhibition of tumor cell growth by a recombinant single-chain antibody-toxin specific for the *erb*B-2 receptor. *Cancer Res.*, **52**, 6310–17.

23. McCartney, J.E., Tai, M.-S., Opperman, H. *et al.* (1993) Refolding of single-chain Fv with C-terminal cystein (sFv′); formation of disulfide-bonded homodimers of anti-c-*erb*B2 and anti-digoxin sFv′. *Miami Short Reports*, **3**, 91.

24. Cumber, A.J., Ward, E.S., Winter, G. *et al.* (1992) Comparative stabilities *in vitro* and *in vivo* of a recombinant mouse antibody FvCys fragment and a bisFvCys conjugate. *J. Immunol.*, **149**, 120–6.

25. Adams, G.P., McCartney, J.E., Tai, M.-S. *et al.* (1993) Highly specific *in vivo* tumor targeting by monovalent and divalent forms of 741F8 sFv, an anti-c-*erb*B2 single-chain Fv molecule. *Cancer Res.*, **53**, 4026–34.

Chapter 35

Carcinoembryonic antigen (CEA) promoter directed tissue specific gene expression in CEA expressing tumour cells

D.F. VIA, J.M. DIMAIO, K.R. BEREND, P.B. JORDAN and H.K. LYERLY

35.1 INTRODUCTION

Transcriptionally directed gene therapy is a promising genetic mechanism for the treatment of cancer [1]. TGT is based on delivery of a gene that will be specifically expressed in cancer cells but not in normal cells by exploiting the transcriptional differences between normal and neoplastic cells. The delivered and expressed gene may then confer selective sensitivity to a chemotherapeutic agent, deliver another gene to enhance the immune response to the tumor or it may correct a genetic defect.

Retroviral vectors provide a highly efficient method for gene transfer into eukaryotic cells and can be engineered to exploit transcriptional differences between normal and neoplastic cells [2]. Furthermore, retrovectors used for gene transfer may only be capable of infecting actively dividing neoplastic cells, while non-dividing non-neoplastic cells would not be infected, thus providing further selectivity in delivered gene expression [3].

In these experiments, the transcriptional regulatory sequence of CEA, which has been shown to direct tissue specific expression in cells producing high levels of this antigen, was used to direct the expression of desired genes [4]. CEA, an oncofetal protein, is often expressed at high levels in gastrointestinal malignancies including colon and pancreatic tumors, but not in normal tissues [5]. The CEA promoter region (CEAP) was utilized to create chimeric genes composed of CEAP linked to the protein coding region of a desired gene.

Secreted alkaline phosphatase (SEAP) is a reporter gene that has been used to measure gene expression in several studies [6,7]. This gene may be linked with cis-acting promoters to measure differential gene expression in various tissues. Herpes simplex virus thymidine kinase (HSV-tk) confers susceptibility to the cytotoxic effects of ganciclovir (GCV) [8]. GCV, an antiviral agent, is phosphorylated by HSV-tk; this intermediate is then further phosphorylated by cellular kinases into a potent DNA synthesis inhibitor. HSV-tk can be used to measure differential gene expression by determining the ^{3}H-thymidine uptake of cells containing the gene following treatment with GCV.

Such transcriptionally directed retroviral gene therapy using CEAP chimeric genes should have several unique features. Firstly, retroviral vectors will only integrate and express their genes in cells which are actively synthesizing DNA. Secondly, the genes will only be expressed in CEA expressing cells;

surrounding non-proliferating, non-CEA expressing normal tissue should not therefore acquire and express the HSV-tk gene and will remain insensitive to GCV. Finally, all of the transduced tumor cells should be killed by the host immune response and/or GCV treatment when the protein, encoded by the delivered gene, is expressed.

35.2 MATERIALS AND METHODS

35.2.1 MATERIALS

Synthetic oligonucleotide PCR primers for amplification of the CEAP, elastase III promoter (ELAP), HSV-tk and SEAP coding regions were designed in our laboratory:

CEAP 5' primer, AATTGGATCCAGCCC-CCAGAGCCACCTCTGTC

CEAP 3' primer, ATTTAAGCTTATG-GTCTCTGCTGTCTGCTCT

ELAP 5' primer, AATTGGATC-CGTTCCAGTGCCCCTGTTC

ELAP 3' primer, ATTTAAGCTTCATCAT-GAGTTTTGTGATG

HSV-tk 5' primer, CCCTCAAGCTTGTA-GAAGCGCGTATGGCTTCG

HSV-tk 3' primer, ATCCATCGATTT-TATTCTGTCTTTTTATTG

SEAP 5' primer, TCGACAAGCTTCTG-CATGCTGCTGCTGCTG

SEAP 3' primer, TAAATCGATGAG-GAAGCAACGCGGGGACCACGGGT-TAAC

Cloning of the CEAP and ELAP PCR products was performed with the TA Cloning® Kit (Invitrogen Corporation, San Diego, CA). Plasmid HSV-106 containing the HSV-tk gene was obtained from Gibco BRL (Gaithersberg, MD). Plasmid BC12/PL/SEAP

containing the SEAP gene was obtained from Bryan Cullen (Duke University Medical Center, Durham, NC) [6]. Plasmid LNCX containing the LNCX retroviral vector was obtained from A. Dusty Miller (The Fred Hutchinson Cancer Research Center, Seattle, WA) [3]. Cloning of the HSV-tk and SEAP plasmid constructs was performed using XL-1 Blue *E. coli* from Stratagene Cloning Systems (La Jolla, CA). DNA products were gel purified using the GeneClean II® kit from BIO 101 Inc. (La Jolla, CA).

35.2.2 CELL LINES

PA 317 (CRL 9078), BxPC3 (CRL 1687) and HeLa (CCL 2.2) cell lines were obtained from the American Type Culture Collection (Rockville, MD).

35.2.3 CONSTRUCTION OF HSV-TK AND SEAP RETROVIRAL SHUTTLE VECTORS

The ELAP region (331 bp) was isolated and amplified by PCR from human genomic DNA; specific primers were designed to insert a 5' *Bam*H I site and a 3' *Hind*III site. PCR primer annealing temperature for this reaction was 63°C and the reaction ran for 40 cycles. This PCR product was cloned into the pCR vector. The CEAP region (504 bp) was prepared in an analogous manner: PCR of human genomic DNA carried out with primers inserting 5' *Bam*HI and 3' *Hind*III sites (primer annealing temperature 63°C; 40 cycle reaction). The HSV-tk (1210 bp) and SEAP (1561 bp) genes were isolated from plasmids (pHSV-106 and pBC12/PL/SEAP, respectively) via PCR (HSV-tk: annealing temperature of 55°C and 25 cycles; SEAP: annealing temperature of 72°C and 40 cycles) using primers designed to insert unique 5' *Hind*III and 3' *Cla*I sites into both genes. These four fragments were digested with the following restriction enzymes: ELAP, *Bam*HI and *Hind*III; CEAP, *Bam*HI and *Hind*III; HSV-tk, *Hind*III and *Cla*I; SEAP, *Hind*III and *Cla*I. They were then purified using the GeneClean II Kit. The pLNCX plasmid vector was linearized with *Bam*HI and *Cla*I and the following chimeras were constructed using the *Bam*HI and *Cla*I sites in the vector: pLN-ELAP/HSV-tk, pLN-ELAP/SEAP, pLN-CEAP/HSV-tk, pLN-CEAP/SEAP (Figure 35.1). The pLNCX plasmid vector was also linearized with *Hind*III and *Cla*I to allow the construction of the pLN-CMVP/HSV-tk and

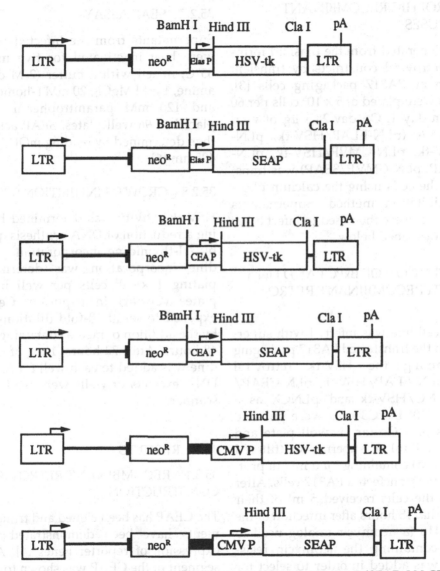

Figure 35.1 Retroviral constructs. Structure of LN-ELAP/HSV-tk, LN-ELAP/SEAP, LN-CEAP/HSV-tk, LN-CEAP/SEAP, LN-CMVP/HSV-tk, LN-CMVP/SEAP. Arrows indicate direction of transcription. LTR, long terminal repeat; neoR, neomycin resistance gene, CMVP, CMV promoter; pA, polyadenylation sites; Elas P, elastase III promoter (ELAP); HSV-tk, HSV thymidine kinase; CEAP, CEA promoter; SEAP, secreted alkaline phosphatase. Restriction enzyme sites as indicated.

359

pLN-CMVP/SEAP chimeras (Figure 35.1). Plasmid DNA of all six retroviral constructs was purified by centrifugation in a cesium chloride gradient containing ethidium bromide.

35.2.4 PRODUCTION OF AMPHOTROPHIC RECOMBINANT RETROVIRUSES

Virus was generated from the plasmid forms of all six retroviral constructs by transient transfection of PA317 packaging cells [3]. PA317 cells were plated at 5×10^5 cells per 60 mm dish on day 1. On day 2, 5 μg of viral plasmid DNA (pLN-ELAP/HSV-tk, pLN-CEAP/HSV-tk, pLN-CMVP/HSV-tk, pLN-CEAP/SEAP, pLN-CMVP/SEAP) was transfected into the cells using the calcium phosphate precipitation method. Supernatants from these cells were then used to infect other cell lines as described below.

35.2.5 INFECTION OF BxPC3 AND HeLa CELLS WITH RECOMBINANT RETRO-VIRUSES

The BxPC3 cell line was infected with supernatants from the transfected PA317 packaging cells containing the HSV-tk retroviral construct (pLN-ELAP/HSV-tk, pLN-CEAP/HSV-tk, pLNC/HSV-tk and pLNCX as a control): 1×10^6 BxPC3 cells were put into single wells of a Costar six-well plate and infected with 1 ml of supernatant (filtered and centrifuged) containing 1 μ u ml^{-1} of protamine from the transfected PA317 cells. After three hours the cells received 5 ml of their required media. 48 hours after infection of the cell lines G418 (a neomycin analog used to select cells containing the neomycin resistance gene) was added in order to select for cells containing each of the retroviral constructs. Cells were washed, counted and placed in fresh media with G418 every three days for a total of 14 days.

35.2.6 INFECTION OF HeLa CELLS WITH SEAP CONSTRUCTS

Supernatants (pLNCX, pLN-CMVP/SEAP and pLN-CEAP/SEAP) from the transfected PA317 cells were used to infect HeLa cells as described above.

35.2.7 SEAP ASSAY

Supernatants from the infected HeLa cells were heat inactivated for five minutes at 65°C, mixed with a buffer (2 M diethanolamine, 1 mM MgCl$_2$, 20 mM L-homoarginine) and 120 mM paranitrophenol and then placed in 96-well plates. SEAP activity was then determined by reading mOD/minute at 405 nm [6].

35.2.8 GROWTH INHIBITION STUDIES

HSV-tk activity was determined by detecting a reduction of DNA synthesis quantified by ^{3}H-thymidine incorporation. ^{3}H-thymidine incorporation was determined by plating 1×10^3 cells per well in 96-well plates (Costar) in triplicate. Cells were exposed to serial 10-fold dilutions of GCV by the addition of media containing GCV for 48 hours. After 72 hours, 1 mg of ^{3}H-thymidine was added to each well for four hours. DNA extracts of wells were read in a beta scanner.

35.3 RESULTS

35.3.1 RECOMBINANT RETROVIRUS CONSTRUCTION

The CEAP has been cloned and truncated elements have been demonstrated to drive expression of reporter genes [4]. A 450 bp segment of the CEAP was shown to drive the highest expression in CEA expressing tissue, suggesting that some cis-acting elements may serve to upregulate CEA expression. This highly active fragment of CEA was utilized to construct recombinant replication defective, amphotrophic retroviruses driven by promoters coupled to HSV-tk and SEAP as seen in Figure 35.1.

The cytomegalovirus immediate early promoter (CMVP), a non-specific constitutive promoter, and the human elastase III promoter (ELAP) were used as control transcriptional regulatory sequences [3,9,10]. CMVP drives non-specific expression in many tissues and ELAP drives expression in pancreatic (acinar) tissue, irrespective of CEA expression. These regulatory/reporter gene constructs allow for the study of differential gene expression in CEA expressing tissue.

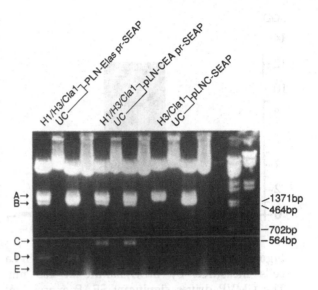

Figure 35.3 Restriction enzyme analysis gel of SEAP constructs. A, 1561 bp *Hind*III/*Cla*I SEAP fragment; B, 1343 bp *Bam*HI/*Cla*I SEAP fragment; C, 504 bp *Bam*HI/*Hind*III CEA promoter fragment; D, 331 bp *Bam*HI/*Cla*I elastase III promoter fragment; E, 218 bp *Hind*III/*Bam*HI SEAP fragment. Lanes 3, 4, 7, 8, 11 and 12 are duplicates, lanes 14 and 15 are molecular weight markers. UC, uncut.

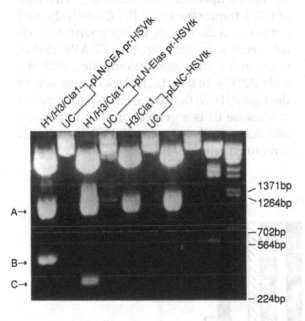

Figure 35.2 Restriction enzyme analysis gel of HSV-tk constructs. A, 1210 bp *Hind*III/*Cla*I HSVtk fragment; B, 504 bp *Bam*HI/*Hind*III CEA promoter fragment; C, 331 bp *Bam*HI/*Hind*III elastase III promoter fragment. Lanes 7 and 8 are duplicates, lanes 9 and 10 are molecular weight markers. UC, uncut.

Restriction mapping of all plasmid constructs confirmed the presence of expected promoters and gene fragments (Figures 35.2 and 35.3). In further studies to define the function of these recombinant retroviruses, a CEA expressing carcinoma cell line (BxPC3) [11] and a non-CEA expressing carcinoma cell line (HeLa) were used to evaluate the tissue specific gene expression levels of retrovirally delivered SEAP and HSV-tk genes transcriptionally regulated by the CEAP, CMVP and ELAP.

35.3.2 SEAP EXPRESSION

Specific CEAP function was determined using a SEAP assay. In Figure 35.4, high OD

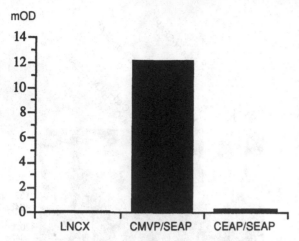

Figure 35.4 SEAP expression in transduced HeLa cells measured by mOD/minute at 405 nm. The CMVP drives significant SEAP expression; however, there is undetectable SEAP expression with the CEAP driving the gene.

values show that infected HeLa cells exhibited high non-specific SEAP expression when coupled to the CMVP but had undetectable SEAP expression with the CEAP; HeLa cells have been previously shown to express constitutively low levels of CEA [4]. This demonstrated that the CEAP was non-

constitutive, although it did not demonstrate tissue specific expression of SEAP. Because *in vivo* as well as *in vitro* expression of the delivered gene was to be documented, the retroviral vector directing expression of HSV-tk with the CEAP was utilized to detect tissue specific transcription directed by the CEAP.

35.3.3 GANCICLOVIR MEDIATED GROWTH INHIBITION

HSV-tk activity was demonstrated in BxPC3 cells transduced with infectious retroviral vector containing the HSV-tk inserts as shown by significant decreases in cell viability when the cells were treated with various concentrations of GCV (Figure 35.5). Mean ^{3}H-thymidine uptake values following extraction of DNA from transduced BxPC3 cells showed a marked reduction in viability with retroviral vectors containing the CEAP/HSV-tk insert and a more modest reduction with the CMVP/HSV-tk insert. The lack of response to the ELAP/HSV-tk insert is an expected result as elastase III is a gene expressed in pancreatic acinar cells whereas BxPC3 is a ductal carcinoma cell line [10].

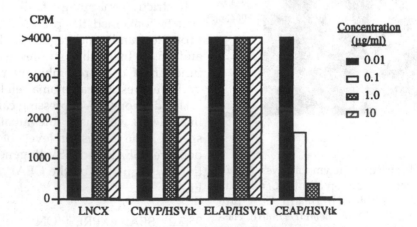

Figure 35.5 Effects of ganciclovir on DNA synthesis in transduced BxPC3 cells measured by ^{3}H-thymidine uptake. Cells containing the HSV-tk insert had significant reduction in DNA synthesis; this effect was marked with the CEAP driving the HSV-tk gene.

In addition to DNA synthesis as detected by thymidine uptake, cell number and viability as detected by vital dye exclusion was performed in parallel experiments. As expected, this demonstrated a significant decrease in cell number and viability in CEA expressing cells transduced with retroviral vectors containing the CEAP/HSV-tk insert and a more modest reduction with the CMVP/HSV-tk insert, when exposed to GCV (data not shown). The concentrations of GCV demonstrating the most marked effect *in vitro* were analogous to serum levels achieved with standard administration GCV to patients.

35.4 DISCUSSION

Transcriptionally directed gene therapy presents a new therapeutic approach to the treatment of patients with otherwise incurable malignant carcinomas. The strategy involves the preferential introduction of a drug susceptibility gene into proliferating tumor tissue, accomplished by transduction of the tumor with a retroviral vector carrying the gene for herpes simplex thymidine kinase, transcriptionally regulated by tumor specific transcriptional response elements. The HSV-tk gene product will only be produced in cells that are mitotically active and are expressing the tumor marker, carcinoembryonic antigen (CEA).

There are three major methods of gene transfer:

1. Chemical (e.g. calcium phosphate precipitation);
2. Physical (e.g. microinjection, electroporation, fusion-liposomes);
3. Viral (e.g. herpes simplex, adenovirus, retrovirus).

Physical and chemical methods have poor gene integration efficiencies, ranging from 1:1000 to 1:100 000, making them impractical for most clinical applications. Adenoviruses and herpes simplex viruses have been used to transfer genes into cells where they can replicate in an extrachromosomal location. They can, therefore, transfer genes into non-replicating tissues (e.g. lung, brain), un-like the murine retroviruses.

In contrast to chemical and physical methods, murine retroviral vectors have proven to be extremely efficient for gene transfer into mammalian cells, with efficiencies as high as 90% in cultured murine fibroblast cell lines. Murine retroviral vectors differ from the adenoviruses and herpes simplex viruses in that the retroviruses will only integrate and subsequently express their genes in proliferating tissues (e.g. tumors). These Moloney murine leukemia virus based (MoMLV) vectors have also been designed to minimize the possibility of recombination resulting in regeneration of a replication competent virus [2,12].

In 1989, the first gene transfer experiment in humans was conducted at the NIH. This study involved the treatment of 10 patients with autologous T cells that had been transduced with a retroviral vector. The vector used in this experiment was LNL6 (constructed by A. Dusty Miller) which has the same general structure and safety modifications as the vector used in our experiments. None of the NIH patients have demonstrated any untoward effects secondary to receiving the genetically altered cells [13].

A protocol for adenosine deaminase deficiency opened in September, 1990, since when two children have been enrolled and 15 intravenous infusions of genetically altered autologous T cells have been administered. These children had significant immunodeficiency before receiving these genetically altered cells, but they have substantially improved after infusions of the gene modified cells. They have been treated with the LASN vector (also constructed by A. Dusty Miller) which, like LNL6, has the same general structure and safety modifications as the vector used in our experiments. Neither child has demonstrated any evidence of adverse effect due to the genetically altered cells.

A number of other gene-marking experiments (e.g. transduction of marrow cells in patients undergoing bone marrow transplantation) and therapy experiments (e.g. insertion of cytokine genes into autologous tumor in an effort to vaccinate a patient) are beginning. No untoward side effects related to retroviral mediated gene transfer have been observed in any patient to date.

Use of the CEAP to drive expression of a delivered gene of interest allows for tumor specific gene expression. CEA expressing cells transduced with retrovector containing the CEAP coupled to the HSV-tk gene expressed higher levels of the HSV-tk gene than did cells containing the HSV-tk gene coupled to the CMVP or ELAP. Non-CEA expressing cells transduced with retrovector containing the CEAP coupled to the SEAP gene did not express the SEAP gene, whereas these cells did express SEAP when the gene was driven by the non-specific CMVP. The CEAP appears to selectively upregulate expression of HSV-tk in CEA expressing cells. In addition, the CEAP appears to inhibit gene expression of SEAP in cells that do not express CEA. This should allow selective targeting of CEA producing cancers in chemosensitizing or immune response enhancing gene therapy systems.

The herpes thymidine kinase gene confers sensitivity upon the cells expressing the gene to the antiviral drug ganciclovir (GCV). GCV is non-toxic to normal tissues but will kill cells (e.g. tumors) expressing this herpes virus enzyme. Other data suggest that bystander tumor cells, not expressing HSV-tk, may also be killed as a consequence of this process, amplifying the antitumor effects of treatment by a process not completely understood.

In animal experiments performed by Culver [14], not all of a tumor's cells were

shown to contain the inserted HSV-tk gene when killed upon ganciclovir challenge. In mice given a subcutaneous tumor in which 100% of the cells carried the HSV-tk gene, complete tumor regressions were seen following GCV treatment. Interestingly, when tumors established from cell mixtures containing 50% HSV-tk gene modified cells and 50% wild type unmodified tumor cells were treated with GCV, almost all tumors regressed. Even in situations where the mixed tumor contained 90% unmodified, wild type tumor cells and only 10% HSV-tk modified tumor cells, complete regression of the cancer was observed with GCV treatment in over half of the animals.

This phenomenon was reproduced *in vitro* when Culver and associates incubated various tumor cell lines with HSV-tk-vector producer cells for 24–72 hours. Following exposure to GCV, the supernatants were removed and transferred to tissue cultures of the wild type tumors (not transduced with the HSV-tk gene). Thymidine incorporation assays revealed that the supernatants significantly inhibited thymidine incorporation in all tumor types. The mechanism of this 'bystander tumor kill' is not yet completely understood. It may involve the production of toxic triphosphates by the interaction of thymidine kinase and GCV leading to inhibition of DNA synthesis and death of replicating cells. It does not seem to involve generalized non-specific cellular toxicity since the overlying skin and other tissues surrounding these HSV-tk treated tumors were not grossly injured while the tumor cells expressing the genes and the admixed wild type tumor cells were completely destroyed.

Since it is unlikely that 100% of tumor cells in the tissues of our patients will be successfully gene modified, this 'bystander' effect is very important for the successful outcome of this treatment approach. Nonetheless, the establishment of transcriptionally directed gene therapy in this tumor cell line may yield significant advances in the understanding of the biology of many malignancies. The ability to selectively express genes in tissues that express CEA can be extended to direct expression of genes in cells expressing the multiple drug resistant gene (MDR), for example. Furthermore, other agents that would have enhanced bystander effects, possibly by secreting toxic metabolites, would enhance the applicability of these methods. This may lead to possible novel treatment modalities for patients with cancers that respond poorly to conventional therapy.

ACKNOWLEDGMENTS

The editorial and administrative assistance of Maureen Coyle and the technical assistance of Salvatore Mungal is gratefully acknowledged. We are grateful for the support of Mr John E. Harris and the Helene Harris Memorial Trust and would like to acknowledge the support and encouragement of Mr Sheldon Milgrom.

REFERENCES

1. Huber, B.E., Richards, C.A. and Krenitsky, T.A. (1991) Retroviral-mediated gene therapy for the treatment of hepatocellular carcinoma: an innovative approach for cancer therapy. *PNAS*, **88**, 8039–43.

2. Miller, A.D. and Rosman, G.J. (1989) Improved retroviral vectors for gene transfer and expression. *Biotechniques*, **7**, 980–8.

3. Miller, D.G., Adam, M.A. and Miller, A.D. (1990) Gene transfer by retrovirus vectors occurs only in cells that are actively replicating at the time of infection. *Mol Cell Biol.*, **10**, 4239–42.

4. Schrewe, H., Thompson, J., Bona, M. *et al.* (1990) Cloning of the complete gene for carcinoembryonic antigen: analysis of its promoter indicates a region conveying cell type-specific expression. *Mol Cell Biol.*, **10**, 2738–48.

5. Warshaw, A.L. and Fernandez del Castillo,C. (1992) Pancreatic c arcinoma. *N. Engl. J. Med.*, **326**, 455–65.

6. Cullen, B. (1986) Trans-activation of human immunodeficiency virus occurs via a bimodal mechanism. *Cell*, **46**, 973–82.

7. Berger, J., Hauber, J., Hauber, R. *et al.* (1988) Secreted placental alkaline phosphatase: a powerful new quantitative indicator of gene expression in eukaryotic cells. *Gene*, **66**, 1–10.

8. Moolten, F.L. (1986) Tumor chemosensitivity conferred by inserted herpes thymidine kinase genes: paradigm for a prospective cancer control study. *Cancer Res.*, **46**, 5276–81.

9. Tani, T., Kawashima, I., Furukawa, H. *et al.* (1987) Characterization of a silent gene for human pancreatic elastase I: structure of the 5' flanking region. *J. Biochem.*, **101**, 591–9.

10. Tani, T., Ohsumi, J., Mita, K. and Takiguchi, Y. (1988) Identification of a novel class of elastase isozyme, human pancreatic elastase III, by cDNA and genomic gene cloning. *J. Biol. Chem.*, **263**, 1231–9.

11. Tan, M.H., Nowak, N.J.., Loor., R. *et al.* (1986) Characterization of a new primary human pancreatic tumor line. *Cancer Invest.*, **4**, 15–23.

12. Miller, A.D. and Buttimore, C. (1986) Redesign of retrovirus packaging cell lines to avoid recombination leading to helper virus production. *Mol. Cell Biol.*, **6**, 2895–902.

13. Rosenberg, S.A., Aebersold, P., Cometta, K. *et al.* (1990) Gene transfer into humans: immunotherapy of patients with advanced melanoma using tumor-infiltrating lymphocytes modified by retroviral gene transduction. *N. Engl. J. Med.*, **323**, 570–8.

14. Culver, K.W., Ram, Z., Wallbridge, S. *et al.* (1992) *In vivo* gene transfer with retroviral vector-producer cells for treatment of experimental brain tumours. *Science*, **256**, 1550–2.

Part Six
Conclusions and Recommendations

Chapter 36

Conclusions and recommendations

36.1 EARLY OVARIAN CANCER AND BORDERLINE TUMOURS

1.1 Early (microscopic) *de novo* ovarian cancer (arising from surface epithelium or its inclusions) can be fatal and may be undetectable by present day screening approaches. Further study of these lesions using the newer molecular based techniques is important, to throw more light on the mechanism of development of these incipient cancers and for the evolution of novel approaches to their detection.

1.2 An unknown proportion of ovarian cancers appears to arise from pre-existent benign tumours or possibly non-neoplastic lesions such as endometriosis. The relationships of malignant, atypical and benign appearing epithelium encountered in both primary and metastatic cancers should be studied. Such investigations should also employ the newer molecular approaches in an attempt to throw some light on the maturation of malignant epithelium into benign appearing epithelium and the origin of malignant epithelium from pre-existing benign epithelium.

1.3 The development of a rat *in vitro* ovarian epithelial cell culture model has been described. The model depends on the collection of epithelial surface cells from the ovary following trypsinization. Resultant cell cultures could then be maintained as continuous confluent cultures and tumourigenicity in nude mice compared with cells passaged through a number of subcultures. This model holds promise for the investigation of ovarian oncogenesis. Preliminary extension of these studies to include human ovarian epithelial surface cells is already underway.

1.4 Normal ovarian surface epithelium has been found to secrete the bioactive cytokines IL-1, IL-6, M-CSF and, rarely, GM-CSF.

1.5 Evidence has been presented suggesting that normal human ovarian surface epithelium expresses little or no E adherin (EC), either in culture or *in vivo*. In contrast, ovarian carcinoma cells acquire an EC positive phenotype.

1.6 EC appears to be an early marker in ovarian carcinogenesis, because it is present in clefts and inclusion cysts of otherwise normal ovaries. Therefore, the microenvironment responsible for the metaplastic changes which take place in these sites is competent to induce or permit EC expression.

1.7 A major comment was made concerning the transition from an EC negative to positive phenotype, which is contrary to other epithelia where neoplastic progression leads to reduced EC expression. However, this is in keeping with the appearance of other characteristics of oviductal, endometrial and cervical epithelia which frequently characterize differentiated epithelial ovarian cancers.

1.8 The implications of the above observations potentially are of considerable significance. Urgent confirmation and extension of these observations is required.

1.9 The biology and natural history of borderline ovarian tumours may be distinct from that of invasive epithelial ovarian cancer.

1.10 Borderline tumours recur as borderline tumours and generally do not transform into invasive ovarian cancer.

1.11 Treatments known to be effective in the management of invasive ovarian cancer are not of proven benefit as adjuvant therapy for borderline tumours.

1.12 The genetic epidemiology and familial risk of borderline tumours are also likely to be distinct from invasive disease but this requires further elucidation.

1.13 Studies are needed to improve our understanding of the unique biology of borderline tumours. Such studies could result in better planning of therapeutic and/or preventive strategies.

1.14 It is possible to identify within women with borderline or low malignant potential ovarian tumours a high risk group, based on staging, ploidy studies and the presence of invasive implants.

1.15 In multivariate analysis of results from the Norwegian Radium Hospital, involving large patient numbers and follow-up to 15 years, DNA ploidy assessment proved to be the most important independent prognostic factor.

1.16 The postprimary surgical identification and optimum management of the high risk

group mentioned above (particularly where invasive implants are present) remain uncertain. There is no proven, effective adjuvant therapy for borderline ovarian tumours. These questions could be resolved by appropriate prospective multicentre trials.

1.17 In the treatment of women with borderline ovarian tumours, reproductive conservation in the appropriate age group should feature highly in management decisions.

1.18 Following surgery for removal of a borderline tumour, there is no evidence for an adverse effect of hormone replacement therapy (HRT). HRT has shown cardiovascular, skeletal and sexual biological benefits and is not contraindicated.

36.2 TUMOUR BIOLOGY

2.1 The growth regulation of ovarian cancer is the result of a complex interaction between its genetic control, presumably via those portions of the genome responsible for the maintenance of normal function, and the abnormal balance of cytokines. Various proto-oncogenes, tumour suppressor genes and some cytokines have been associated with growth control. These can be amplified and/or mutated which can be associated with a malignant phenotype.

2.2 There may be a dynamic interaction between the expression of oncogenes or mutation of a tumour suppressor gene and the production of several cytokines. The receptors for several of these cytokines may be encoded by certain oncogene loci. For example, her-2/*neu* encodes an EGF-like receptor and a region homologous to c-*fos* is also a portion of the transcription binding site for the IL-6 receptor.

2.3 In retrospective studies, persistence of EGFR, overexpression of her-2/*neu* and novel expression of *fms* in tumour tissue have been factors that predict a poor prognosis for patients with epithelial ovarian cancer. TGFα occurs in most ovarian cancers and the ratio of EGFR/TGFα might be of prognostic value. TGFα is present in all EGFR positive tumours.

2.4 Activity of transmembrane growth factor receptor tyrosine kinases can be upregulated by phosphorylation of tyrosine residues on their intracellular domains. Tyrosine phosphatases can downregulate kinase activity or neutralize effects on downstream substrates. At least a dozen protein tyrosine phosphatases (PTPases) can be detected in human ovarian cancers. PTP1B protein is expressed at very low levels in normal ovarian epithelium but is overexpressed in 80% of ovarian cancers. Marked overexpression of PTP1B has correlated with continued expression of EGFR, overexpression of her-2/*neu* and expression of *fms*. PTPases might either offset kinase effects or reprime kinases for additional signalling. In either case, co-expression of PTPases and kinases might modify prognosis and affect tumour growth, invasiveness or drug resistance.

2.5 TNF, IL-1 and IL-6 can stimulate proliferation of a fraction of ovarian cancer cell lines. TNFα may function as a viability/growth sustaining factor for ovarian cancers. TNF or IL-1 produced by macrophages may stimulate endogenous expression of TNF in ovarian cancers which could cause tumour cell proliferation. TNFα mRNA and protein are present in a majority of human ovarian cancers and the level of expression correlates with tumour grade. Antibodies against TNF or soluble TNF receptor can block proliferation induced with TNF or IL-1. Antisense RNA against TNF can block stimulation with IL-1 but not TNF. These data suggest that paracrine stimulation by TNF and IL-1 can induce autocrine stimulation of TNF which is critical to proliferation. This may apply to 10–15% of cases in the absence of exogenous EGF/TGFα and to 30–40% of cases in the presence of these growth factors which have been found in ovarian cancer tissue and in ascitic fluid. Repeated injections of TNF can stimulate growth of ovarian cancer heterografts in nude or scid mice and invasion of peritoneal surfaces. Enhanced formation of tumour nodules has been observed and increased invasion of matrigel membranes observed *in vitro* in the presence of TNF.

2.6 Many ovarian cancers express TNF/LT soluble membrane receptors. The level of expression appears to correlate with disease status and tumour burden. Studies have focused on the use of circulating TNF/LT as a tumour marker, as there is some complementarity with CA125.

2.7 Therapeutic intervention could involve blocking TNF production or action in those patients whose tumours are stimulated by TNF or, conversely, administering TNF in those patients whose tumours are inhibited by the cytokine. Xenograft studies of ovarian cancer suggest that the most important actions of interferon-γ are directly on the ovarian tumour cells and that it is a cytostatic/cytotoxic cytokine in the absence of exogenous TNF. In other cell lines cytokines such as TNFα may induce apoptosis, possibly by upregulation of a mutant tumour suppressor gene, p53. TNFα also has been used in combination with anthracyclines in those patients whose tumours are inhibited by this cytokine.

2.8 Several other cytokines, e.g. IL-6, may function as paracrine growth factors, downregulating p53. IL-6 may also function as a viability enhancing factor, inhibiting apoptosis (programmed cell death).

2.9 The context in which TNF acts in animal models and in human cancers will determine its ultimate action. Its function in stimulating tumour cell proliferation, tumour stroma formation or tumour cell death will be determined by many other factors in the local environment.

2.10 Ascitic fluid may provide a window to characterize the environment of the ovarian cancer cell. Ascitic fluid contains potent growth supporting activity *in vitro* and in the peritoneal cavity of nude mice.

2.11 In addition to the large number of polypeptide growth factors described therein, ascitic fluid contains at least one unique lipid designated OCAF. This lipid appears to be a highly acidic, polar phospholipid with a glycerol backbone. OCAF signals cells through phosphatidyl inositol hydrolysis and increases in cytosolic free calcium. Non-hydrolysable lipids are currently in clinical trials for a variety of cancers. Derivatives of OCAF may prevent functional activation of the receptor and play a role in therapy. In addition, the signal transduction pathway activated by OCAF is target for anticancer drugs such as CA1 and inhibitors of isoprenylation.

2.12 An understanding of the mechanisms that regulate the growth of ovarian cancer should permit the development of therapeutic strategies that exploit these pathways.

36.3 THERAPY

3.1 There exists a hierarchy of sensitivity and resistance of ovarian tumour cell lines to cytotoxicity initiated by a variety of agents delivered invasively or non-invasively.

3.2 Ovarian cancer cell lines resistant to drugs, TNF or toxins, whether MDR+ or MDR–, are rendered sensitive to combination treatments with (i) TNFα + drug (CDDP, ADR), (ii) TNFα + toxin (DTX), and (iii) anti-*fas* antibody + drug/toxin. Both additive and synergistic cytotoxic effects are obtained with very low concentrations.

3.3 Studies of the mechanism of overriding resistance show (i) no effect on the MDR phenotype, (ii) downregulation of constitutive and induced TNF mRNA, (iii) downregula-

tion of glutathione levels and (iv) shifting of the TNF mediated cytotoxic pathway.

3.4 Overriding resistance by subtoxic, low concentrations of combination treatments now requires preclinical and clinical study.

3.5 Cisplatin resistance is an important clinical problem. To identify the fullest possible range of mechanisms potentially responsible for cisplatin resistance and the cross resistance characteristic of cisplatin refractory patients, models with high levels of primary cisplatin resistance may be most relevant.

3.6 Cisplatin resistance is accompanied by changes in three major categories of resistance: (i) decreased cell associated drug levels, (ii) increased potential for drug inactivation, (iii) alterations in DNA damage and repair.

3.7 Preclinical studies have shown the ability to circumvent cytoplasmic and nuclear drug inactivation by GSH through buthionein sulphoximine (BSO) treatment and also through inhibition of DNA repair by aphidicolin. In both cases the activity of the primary cytotoxic drug is increased.

3.8 A phase I clinical trial of BSO and melphalan reveals that it is possible to substantially decrease WBC and tumour cell GSH at a BSO dose of 13g m^{-2} every six hours for six doses.

3.9 Meta-analysis of studies investigating the use of chemotherapy in ovarian cancer-suggests multiagent cisplatin enhancing regimens produce a better response that cisplatin alone for a given fixed dose of cisplatin.

3.10 This dose intensity effect for cisplatin on response is less obvious at doses >25 mg m^{-2} week^{-1} within multiagent regimens or >30 mg m^{-2} week^{-1} when used as a single agent. The extent to which outcome is predicted on dose intensity *vs* total dose received remains conjectural. The incorporation of dose intensity or the presence or absence of cisplatin in a large multivariate analysis showed both to be independent prognostic variables and, together with stage (III *vs* IV), displaced maximum cytoreductive surgery (MCS) as an independent variable. This provides ethical justification for prospectively testing the role of MCS for patients with advanced disease who receive multiagent platinum containing chemotherapy, with appropriate attention to the dose intensity considerations mentioned above.

3.11 Platinum based chemotherapy remains an important component in the management of advanced ovarian cancer. Strategies to optimize the therapeutic benefits of carboplatin include utilization of a targeted AVC dosage formula (after Calvert), combinations with other drugs including Taxol and experimental programmes designed to overcome drug resistance and safely achieve higher levels of dose intensity.

3.12 The major dose limiting toxicity of carboplatin is thrombocytopenia. Previous clinical studies with high dose carboplatin and GM-CSF showed no protective benefit. By contrast, other studies have suggested that IL-3 or IL-1 may reduce the extent of thrombocytopenia. However, when patients received dose intense therapy without IL-1 followed by identical therapy with IL-1, no protective benefit could be demonstrated. Further studies with IL-1, IL-3 and other haematopoietic growth factors are indicated to re-solve this question.

3.13 Another approach under investigation is the use of autologous bone marrow or peripheral blood progenitor cell supports. Preliminary studies have demonstrated that these approaches are feasible, but they have only limited benefit in patients with recurrent disease. Ongoing studies are applying these techniques as a component of initial therapy for previously untreated patients.

3.14 Radiotherapy has proven efficacy as a curative modality when used a sole postoperative therapy in a selected group of patients with ovarian cancer.

3.15 After chemotherapy of advanced disease 50–60% of patients who have negative second look laparotomy will relapse (75–100% in peritoneum).

3.16 Consolidation with salvage therapy directed at the peritoneal cavity seems appropriate and radiotherapy is one such possibility.

3.17 The value of addition of sequential radiotherapy after chemotherapy is unknown, since large randomized trials in appropriately selected patients have not been performed.

3.18 The strategy needs to be tested with appropriate radiotherapy (that is, with acceptable toxicity) in controlled trials. Patients who might benefit would include (i) those with microscopic residual disease (grades 1 and 2) and (ii) those with negative second look laparotomy but with a high risk of relapse (for example, grade 3, age >50 years, or with a large residuum prior to chemotherapy).

3.19 New active cytotoxic agents, preferably showing a lack of cross resistance with cisplatin and carboplatin, are needed for the treatment of epithelial ovarian cancer.

3.20 The taxane family is a new class of anti-cancer drugs with an original chemical structure and an unusual mechanism of action at the microtubule level. Taxol, the parent drug, has recently been registered in the US for use in platinum refractory ovarian cancer patients. In patients with progressive disease during or shortly after platinum therapy, Taxol induces an objective response rate of 20–30%, which is double the response rate obtained with other chemotherapeutic agents in this very unfavourable patient subset.

3.21 Future directions for Taxol in the treatment of advanced ovarian cancer include incorporation of the drug into existing chemotherapy regimens, administration via the intraperitoneal route for small volume residual disease and perhaps use as a radiosensitizer.

3.22 In the meantime, the search for second generation taxoid compounds is being actively pursued in the hope of discovering Taxol related drugs with an improved therapeutic index and showing no cross resistance with the parent drug.

3.23 Taxotere (docetaxel, RP56976) is the first semisynthetic taxoid compound to have been used in clinical trials. The toxicity profiles of Taxol and Taxotere are not superimposable. Early phase II results show at least the same level of activity for Taxotere compared with Taxol. The current challenge in the clinical development of this very active second generation taxoid drug is understanding and possibly circumventing its dose related and dose limiting side effect, namely fluid retention.

3.24 Data have been presented on studies of dose and infusion time for paclitaxel in ovarian cancer. Patients receiving the higher dose (175 mg m^{-2} *vs* 135 mg m^{-2}) experienced more neurosensory toxicity and arthromyalgia. Those randomized to the three hour infusion demonstrated significantly less haematological toxicity (particularly neutropenia and infection) without an increase in hypersensitivity reactions.

3.25 The best toxicity index appears to be achieved with the shorter infusion. The fact that paclitaxel can be given safely in an outpatient study will reduce the costs and inconvenience of treatment. While the overall response rate is modest, a proportion of patients with truly platinum resistant tumours will respond, indicating a poten-tially important degree of therapeutic non-cross resistance.

3.26 Tamoxifen as a second line treatment appears to have a clinical response in ovarian cancer of the order 8–20%. The potential benefits from the point of view of quality of life make this drug an attractive option for further study.

3.27 Issues concerning ethical decision making in the care of the seriously ill and dying patient have been considered. Such patients with ovarian cancer have needs for: information about the illness and management options, which is accurate and gently conveyed; effective symptom control directed to the alleviation of pain and suffering; ongoing supportive care and information for the patient and her family; accompaniment and continued support by physicians and health care teams; opportunities to emphasize life and living; acknowledgement of themselves as unique individuals; opportunities for choice in options for their care and the development of goals of their care.

3.28 Ethical decision making must involve patients and their families. The physician must be ethical in his/her qualities and motivations and utilize a combination of biomedical principles and the ethics of caring.

3.29 Decisions reached should be made on an individual basis according to the wishes and circumstances of the individual woman and within an appropriate clinical context (illness and likely prognosis, etc.).

3.30 Potentially ethically defensible medical practices may include (i) cessation of treatment, (ii) non-initiation of treatment and (iii) morally required treatments that may shorten life (treatment of symptom crises).

3.31 These practices can be distinguished from euthanasia (acting with the intention to take life), which is not part of medical or health care practice and is a subject of considerable controversy.

3.32 Serum markers might be used in combination with transvaginal sonography for early detection of ovarian cancer. In studies to date, CA125 detected only about 50% of stage I ovarian cancers.

3.33 When sera from 46 patients with stage I ovarian cancer were tested for three markers – CA125, M-CSF and OVX1 – 98% had an elevation of at least one marker. Similar screening of 204 sera from patients who did not develop ovarian cancer within a two year period indicated a specificity of 89% for the three marker panel. Among 18 patients who had been missed by CA125 in a screening trial but subsequently developed ovarian cancer within two years, 40% had an elevation of M-CSF or OVX1.

3.34 Consequently, the three marker panel might be considered to be a trigger to prompt screening with transvaginal ultrasound. In addition to eliminating 89% of ultrasound scans needed for screening, the specificity of the panel is 50% for distinguishing benign from malignant pelvic masses, reducing the number of patients likely to be false-positives on transvaginal scanning.

3.35 Additional specificity might be attained by using additional markers. In a study of pelvic masses using eight markers and subsequent analysis with classification and regression free analysis, this proved superior to the use of CA125 alone or analysis with covariant analysis or with different panels.

3.36 Intraperitoneal interferonγ is an effective treatment of residual ovarian carcinoma after chemotherapy. IFNα achieves a 40% CR in residual lesions less that 5 mm and a 20% CR when tumour size is between 5 and 20 mm. Response rate is higher in younger patients. Median duration of response is 21 months and two year survival of responder patients is 80%.

3.37 Intraperitoneal IFNα is equally active in chemoresistant and chemosensitive ovarian tumours and is thus a suitable complementary treatment to chemotherapy in the therapeutic strategy for ovarian cancer.

3.38 High levels of matrix metalloproteinases (MMPs) in active and inactive form can be found in human ovarian cancer biopsies. There was no correlation with tumour grade, unlike findings in breast and bladder cancer biopsies. mRNA for these MMPs and their tissue inhibitors is found in stromal cells immediately adjacent to the tumour cells. Thus the tumour cells appear to induce proteases and their inhibitors in the surrounding stroma, but the inducing signals have not been identified. A synthetic MMP inhibitor increased survival of mice bearing ovarian cancer ascitic xenografts approximately six-fold, resolved ascites, decreased tumour burden and encouraged the development of a poorly vascularized solid tumour. It is suggested that endogenous MMP activity in the peritoneum keeps the tumour in ascitic form and prevents formation of extracellular matrix and stroma. MMP inhibitors may have clinical application in ascitic ovarian cancer.

3.39 The use of alternative targets for drug development has led to the identification of a new category of agents, those which inhibit signal transduction. By inhibition of calcium influx with agents such as CA1, or targeting other signalling pathways such as isoprenylation, less toxic therapeutic approaches may be identified. CA1 is a small hydrophobic compound used orally with minimal toxicity. It is currently in phase I clinical trial and phase II trials are planned in ovarian cancer.

3.40 Tumour associated antigens are potential targets for the immune system. Some of these have recognized monoclonal antibodies

(CA125, PEM and MOV18). Some may be mutated oncogenes (p53). Molecules recognized by cytotoxic T cells can also be identified. Therapy may be considered using antibodies/antigens. Monoclonal antibodies may be used alone, carrying toxic agents, or used in a modified form (single chain FUs, humanized bispecific). Where DNAs coding for antigens have been cloned, the antigens can be used as immunogens and here effective antigen presentation needs to be considered, since tumours expressing the antigens are not rejected. Antibodies may also act as antigens inducing anti-idiotype response (Ab2), where Ab2 resembles the antigen to which the first antibody is directed. This action could improve survival of ovarian cancer patients given antibodies to the polymorphic epithelial mucin (PEM).

3.41   Antibodies can also be used to target T cells to tumour cells when one arm of the antibody is directed to the tumour associated antigen and the other to the CD3 T cell receptor. Such a bispecific antibody directed to the MOV18 antigen has been shown to mediate target cell lysis *in vitro* with T cell clones or preactivated PBL from ovarian cancer patients. Preclinical studies with ovarian cancer xenografts in nude mice showed protection of 30% mice by human PBL armed with the bispecific antibody.

3.42   Clinical trials with advanced ovarian cancer patients resistant to chemotherapy suggest the above approach is promising, since complete or partial responses were seen in 60% of patients. It may be that humanized antibodies should be used in future to avoid the human antimouse antibody (HAMA) response. It will also be preferable to develop methods where T cells are activated *in vivo* rather than *in vitro*.

3.43   The antigen PEM is coded for by the MUC1 gene and is expressed by more than 90% of ovarian cancers. PEM is a transmembrane molecule with an extracellular domain containing many tandem repeats which are differentially glycosylated in tumours. The repetitive structure makes the molecule highly immunogenic. Humoral and cellular responses to PEM have been noted in ovarian and breast cancer patients.

3.44   Cytotoxic T cells can be isolated from leucocytes infiltrating ovarian malignant ascites, which proliferate in the presence of IL-2 and autologous tumour cells. CD3+ CD8+ lines were isolated which kill autologous tumour cells as well as allogeneic PEM expressing targets. Killing of MUC1 transfected targets confirms that the target antigen is PEM. The T cell receptor phenotype repertoire of these cells shows a more restricted usage, particularly where killing is non-restricted. Non-restricted cell killing could make the PEM antigen an important target for the immune system, since HLA class I expression can be lost in tumours.

3.45   Model systems for evaluating methods of antigen presentation have been developed. Based on results from the Ta3H mouse model, clinical trials in breast and ovarian cancer using synthetic carbohydrates (corresponding to the short oligosaccharide side chains seen in tumours) have begun. This active specific immunotherapy (ASI) is well tolerated with responses and, more importantly, disease stabilization noted. To counteract possible immunosuppressive effects of the antigen, low dose cyclophosphamide is also administered. Several centres are involved in trials.

3.46   There are many possible immunogens based on PEM which could be developed. For comparison of efficacy a syngeneic mouse model using a mouse mammary tumour cell line transfected with MUC1 is used. Polypeptides, recombined vaccinia and transfected cells can all inhibit tumour growth.

The system will be useful for evaluating the importance of costimulating molecules (B7, IL-2).

3.47 The most appropriate model to date for preclinical studies is a transgenic mouse expressing the human MUC1 gene. Spontaneous mammary tumours can be developed in this mouse allowing testing of vaccination protocols.

3.48 For delivery of costimulatory molecules and/or antigens, tissue specific promoters are important and the promoter region of the MUC1 gene has been analysed to identify elements necessary for tissue specific expression. The promoter can also be used coupled to an oncogene to obtain PEM expressing epithelial tumours, possibly ovarian, in the transgenic mouse.

3.49 Immunotherapy has great potential. The challenge is to identify methods of antigen presentation which are efficacious and feasible.

36.4 GENETICS

4.1 Systemic epidemiological studies of ovarian cancer have shown it to be two- to three-fold commoner in first degree relatives of affected women than in the general population.

4.2 There is also a familial association with breast, colorectal and stomach cancers. The association in families between ovarian and breast cancer may be largely explained by the autosomal dominant 'breast–ovarian' cancer families, while the association with colorectal cancer is probably due to certain hereditary non-polyposis colon cancer (HNPCC, also sometimes called Lynch II syndrome) families which have recently been shown to map to a gene on chromosome 2p. In these families, however, colorectal cancer is at least 10 times as frequent as ovarian cancer.

4.3 Most but not all ovarian cancer families are probably included in the high penetrance breast–ovarian cancer families. These have been shown by extensive DNA marker linkage studies to map to a position on chromosome 17q21 and the corresponding gene has been called BRCA1.

4.4 In extensive collaborative studies involving many groups in Europe and North America it has been shown that approximately a quarter of the breast cancer families showing linkage to 17q21 are breast–ovarian families while it is clear that less than half of breast cancer families without ovarian cancer, even involving an early age of onset, are linked to 17q21.

4.5 BRCA1 has been localized to the interval between RARA and D17S78, a region of approximately 3 Mb. Allele studies on tumours further suggest that BRCA1 may lie between RNU2 and D17S78, raising the hope that the gene itself may soon be identified by testing candidates within a region of less than 1 Mb.

4.6 Females presumed to be BRCA1 mutation carriers are estimated to have a lifetime risk by age 70 years of about 70% for breast cancer and 40% for ovarian cancer. There is, however, evidence for some heterogeneity of risk between families, especially for ovarian cancer.

4.7 The ovarian cancer risk is very low below age 40 and has a similar distribution of age of onset to that in the general population. By contrast, breast cancer in BRCA1 mutation carriers appears to have an age of onset which peaks much earlier that the general population, at age 45, suggesting that the effect of the gene is particularly on increasing the risk of premenopausal as opposed to postmenopausal breast cancer.

4.8 BRCA1 germ line mutations may account for as much as 10% of all ovarian cancers but probably for no more that 1–2%

of breast cancers. A comparison between affected and unaffected BRCA1 mutation carriers should help to identify risk factors in predisposed individuals and these need to be evaluated in collaborative studies. Data so far indicate that parity does not have an effect on BRCA1 mutation carriers and cancer risk for such carriers has increased for those born after 1930 compared to those born earlier.

4.9 Evidence for the existence of ovarian cancer families with and without breast cancer not linked to 17q21 has come particularly from extensive studies in Utah of the descendants of the Mormon pioneers.

4.10 With regard to BRCA1 mutation carrier families, further discussion is needed on how at present to advise known carriers. When, if at all, should mastectomy or oophorectomy be recommended? Should carriers take oral contraceptives and what should they be advised with respect to hormone replacement therapy? All studies on these families should take into account psychological factors and the importance of appropriate counselling.

4.11 Studies of the role of ultrasound and tumour marker screening for BRCA1 mutation carriers must continue.

4.12 Genetic heterogeneity within and between families could indicate the presence of significant modifier genes. Such studies will be greatly enhanced once the BRCA1 gene itself has been identified. In anticipation of this, it is recommended that a register of all BRCA1 carriers should be established internationally to carry out such collaborative investigations.

4.13 Once the BRCA1 gene has been identified it may be possible to establish more directly the proportion of ovarian cancer cases in the population due to germ line BRCA1 mutations and their associated penetrance.

4.14 The role of the recently identified gene on chromosome 2 in ovarian cancer needs to be identified.

4.15 Allele loss at 17p seems to be almost if not entirely explained by mutations in the p53 gene. Immunohistology suggests that approximately 50% of ovarian cancers express elevated levels of p53 and sequencing indicates that essentially all of these are due to mutations in the gene. The distribution is similar to the germ line mutations that have been observed in other genes.

4.16 While some allele loss data suggest the focus of loss around 17q21, other data suggest that the major event may be loss of the whole chromosome 17, namely non-disjunction. In that case there would be no clear evidence of allele loss around 17q21.

4.17 Some evidence suggests that the p53 mutations may be associated with more advanced and aggressive cancers while those involving 17q occur earlier.

4.18 Significant allele losses have been described on several other chromosomes. Clearest evidence for this exists for 6q (probably q27-ter), 11p (probably 11p15.5 and not 11p13.3, as the Wilms' tumour gene seems not to be mutated in ovarian cancer), 13q (apparently not Rb) and 18q (possibly the DCC gene). Additional evidence for allele loss has been found for 4q, 5q (not APC), 11p and Xq. There is obviously much further work to be done to identify potential tumour suppressor genes involved in ovarian cancer.

4.19 A number of associations have been found between the extent of allele loss and tumour grade. There is more extensive genetic change, as is to be expected, in high grade carcinoma. The extent to which the general background of allele loss found in high grade tumour is non-specific and associated with a general increase in aneuploidy is not clear. Specific genetic changes such as in p53 could be associated with an increase in this general loss of heterozygosity.

4.20 Careful comparisons of cystadenomas, low malignant potential (LMP) tumours and low and high grade carcinomas suggest qualitative differences in their genetic changes. Low grade or histologically benign cysts adjacent to high grade carcinomas seem to share genetic changes such as in p53 or 11p allele loss indicating that the low aggressive portions of such tumours were not typical cystadenomas or low grade carcinomas. This suggests that if there is progression from low to high aggressive lesions then it is only a very small proportion of the low aggressive lesions which progress. Chromosome Xq allele loss may be particularly important in the genesis of LMPs and these when combined with other losses may lead to higher grade cancers.

4.21 In evaluating genetic changes in ovarian cancers, as in other cancers, it is important to surmount the problem of contamination with normal tissues. One approach uses the elegant technique of marking areas on a slide to protect them from UV irradiation and then eliminating other material by extensive UV treatment to disable it as a substrate for PCR.

4.22 Other approaches include the use of cell lines established from carcinomas or cells from pleural effusions from which epithelial cells can be purified by a variety of approaches. Flow cytometry could also be used for selecting aneuploid nuclei that could be analysed by PCR.

4.23 Detection of mutant cells from ovarian cancers shed into the blood or bone marrow may be a valuable approach for early detection of ovarian cancers. Some studies suggest that as many as 20–30% of bone marrows of ovarian cancer patients being considered for autologous bone marrow transplants were positive for cancer cells.

4.24 Recent data suggest that as many as 50% of borderline mucinous tumours carry *ras* mutations. It is important to confirm these observations.

4.25 Monoclonal antibody based therapy of ovarian cancer could be improved by identifying the functions of targeted antigens. For example, MOV18 has been identified and shown to recognize the folate receptor coded by the gene located on 11q13.3, suggesting the use of antifolate therapy. OVTL-3 and G253 recognize different members of the immunoglobulin supergene family, the former a channel mapping to 3q 12-13 and the latter an adhesion molecule with homology to MUC18 found in melanomas mapping to 19q13.3. OVTL30 is ICAM1, suggesting that ovarian cancer cells may in some sense be activated and there is an intriguing gene, possibly CA125 related, that maps to 17q21.1. So far no mutations in any of these genes have been found in ovarian cancer cells.

4.28 Another approach to improving monoclonal antibody reagents for therapy is through the production of genetically engineered derivatives that may overcome the problems of tumour penetration and immunogenicity. Recombinant single chain Fv (sFv) fragments penetrate tumours more rapidly and are also cleared more rapidly from the circulation and so are less immunogenic. Engineered sFv conjugates or chimeric proteins may be promising as therapeutic agents, particularly if methods can be identified to enhance tumour retention. Approaches include the construction of multivalent or bispecific reagents and the use of a biotin–avidin sequential amplification scheme. Patterns of antigen internalization and catabolism influence the efficacy of toxin conjugated whole Ig and sFv reagents in therapy. This needs to be considered in the choice of reagents. Targeting of radioactivity, for example yttrium 90, may not be influenced to the same extent by antigen internalization.

4.29 Gene therapy offers the prospect of some highly novel approaches to the treatment of ovarian cancers. Appropriate retrovirally based vectors using tissue specific promoters, such as thromcap A, can target genes to particular cells or cell types. This approach can be used to sensitize cancers, for example, to ganciclovir by inserting the HSV-tk gene into the tumour. Though it is hard to envisage that a sufficiently high proportion of tumour cells can be targeted in this way, the approach may be useful in localized treatment and there may be an extension to untargeted cells by bystander effects.

4.30 A more promising application is the targeting of genes that stimulate immune response to tumour cells such as IL-2 and other cytokines, as well as accessory molecules such as B7. Animal models using IL-2, interferonγ and other cytokine ·transfected cells have shown dramatic immune protection to subsequent challenge. These approaches offer totally new opportunities for development of cancer immunotherapy even when the potential target antigens are not yet defined.

Index